Irish Medical Education and Student Culture, c.1850–1950

Reappraisals in Irish History

Editors
Enda Delaney (University of Edinburgh)
Maria Luddy (University of Warwick)

Reappraisals in Irish History offers new insights into Irish history, society and culture from 1750. Recognising the many methodologies that make up historical research, the series presents innovative and interdisciplinary work that is conceptual and interpretative, and expands and challenges the common understandings of the Irish past. It showcases new and exciting scholarship on subjects such as the history of gender, power, class, the body, landscape, memory and social and cultural change. It also reflects the diversity of Irish historical writing, since it includes titles that are empirically sophisticated together with conceptually driven synoptic studies.

1. Jonathan Jeffrey Wright, *The 'Natural Leaders' and their World: Politics, Culture and Society in Belfast, c.1801–1832*

2. Gerardine Meaney, Mary O'Dowd and Bernadette Whelan, *Reading the Irish Woman: Studies in Cultural Encounters and Exchange, 1714–1960*

3. Emily Mark-FitzGerald, *Commemorating the Irish Famine: Memory and the Monument*

4. Virginia Crossman, *Poverty and the Poor Law in Ireland 1850–1914*

5. Paul Taylor, *Heroes or Traitors? Experiences of Southern Irish Soldiers Returning from the Great War 1919–39*

6. Paul Huddie, *The Crimean War and Irish Society*

7. Brian Hughes, *Defying the IRA? Intimidation, coercion, and communities during the Irish Revolution*

Irish Medical Education and Student Culture, *c*.1850–1950

LAURA KELLY

LIVERPOOL UNIVERSITY PRESS

First published 2017 by
Liverpool University Press
4 Cambridge Street
Liverpool
L69 7ZU
www.liverpooluniversitypress.co.uk

This paperback edition published 2020

British Library Cataloguing-in-Publication data
A British Library CIP record is available

ISBN 978-1-78962-816-6

Typeset by Carnegie Book Production, Lancaster
Printed and bound by CPI Group (UK) Ltd, Croydon CR0 4YY

Contents

Figures

Cover image: Man seated, possibly J.J. Clarke, with skeleton,
    c.1897–1904. From the Clarke Photographic Collection.
    Courtesy of the National Library of Ireland.

Tables

Acknowledgements

I am grateful to many individuals who helped at various stages with this project. Without their support and encouragement this book would not have been written. I was very fortunate to be awarded an Irish Research Council postdoctoral research fellowship between 2012 and 2014 which made the research for this book possible. I am thankful to the IRC for this support. I am also grateful to the Wellcome Trust which provided a small grant in the first year of the project which enabled me to undertake archival research in London.

I undertook the fellowship at the Centre for the History of Medicine in Ireland (CHOMI) at University College Dublin and am extremely grateful to my mentor there, and centre director, Catherine Cox. The two years I spent at UCD were extremely enjoyable, intellectually stimulating and fun, and I learnt a great deal under Catherine's guidance. Intellectually and socially, being part of CHOMI was an excellent experience, and I am thankful to Catherine and my former colleagues there, including Stephen Bance, Fiachra Byrne and David Durnin. My time at UCD was also made extra enjoyable owing to the support of a fantastic group of postdocs in the School of History and Archives, which included Edward Collins, Niamh Cullen, Selena Daly, Aaron Donaghy, Maria Falina, Susan Grant, Carole Holohan, Mark Jones, Eoin Kinsella, Matthew Lewis, Sarah McCann, James Matthews, Mercedes Peñalba, Dmitar Tasić, Patrick Walsh, Niamh Wycherley, many of whom I now count as good friends and with whom I shared lots of fun times both inside and outside of UCD. In particular, Patrick, Eoin and later Sarah, had the joy of getting to share an office with me – and I am grateful to them for putting up with me. I am also thankful for the support of other colleagues in the School of History at UCD, including Judith Devlin, Lindsey Earner-Byrne, Tadhg O hAnnrachain, Susannah Riordan and Jennifer Wellington. While at UCD, I held a workshop on the history of medical education supported by CHOMI and funded by the Irish Research Council and the Wellcome Trust, and I am most grateful to the participants at this workshop, in particular the keynote speaker, John Harley Warner, who all helped me to rethink aspects of my own work.

This book draws on a significant amount of archival research. I am therefore thankful to all of the archivists and librarians who provided assistance with this project, in particular, Annaig Boyer and staff at the Medical Missions Sisters Archives, Brian Donnelly (National Archives of Ireland), Noelle Dowling (Dublin Diocesan Archives), Stanley Hawkins (Royal Victoria Hospital, Belfast), Barry Houlihan and Kieran Hoare (NUI Galway Archives and Special Collections), Ursula Mitchell (QUB Special Collections), Caitriona Mulcahy (UCC University archives), Meadhbh Murphy and Mary O'Doherty (RCSI Heritage Collections), Eugene Roche and staff at UCD archives and Special Collections, and Harriet Wheelock (RCPI Heritage Centre). I would also like to thank the staff at the National Library of Ireland, TCD Manuscripts Department and Early Printed Books and the Wellcome Library. All of the above were very kind in photographing images from their collections for me to reproduce here while Juliana Adelman kindly alerted me to the existence of the wonderful cover image from the Clarke Collection of the National Library of Ireland. I am also indebted to the 24 men and women who graduated from Irish medical schools in the 1940s and 1950s who gave up their time to be interviewed by me about their experiences. This, for me, was the most enjoyable and interesting part of the project and I am very grateful to all of them for speaking to me about their student days.

I am very thankful to Greta Jones who has always provided encouragement to me at different stages of my career, and who kindly read over some of the book before submission and provided useful comments. Thanks also to Aileen Fyfe and Marguerite Dupree who continue to be inspiring mentors, and to my good friends and former colleagues at NUI Galway, in particular, Rebecca Anne Barr, Sarah-Anne Buckley, Caitriona Clear, Tomás Finn and Kevin O'Sullivan. Thanks also to Patrick Bourke, Michael Brown, Catherine Cox, Susan Grant, Carole Holohan, Eoin Kinsella, Maeve O'Brien and Matt Smith who each kindly read chapters of the book and provided helpful feedback. Thanks to Michelle Smith for her excellent transcription work. The staff of Liverpool University Press have been wonderful to work with. I am especially grateful to Alison Welsby, editorial director, for her support with this project, to Enda Delaney and Maria Luddy, the series editors, and to the two anonymous reviewers for their insightful and constructive feedback. Thanks to Conor Reidy for creating the index. A selection of Chapter 5 was published in the journal *History of Education* and I am thankful to the publishers and editor for granting me permission to republish that material here.[1]

---

1 Laura Kelly, 'Irish medical student culture and the performance of masculinity, c.1880–1930', *History of Education* 46(1) (2017): 39–57.

This book was written partly in Dublin and partly in Glasgow, where I took up a lectureship at the University of Strathclyde in February 2015. I am therefore also very grateful to my wonderful colleagues in the School of Humanities and Social Sciences, the support team in the School, and colleagues in the Centre for the Social History of Health and Healthcare and the Scottish Oral History Centre, who have all made me feel very welcome. In particular, I would like to thank Patricia Barton, Stephen Mawdsley, Jim Mills, Arthur McIvor, Emma Newlands, Linsey Robb, Matt Smith and Manuela Williams, who have all been exceptional colleagues. The Section of the History of Medicine at Yale University was the ideal environment for completing my book revisions in the autumn of 2016 and I am most grateful to Naomi Rogers, John Harley Warner, and the academic and graduate student community there.

Several friends provided support and fun times away from academia – among them I am especially grateful to Lucy, Maeve and Sarah for many years of friendship. Finally, a huge thank you to Patrick for his love, kindness and companionship, and to my family – my brothers Seán and Ciarán and most of all, my parents, John and Angela – for their constant encouragement and support.

Abbreviations

Irish medical schools, examining institutions and licensing bodies
KQCPI   King and Queen's College of Physicians in Ireland
NUI   National University of Ireland
QCB   Queen's College Belfast
QCC   Queen's College Cork
QCG   Queen's College Galway
QUB   Queen's University Belfast
RCPI   Royal College of Physicians of Ireland
RCSI   Royal College of Surgeons in Ireland
RUI   Royal University of Ireland
TCD   Trinity College Dublin
UCC   University College Cork
UCD   University College Dublin
UCG   University College Galway

Medical journals
BMJ   *British Medical Journal*
DMP   *Dublin Medical Press*

Medical organisations
GMC   General Medical Council
RAMC   Royal Army Medical Corps

Student societies and organisations
BMSA   Belfast Medical Students' Association
British MSA British Medical Students' Association
IMSA   Irish Medical Students' Association
OTC   Officers' Training Corps
QCCMSA   Queen's College Cork Medical Students Association

Introduction

In 1853, after some years of consideration about entering the medical profession, 16-year-old James Little (1837–1916) commenced his medical studies. After a family council, 'the best bargain was made' for Little to be assigned as an apprentice to Dr Cohan in Armagh before commencing his studies in Dublin. In November of that year, 'an offer of becoming an inmate in William Stephen's Family was at last made and at once embraced and thither I sent with my father – I went round to the different professors – took out my tickets and entered upon my 1st year as a Dublin Medical Student at the Royal College of Surgeons'.[1]

Little does not live up to the stereotype that has often been presented of the nineteenth-century medical student. He found student life lonely, did not mix with other medical students, and studied alone, stating 'this may have kept me from dissipation but I would not advise such a course'.[2] Little also struggled financially as he was not sent enough money by his father. However, by his second session of study, he 'felt more a man' and now had the courage to ask his father for money for his sundry expenses. At the same time, considering matters retrospectively, Little regretted that he had not socialised more with his fellow students, stating that if he had he 'might have done some things which were wrong', but that he would have been 'more manly – I would have studied better, I would have got on faster and some bad habits would have been corrected', and that his want of money for recreations did him much harm.[3]

The experiences of medical students of the past, like James Little, have received surprisingly little attention from historians.[4] In his ambitious

1 Diary of James Little, p. iv [RCPI Heritage Centre, TPCK/6/5/10].
2 Diary of James Little, p. 5.
3 Diary of James Little, pp. 5–6.
4 There have been a number of studies on the history of medical education since the 1920s. While these have comprehensively shown how medical education developed in the nineteenth and twentieth centuries, they have generally failed to illuminate the experiences of medical students. For example, Abraham Flexner, *Medical education:*

comparative study of medical education in Britain, France, the United States and Germany, Thomas Neville Bonner asserted that 'the lives and experiences of students in general and their impact on medical education have been too little studied'.[5] Similarly, echoing such sentiments more recently, Keir Waddington has commented that 'in the historiography of medical education, students are largely absent or silent consumers'.[6] This book aims to address this historiographical gap through an exploration of the experiences of medical students who trained at Irish institutions in roughly the 100-year period between the mid-nineteenth to mid-twentieth century. I endeavour also to provide a history of student life and culture in Ireland. While there have been numerous useful institutional histories of Irish universities, these have tended to take a 'top-down' approach, focusing on the administration, financing and professors in these institutions, with the voices of students often missing.[7] The professional identity of Irish students,

a comparative study (New York: Macmillan, 1925); Charles Newman, The evolution of medical education in the nineteenth century (Oxford: Oxford University Press, 1957); Theodor Puschmann, A history of medical education (New York: Hafner, 1966); C.D. O'Malley (ed.), The history of medical education (Berkeley: University of California Press, 1970). In recent years, studies of medical education have begun to address this gap in the historiography. Histories of medical education in Edinburgh and London have been joined by research on medical education and student experience elsewhere in Britain, America and Europe. See, for example, S.C. Lawrence, Charitable knowledge: hospital pupils and practitioners in eighteenth-century London (Cambridge: Cambridge University Press, 1986); Lisa Rosner, Medical education in the age of enlightenment: Edinburgh students and apprentices, 1760–1826 (Edinburgh: Edinburgh University Press, 1991); E.A. Heaman, St Mary's: the history of a London teaching hospital (Liverpool: Liverpool University Press, 2003); Jonathan Reinarz, Health care in Birmingham: the Birmingham teaching hospitals, 1779–1939 (Woodbridge: Boydell Press, 2009); Lisa Rosner, 'Student culture at the turn of the nineteenth century', Caduceus 10(2) (1994): 65–86; Colin Jones, 'Montpellier medical students and the medicalisation of eighteenth-century France', in Roy Porter and Andrew Wear (eds), Problems and methods in the history of medicine (London: Croom Helm, 1987), pp. 57–80; Keir Waddington, Medical education at St Bartholomew's Hospital, 1123–1995 (Woodbridge: Boydell Press, 2003); Mark. W. Weatherall, Gentlemen, scientists and doctors: medicine at Cambridge, 1800–1940 (Woodbridge: Boydell Press, 2000).
5 Thomas Neville Bonner, Becoming a physician: medical education in Britain, France, Germany and the United States, 1750–1945 (Oxford: Oxford University Press, 1995), p. 7.
6 Keir Waddington, 'Mayhem and medical students: image, conduct, and control in the Victorian and Edwardian London teaching hospital', Social History of Medicine 15(1) (2002), p. 45.
7 See, for instance, R.B. McDowell and D.A. Webb, Trinity College Dublin, 1592–1952: an academic history (Cambridge: Cambridge University Press, 2004); Tadhg Foley (ed.), From Queen's College to National University: essays on the academic history of QCG/UCG/NUI Galway (Dublin: Four Courts Press, 1999); John A. Murphy, The College: a history of Queen's/University College, Cork, 1845–1995 (Cork: Cork University Press, 1996); Donal McCartney, UCD: a national idea: the history of University College,

like their counterparts in Britain, America and elsewhere, was cemented through shared experiences. Irish medical education was additionally shaped by local, economic and gendered concerns, and the country's distinctive religious and political context further influenced student life and experience. Through a focus on educational and extra-curricular experiences and the formation of professional identity, this book seeks to reinstate the student's voice in the history of medical education in Ireland and to improve our understanding of the history of the Irish medical profession.

Dissecting the history of the medical profession and medical education in Ireland

The history of the medical profession is crucial to understanding the history of medical education. For most of the period under consideration in this book, Ireland was part of the United Kingdom, and thus the Irish and British medical professions were intertwined. The Irish Free State was established in December 1922, but even after this the Irish medical profession remained deeply influenced by its British counterpart and Irish medical schools continued to be monitored by the General Medical Council in London.

The process of professionalisation, it has been argued, is a significant factor in the emergence of modern society.[8] The period from 1750 to 1850 was crucial not only for the medical profession, but for other professions which were beginning to organise and regulate themselves and experience changes with their relationship to society in general.[9] In the early nineteenth century, the British medical profession had a tripartite structure, composed broadly of physicians, surgeons and apothecaries, with each of these having their own functions, forms of education, tests of competence and corporate bodies.[10] Physicians, who comprised the first estate, were concerned with the treatment of internal diseases by medical means with diagnoses resulting from gathering the detailed history of the illness, details of the patient's constitution and way of life, through observation of the patient and his urine and by feeling

---

Dublin (Dublin: Gill & Macmillan, 1999); T.W. Moody and J.C. Beckett, *Queen's, Belfast, 1845–1949: the history of a university* (London: Faber & Faber, 1959).

8 Harold Perkin, *The rise of professional society: England since 1880* (London and New York: Routledge, 1989) cited in Marcus Ackroyd, Laurence Brockliss, Michael Moss, Kate Retford and John Stevenson, *Advancing with the army: medicine, the professions and social mobility in the British Isles, 1790–1850* (Oxford: Oxford University Press, 2007), p. 1.

9 Ackroyd et al., *Advancing with the army*, p. 1.

10 Noel Parry and José Parry, *The rise of the medical profession: a study of collective social mobility* (London: Croom Helm, 1976), p. 104.

the pulse.[11] Surgery was concerned with the treatment of external disorders, especially ones which required 'manual interference' such as wound-dressing, the setting of fractures, reduction of dislocations and operations which required incisions.[12] Apothecaries, the third estate of the medical profession, were concerned with the dispensing of prescriptions written by physicians.[13] Although Anne Digby has argued for a more nuanced approach to such a categorisation of the medical profession, and many studies have emphasised the dominance of general practice rather than a strict tripartite structure, the strains between these different practitioners, in addition to the rise of unlicensed 'quacks' and druggists in the period, resulted in great tensions within the medical profession.[14] Meanwhile, although medical education had become more institutionalised and had integrated ideas of the profession from the early nineteenth century, with students coming under the control of an elite group of teachers, the organisational structure of medical education was in a chaotic state.[15] A medical licence in Britain could be obtained from one of nineteen different licensing bodies, while 'the rules governing their recognition were a tangle of conflicting rights and powers', with medical men practising with 'university degrees, various forms of medical licences, sometimes a combination of these and sometimes with none at all'.[16] Changes were introduced in the nineteenth century with regard to the subjects on the curriculum for a medical education as a result of the effects of the scientific revolution of the preceding century.[17] Medical curricula also differed from one university to another: for example, a medical student at Cambridge in the first half of the nineteenth century would receive an education rooted in the study of classic texts of literature and medicine,[18] while a student at Glasgow or Edinburgh would receive an education which was more akin to courses on the Continent and which would integrate him in the practical work of the clinic as well as introducing him to scientific subjects such as anatomy and chemistry.[19]

11   Irvine Loudon, *Medical care and the general practitioner, 1750–1850* (Oxford: Oxford University Press, 1986), p. 19.
12   Loudon, *Medical care and the general practitioner*, p. 19.
13   Loudon, *Medical care and the general practitioner*, p. 19.
14   Anne Digby, *Making a medical living: doctors and patients in the English market for medicine, 1720–1911* (Cambridge: Cambridge University Press, 1994), pp. 28–9.
15   See, for example, S.C. Lawrence, *Charitable knowledge: hospital pupils and practitioners in eighteenth-century London* (Cambridge: Cambridge University Press, 1986); Ivan Waddington, *The medical profession in the industrial revolution* (Dublin: Gill & Macmillan, 1984); M. Jeanne Peterson, *The medical profession in mid-Victorian London* (Berkeley: University of California Press, 1978), p. 5.
16   Peterson, *The medical profession in mid-Victorian London*, p. 5.
17   Bonner, *Becoming a physician*, p. 14.
18   Bonner, *Becoming a physician*, p. 40.
19   Bonner, *Becoming a physician*, p. 41.

The Medical Act was an important landmark in the history of the British medical profession. It was introduced in 1858 in an attempt to put an end to frictions within the profession. The Act established the General Medical Council of Medical Registration and Education (GMC) in order to distinguish qualified practitioners from unqualified ones in addition to implementing the legal rights of the profession.[20] The GMC regulated medical education in Britain and Ireland, with reform of education being an important priority of not just the medical profession but of other professions in this period.[21] The Act stipulated that in order to appear on the newly established *Medical Register*, a list of all registered medical practitioners in the United Kingdom, a doctor had to possess a licence or medical degree from one of the nineteen registered bodies in Britain and Ireland. This also meant that women doctors now had no means of placing their names on the *Medical Register* because they were unable to obtain qualifications from these bodies.[22] However, the Medical Act ultimately did not succeed in putting an end to the rigid divisions within the medical profession: instead, it replaced the tripartite structure of the profession with a new type of medical hierarchy of hospital consultants and general practitioners. During the Victorian era, the combination of divisions within the medical profession and competition for patients resulted in professional tensions and an increasingly competitive medical marketplace.[23] Moreover, despite its intentions, historians have largely agreed that the Act 'failed to integrate medicine and to specify a single means of entry to it'.[24] From the mid-1860s, medical schools became increasingly important as an agent of profession-alisation.[25] Students were 'initiated into the social mores of the profession

---

20 Mark Weatherall, 'Making medicine scientific: empiricism, rationality and quackery in mid-Victorian Britain', *Social History of Medicine* 9(2) (1996), p. 176.

21 Parry and Parry, *The rise of the medical profession*, p. 133.

22 Anne Witz, *Professions and patriarchy* (London: Routledge, 1992), pp. 79–80. This remained the case until the King and Queen's College of Physicians in Ireland took advantage of the 1876 Enabling Act and allowed British women who had studied abroad to take their licentiate examinations and thus have a means of registering themselves as medical practitioners. See Laura Kelly, '"The turning point in the whole struggle": the admission of women to the King and Queen's College of Physicians in Ireland', *Women's History Review* 22(1) (2013): 97.

23 See Peterson, *The medical profession in mid-Victorian London* and Anne Digby, *Making a medical living: doctors and patients in the English market for medicine, 1720–1911* (Cambridge: Cambridge University Press, 1994).

24 Digby, *Making a medical living*, p. 31.

25 As Waddington has pointed out, there have been a number of studies which have focused on the structure of medical training as part of a history of professionalisation, and more recently attention has been directed at the move away from book learning and apprenticeship to the institutionalisation of teaching in the eighteenth century and the impact of Paris medicine. Such studies depict medical schools as 'agents of

by the culture of the classroom, laboratory, and sports field rather than through the personal example of a single professional'.[26] Yet, it is clear that the type and quality of education provided varied from one medical school to another. Efforts to standardise medical education were not made until the Medical Amendment Act of 1886 which set out that all medical students were required to have a qualification in surgery, midwifery and medicine, while apprenticeship was formally abolished by the GMC in 1892.[27]

The Irish medical schools

From the eighteenth century, Dublin developed into a major centre of medical education and by the mid-nineteenth century there existed a large number of teaching hospitals and medical schools.[28] Dublin achieved international renown in the first half of the nineteenth century for its system of bedside clinical teaching, which was made famous by Robert Graves and William Stokes, physicians at the Meath Hospital. Graves, Stokes, Abraham Colles and others generated an outstanding reputation as a result of their 'exceptional personal skills of rigorous observation, forensic investigation and a humane patient-centred ethic'.[29] Robert Jones, who came from Wales to study at the Meath Hospital in 1836–7 remarked on the impression that Robert Graves made on him, stating in a diary entry:

> Visited the Meath Hospital this morning to the Medical and Surgical Practice of which I have entered as a pupil for six months – went round the ward with Surgeon Colles and saw some interesting cases of Pneumonia and was much pleased with the Clinical remarks of Dr. Graves who visits the Hospital early in the morning, he seems to be a very sharp man and full of practical information, his manner is

professionalisation and socialisation or a source of income, with medical education either part of a mechanism that made hospitals central to the hierarchy of medicine, or a vehicle for the laboratory' ('Mayhem and medical students', pp. 45–6).

26 Stella V.F. Butler, 'A transformation in training: the formation of university medical faculties in Manchester, Leeds and Liverpool, 1870–84', *Medical History* 30 (1986), p. 131.

27 Digby, *Making a medical living*, p. 31 and Butler, 'A transformation in training', p. 131.

28 Greta Jones and Elizabeth Malcolm, 'Introduction: an anatomy of Irish medical history', in Greta Jones and Elizabeth Malcolm (eds), *Medicine, disease and the state in Ireland, 1650–1940* (Cork: Cork University Press, 1998), p. 1.

29 David Dickson, *Dublin: the making of a capital city* (London: Profile Books, 2014), p. 313.

pleasing and communicative to the pupils, he is decidedly the most gentlemanly lecturer I have yet met with among the Dublin Teachers.[30]

On the strength of the reputation of Graves and this group of less than a dozen practitioners who were famed for their teaching and advocacy of new medical instruments such as the stethoscope, the city of Dublin 'shifted from its old dependence on universities abroad for medical education (in Scotland, Holland and France) to becoming a centre in its own right'.[31] Medical journals, another important symbol of medical professionalisation, were also founded, including the *Dublin Journal of Medicine and Chemistry* in 1832 and the *Dublin Medical Press* in 1839.[32] However, this is not to suggest that Irish medical practitioners were united; indeed, religious sectarianism was rife in the Irish medical profession in the nineteenth century.[33] Irish medical students were not only hampered by the disorganised system of education they had in common with their British neighbours, but religious affiliation further affected the choice of medical school in Ireland well into the twentieth century. Catholic and Dissenter students were excluded from Trinity College Dublin by the extension of religious tests from 1637.[34] From 1793, Catholic students were permitted to take degrees at Trinity College; however, they

30 Notes made by Robert Jones, Dublin, 1 November 1836, p. 37. From Papers of Robert Jones relating to his studies in Dublin at the Royal College of Surgeons in Ireland and the Meath Hospital 1836–1837 [Wellcome Library, MSS 6061–6062].
31 Dickson, *Dublin: the making of a capital city*, p. 313.
32 Dickson, *Dublin: the making of a capital city*, p. 314. For more on the history of the Dublin Medical Press, see Ann Daly, 'The Dublin Medical Press and medical authority in Ireland, 1850–1890' (unpublished PhD thesis, National University of Ireland Maynooth 2008).
33 There was prejudice against Catholic doctors in the nineteenth century with regard to public appointments. In his evidence to the 1843 Committee on Medical Charities, Dominic Corrigan, an eminent Catholic physician in Dublin, estimated that there were 107 public medical positions in Dublin, of which only 13 were filled by Catholics. Another physician, William Smith O'Brien, claimed that the system of filling hospital vacancies in Dublin was one of 'bargain and sale' and that it was heavily influenced by familial, professional and religious favouritism. See Geary, *Medicine and charity in Ireland, 1718–1851* (Dublin: University College Dublin Press, 2005), p. 130. Similarly, in the 1850s, with the establishment of the dispensary service, allegations were made that these appointments depended on the candidate's sectarian and political allegiances. See Catherine Cox, 'Access and engagement: the medical dispensary service in post-Famine Ireland', in Catherine Cox and Maria Luddy (eds), *Cultures of care in Irish medical history, 1750–1950* (Basingstoke: Palgrave Macmillan, 2010), p. 62. In the nineteenth century, despite representing the majority of the population, Catholic doctors were often excluded from medical posts, while in the early twentieth century, following the establishment of the Irish Free State, there was prejudice against Protestant doctors, now in the minority.
34 F.O.C. Meenan, *Cecilia Street: the Catholic University School of Medicine, 1855–1931* (Dublin: Gill & Macmillan, 1987), p. 2.

could not hold fellowships or scholarships without having to take an oath which was against the Catholic faith. In 1873, Fawcett's Act removed the requirement to take these oaths, and religious tests, with the exception of those connected with the School of Divinity, were banned. However, the Catholic hierarchy condemned this measure as 'an act of secularisation' and continued to warn Catholic students against entering Trinity College.[35] Furthermore, Catholic bishops believed that through attendance at Trinity College, Catholic students would be drawn into conformity or conversion to Protestantism.[36] An episcopal ban on Catholic students entering Trinity College Dublin was in existence until 1970.[37] As a result, numbers of Catholic students at Trinity College Dublin in the nineteenth century were low. As the nineteenth century went on, the proportion of Protestant Dissenter students rose steadily; however, the proportion of Catholic students varied more irregularly.[38] Up until 1900, Catholic students comprised only between 5 per cent and 10 per cent of students at Trinity College. Between 1923 and 1930, numbers rose to 20 per cent, with a sudden decline in the mid-1930s, to 8 per cent, this probably a result of increased ecclesiastical discouragement. By 1950, Catholic students comprised 23 per cent of students.[39]

As a consequence, Irish Catholic doctors in the first half of the nineteenth century tended to have been educated at one of the private Dublin medical schools, the Royal College of Surgeons or at one of the European medical schools, such as Leiden, Edinburgh or Glasgow. There were a number of private medical schools in existence in Ireland in the period, with the majority of these declining by the 1850s, or being absorbed into the larger medical schools.[40] These schools did not have the authority to grant degrees

35 Senia Pašeta, 'Trinity College, Dublin, and the education of Irish Catholics, 1873–1908', *Studia Hibernica* 30 (1998–9), p. 10.
36 Gearoid O'Tuathaigh, 'The establishment of the Queen's Colleges: ideological and political background', in Tadhg Foley (ed.), *From Queen's College to National University: essays on the academic history of QCG/UCG/NUI Galway* (Dublin: Four Courts Press, 1999), pp. 9 and 15.
37 Dermot Moran, 'Nationalism, religion and the education question', *Crane Bag* 7(2) (1983), p. 82.
38 R.B. McDowell and D.A. Webb, *Trinity College Dublin, 1592–1952: an academic history* (Cambridge: Cambridge University Press, 2004), p. 247.
39 McDowell and Webb, *Trinity College Dublin, 1592–1952*, p. 504.
40 For example, in Dublin, there was Crampton's School of Anatomy (established in 1804), Kirby's School (established in 1809), the Medical School of the House of Industry Hospitals (1812), The Theatre of Anatomy, subsequently the Anatomico-Medical School, Moore Street (1820), the first School of Anatomy and Surgery, Eccles Street (1822), the Park Street School (1824) and the Ledwich (1836), in addition to several private anatomy schools (see Sir Charles A. Cameron, *History of the Royal College of Surgeons in Ireland and of the Irish Schools of Medicine including numerous biographical sketches; also a medical bibliography* (Dublin: Fannin & Co., 1886), pp. 513–35). In

or licences but prepared medical students for the examinations of the various licensing bodies.[41]

In 1845, the three Queen's Colleges were founded by Robert Peel's Colleges Act in order to provide non-denominational education. These three colleges, in Cork, Belfast and Galway, opened in 1849. Through this early form of constructive unionism, Peel answered the occasional demands for university education for middle-class Catholics, and in the case of Belfast, for Dissenters.[42] Pressure for a state-funded Catholic university, or the Irish university question, was one of the most pressing political issues of the nineteenth century, capturing 'the attention of the Catholic church, British legislators and influential lay people, all of whom were aware of its potential impact on its beneficiaries, the future ruling class of Ireland'.[43] The Catholic hierarchy forbade Catholic students from attending the 'godless' Queen's colleges and the Catholic University opened in 1854 in order to fill the demand for a Catholic institution.[44] The medical school of the Catholic University was formally opened in November 1855.[45] The Catholic University did not possess a charter and therefore could not award degrees, and it suffered from financial difficulties. As a result, medical students who were educated there tended to take the licences of the Royal College of Surgeons, the King and Queen's College of Physicians or Apothecaries' Hall. Irish universities were beset with similar difficulties to British ones, such as the underdevelopment of secondary schools and a narrow demand for anything other than vocational education, problems which were compounded by religion and politics.[46] The medical schools were the most successful parts of the Catholic University and the Queen's Colleges.[47]

Belfast, students were educated at the medical school of the Royal Belfast Academical Institution (established in 1835) (see Peter Froggatt, 'Competing philosophies', in Jones and Malcolm, *Medicine, disease and the state in Ireland*, pp. 59–84 and Peter Froggatt, 'The first medical school in Belfast, 1835–49', *Medical History* 22 (1978): 237–66). There also existed four private medical schools in Cork in the early nineteenth century, including John Woodroffe's School of Anatomy, founded in 1811 ('New exhibition celebrates Cork anatomists', *Cork News*, 15 September 2011).

41   Meenan, *Cecilia Street*, p. 4.
42   O'Tuathaigh, 'The establishment of the Queen's Colleges', pp. 9 and 15.
43   Senia Pašeta, 'The Catholic hierarchy and the Irish university question, 1880–1908', *History* 85(278) (2000), p. 268.
44   In 1881, the university was reorganised as University College Dublin (UCD). By the 1940s, UCD had become the largest university in the state. The Queen's Colleges became University College Cork, University College Galway and Queen's University Belfast in 1908.
45   Meenan, *Cecilia Street*, p. 13.
46   R.D. Anderson, *Universities and elites in Britain since 1800* (Cambridge: Cambridge University Press, 1992), p. 28.
47   Anderson, *Universities and elites in Britain since 1800*, p. 28.

In 1879, the Royal University of Ireland (RUI) was founded. The RUI had the authority to award degrees to students who passed its annual examinations, with students being able to choose their place of education. University prizes and scholarships were also open to students of all denominations. In 1885, 2,890 students presented themselves for examination, with this number rising to 3,745 in 1905.[48] In 1881, the Catholic University was reorganised as University College Dublin (UCD) and medical students began to take the examinations of the RUI. The Irish Universities Act of 1908 dissolved the RUI and created two separate examining institutions: The National University of Ireland, with three constituent colleges, University College Dublin, University College Galway, University College Cork, and Queen's University Belfast. Chapter 1 explores this complex medical school marketplace of mid- to late nineteenth-century Ireland, highlighting not only the range of options for qualification available to Irish medical students but also the problems with Irish medical schools which have not hitherto been explored by historians. Irish schools were plagued by economic difficulties, poor conditions, the sham certificate system, night lectures and 'grinding', all of which affected students' experiences in different ways. Furthermore, intense competition between medical schools essentially meant that students wielded a great deal of power as consumers. This period also witnessed complaints by medical students about the quality of the education they were receiving, resulting, for example, in a series of visitations, or regulatory inspections, to Queen's College Cork and Queen's College Galway. Andrew Smith Melville, a medical student at Queen's College Galway, made a series of complaints to the *Lancet* medical journal about the quality of clinical instruction in Galway, resulting in an Extraordinary Visitation in 1870 by the vice-chancellor of the Queen's University, as well as the Presidents of the Royal College of Surgeons and Royal College of Physicians in Ireland. As the medical profession became increasingly professionalised student behaviour improved, but disturbances and protests in relation to professional matters or standards of education were not uncommon.

The university was crucial in providing students with a sense of identity. As Tomás Irish has suggested, universities, in a sense, may be described as families.[49] Students had a limited choice of colleagues and lived and socialised with members of the same group, in the same way that family members do, while the university community became a surrogate family.[50] Moreover, kinship could be established not only through membership of

---

48   Pašeta, 'Trinity College, Dublin, and the Education of Irish Catholics, 1873–1908', p. 8.
49   Tomás Irish, 'Fractured families: educated elites in Britain and France and the challenge of the Great War', *Historical Journal* 57(2) (2014), p. 511.
50   Irish, 'Fractured families', pp. 511–12.

the university, but also through university societies and sports clubs.[51] The overall result was 'an intimate network of men who were friends, enemies, and many shades in between, but inextricably linked by this association for the rest of their lives'.[52]

According to Manuel Castells, 'identity' 'is people's source of meaning and experience'.[53] Crucially, as Digby has argued, 'medical schools helped individuals internalise a medical culture and so construct a professional identity, not least by supplying role models of how doctors might present themselves to the world, providing templates for how things should be done, and indicating how situations could be tackled without losing face'.[54] Medical schools imbued students with a sense of identity and status and created robust networks not only amongst the students themselves but also between students and their teachers.[55] Medical schools also played a central role in encouraging professional ideals such as hard work and discipline.[56] Chapter 2 investigates how Irish medical schools from the mid-nineteenth century attempted to inculcate students with the ideals of the profession and reform the reputation of the rowdy medical student in order to help improve the status of the profession. Addresses to students have captured important themes in the history of medical education and these will also be utilised in order to illuminate the qualities that were expected of Irish medical students in the period.[57] The nineteenth century was also an important period in the transformation of the image of the medical student from 'urban pariah to a hardworking individual training for a respectable profession'.[58] This chapter shows how representations of medical students changed in Ireland over the period, examining the importance of class, religious affiliation and the appropriate traits that students were expected to possess.

The issue of class and social mobility is an important consideration of this book. Medical education offered a means of social mobility to those who undertook it in Ireland in the nineteenth and twentieth centuries.

---

51 Irish, 'Fractured families', pp. 511–12.
52 Irish, 'Fractured families', p. 512.
53 Manuel Castells, *The power of identity* (Oxford: Blackwell, 1997), p. 6.
54 Anne Digby, 'Shaping new identities: general practitioners in Britain and South Africa', in Kent Maynard (ed.), *Medical identities: health, well-being and personhood* (New York: Berghahn Books, 2007), p. 20.
55 Loudon, *Medical care and the general practitioner*, p. 41, cited in Marguerite Dupree and Anne Crowther, *Medical lives in the age of surgical revolution* (Cambridge: Cambridge University Press, 2007), p. 2.
56 Waddington, 'Mayhem and medical students', p. 47.
57 See, for example, Michael Brown, 'Like a devoted army: medicine, heroic masculinity and the military paradigm in Victorian Britain', *Journal of British Studies* 49(3) (2010): 592–622.
58 Waddington, 'Mayhem and medical students', p. 63.

Recent research has honed in on the social backgrounds of medical students, illustrating how medical education could be used as a tool for upward mobility.[59] Chapter 3, through an exploration of the social and religious backgrounds of a sample of Irish medical students, illustrates the dominance of the middle classes in Irish medical schools from the mid-nineteenth to the early twentieth century, while also outlining institutional differences, the reasons underpinning students' decisions to pursue medical education and the cost of education and living arrangements.

Bonner, Waddington, Reinarz and van Heteren, amongst others, have shown how medical education can vary widely and how students' experiences are shaped by local and national differences.[60] We know very little about the educational experiences of Irish medical students while at university. Although there have been a number of institutional histories of Irish medical schools, these tend to focus on the background behind the founding of the schools, the main events in the schools' histories and the historical actors

---

59 See, for example, Dupree and Crowther, *Medical lives*; Florent Palluault, 'Medical students in England and France 1815–58: a comparative study' (unpublished DPhil. thesis, University of Oxford, 2003); Laura Kelly, 'Migration and medical education: Irish medical students at the University of Glasgow, 1859–1900', *Irish Economic and Social History* 39(1) (2012): 39–55. Dupree and Crowther, for example, in their comprehensive study of the social backgrounds and careers of medical students at Glasgow and Edinburgh in the nineteenth century, have illuminated themes such as social mobility as well as addressing aspects of medical student life such as living conditions and extra-curricular activities.

60 See Bonner, *Becoming a physician*; Keir Waddington, *Medical education at St Bartholomew's Hospital, 1123–1995* (Woodbridge: Boydell Press, 2003); Jonathan Reinarz, *Health care in Birmingham: the Birmingham teaching hospitals, 1779–1939* (Woodbridge: Boydell Press, 2009); and G. van Heteren, 'Students facing boundaries: the shift of nineteenth-century British student travel to German universities and the flexible boundaries of a medical educational system', in V. Nutton and R. Porter (eds), *The history of medical education in Britain* (Amsterdam: Rodopi, 1995). Bonner has also pointed out the 'persistence of national differences in shaping the outcome of social and scientific movements in medical teaching' (*Becoming a physician*, p. 10). Complementing this, Christopher Lawrence's work illustrates the potential for investigating how modern national identity informs medical education systems (Lawrence, 'The shaping of things to come: Scottish medical education, 1700–1939', *Medical Education* 40(3) (2006): 212–18). Research on the Birmingham teaching hospitals has illustrated how histories of provincial medical education can provide new perspectives by rethinking the London model of education that was previously believed to be dominant (Reinarz, *Health care in Birmingham*). Likewise, in the American context, Warner has shown how in the Southern states of the United States, physicians claimed that Southern medical practice was distinctive and that therefore medical students ought to be educated in Southern medical institutions. Furthermore, 'clinical training both gave Southern medical education its identity and drew attention to the inadequacies of Northern schools' (see John Harley Warner, 'A Southern medical reform: the meaning of the antebellum argument for Southern medical education', *Bulletin of the History of Medicine* 57(3) (1984): 364–81).

and professors that were involved in these events.[61] Chapter 4 explores what students studied at Irish medical schools from the late nineteenth century to the early years of the twentieth. It examines the importance of educational tools such as medical museums, laboratories and medical student societies in the context of students' educational experiences and whether the role of science in medical curricula was affected by the differing philosophies of Irish universities. The transition from the lecture theatre to the hospital ward was a turning point in the educational experiences of many Irish doctors. Drawing primarily on doctors' memoirs, student magazines and the surviving records of Irish hospitals relating to clinical education, this chapter illuminates this important facet of medical students' experiences and how it helped to shape professional identity.[62]

61 See, for example, on Queen's College Cork: Denis J. O'Sullivan, *The Cork School of Medicine: a history* (Cork: UCC Medical Alumni Association, University College Cork, 2007) and Ronan O'Rahilly, *A history of the Cork medical school, 1849–1949* (Cork: Cork University Press, 1949); Queen's College Galway: James Murray, *Galway: a medico-social history* (Galway: Kenny's Bookshop and Art Gallery, 1994); Queen's College Belfast: Peter Froggatt, 'The distinctiveness of Belfast medicine and its medical school', *Ulster Medical Journal* 54(2) (1985): 89–108; Royal College of Surgeons: J.B. Lyons, *The irresistible rise of the RCSI* (Dublin: Royal College of Surgeons, 1984); Eoin O'Brien, *The Royal College of Surgeons in Ireland: 1784–1984* (Dublin: Eason, 1984); J.D.H. Widdess, *The Royal College of Surgeons in Ireland and its medical school* (Edinburgh: E. & S. Livingstone, 1967); Charles A. Cameron, *History of the Royal College of Surgeons in Ireland and of the Irish Schools of Medicine, including numerous biographical sketches; also a medical bibliography* (Dublin: Fannin & Co., 1886); Royal College of Physicians: J.D.H. Widdess, *A history of the Royal College of Physicians of Ireland, 1654–1963* (Edinburgh: E. & S. Livingstone, 1964); Trinity College Dublin: T.P.C. Kirkpatrick, *History of the medical teaching in Trinity College Dublin and of the School of Physic in Ireland* (Dublin: Hanna and Neale, 1912); the Catholic University: Meenan, *Cecilia Street*; Ronan O'Rahilly, *Benjamin Alcock: the first professor of anatomy and physiology in Queen's College Cork* (Cork: Cork University Press, 1948).

62 Student magazines are useful in illuminating what it was like to be a student in the nineteenth and twentieth centuries. See, for instance, Janet Browne, 'Squibs and snobs: science in humorous British undergraduate magazines around 1830', *History of Science* 30(3) (1992): 165–97. Irish student magazines I will draw on include *Q.C.C., The Quarryman* (Cork), *Q.C.B., Snakes Alive, The Northman* (Belfast), *Q.C.G.* (Galway), *Mistura, R.C.S.I.: A Students' Quarterly* (Royal College of Surgeons), *The National Student, St. Stephen's: A Record of University Life* (Catholic University, later University College Dublin), and *T.C.D.: A College Miscellany* (Trinity College Dublin), most of which began to be produced from the early 1900s. My methodology is also influenced by historians who have effectively utilised personal sources such as student diaries and letters, photographs and doctors' memoirs. See, for example, John Harley Warner, *The therapeutic perspective: medical practice, knowledge and identity in America, 1820–1885* (Princeton, NJ: Princeton University Press, 1997); Lisa Rosner, 'Student culture at the turn of the nineteenth century', *Caduceus* 10(2) (1994): 65–86; John Harley Warner and James M. Edmondson, *Dissection: photographs of a rite of passage in American medicine, 1880–1930* (New York: Blast Books, 2009) and Crowther and Dupree, *Medical lives*.

The period under study in this book was a politically fraught one, with twentieth-century Ireland witness to the Easter Rising, the Irish War of Independence, the Civil War and the First and Second World Wars. The First World War, for instance, has been described as 'the greatest caesura in the life of Trinity College Dublin', with almost one-third of the 3,000 members of the college involved in the war serving in the Royal Army Medical Corps.[63] Approximately 320 former students of the Catholic University Medical School served in the British armed forces during the First World War, with sixteen of these dying in action or while on active service. Students from UCD were, however, less enthusiastic for supporting the war effort and there was more support for 'breaking the connection with England'. However, when the actual fighting began, during Easter 1916, 'the medical school did not appear to be strongly represented in Dublin'.[64] Overall, however, it does not appear that medical students' day-to-day lives or educational experiences, for the most part, were affected significantly by these political events. However, Irish medical education following the establishment of the Free State was fraught with a number of problems, including sectarianism, lack of adequate scientific research and an over-supply of medical schools.[65]

Gender is another important focus of this book. It is clear that the identity of medical students was not only bound up with concepts of class, but also centred on ideas of manliness and masculinity. Chapter 5 explores this issue through particular focus on 'rites of passage' in different educational spheres from the late nineteenth to the early twentieth century, and through an examination of students' extra-curricular activities. Importantly, these activities represent an aspect of student life that is often overlooked but which was equally important in the development of the Irish medical practitioner. The late nineteenth century is a significant point in the history of Irish medical education as this was when women began to enter Irish medical schools and Irish medical institutions played a key role in the registration of women practitioners in this period. In 1877, the King and Queen's College of Physicians in Ireland (KQCPI) became the first institution to take advantage of the Enabling Act, which allowed women doctors who had attained foreign qualifications to obtain the licence which would allow them to practise as physicians in Britain. Women began to enter Irish medical schools as students from the 1880s, and by 1904 women were

---

63 Tomás Irish, *Trinity in war and revolution, 1912–1923* (Dublin: Royal Irish Academy, 2015), pp. 79 and 101.

64 Meenan, *Cecilia Street*, p. 93.

65 Greta Jones, 'The Rockefeller Foundation and medical education in Ireland in the 1920s', *Irish Historical Studies* 30(120) (1997): 564–80.

able to enter all of the Irish medical schools. Nonetheless, in spite of the seemingly egalitarian attitudes towards women students in Irish medical schools, extra-curricular activities and educational rites of passage helped to preserve medicine as a predominantly masculine sphere of practice. While women students are discussed throughout the book, Chapter 6 focuses exclusively on their experiences, and suggests that although they were readily integrated into Irish medical schools and hospitals, women medical students occupied a separate sphere from the male students with regard to their social experiences and were also represented in a particular way.[66]

The final chapter of the book explores medical student life from the 1920s to the 1950s. The chapter draws on 24 revealing oral history interviews conducted by the author with Irish physicians who trained at Irish medical schools in the 1940s and 1950s. Oral history is a valuable means of investigating the experiences of students of the past and is different from other sources in that 'it tells us less about *events* than about their *meaning*'.[67] Moreover, as sociologist Maurice Halbwachs has argued, 'an individual's memory is always situated within a collective or group consciousness of an event or experience', with individual memory being viewed as inseparable from the collective.[68] Of course, there are issues with memory, and, given the ages of the participants, changes in their socio-economic standing or in their personal subjective consciousness may have affected how they recalled their student days.[69] However, these sources are arguably invaluable in providing an insight into personal experience. As Alessandro Portelli has eloquently surmised, 'Oral sources tell us not just what people did, but what they wanted to do, what they believed they were doing, and what they now think they did'.[70] These interviews provide first-hand accounts of the experiences of Irish medical students during a time of an increasingly conservative Irish society. They highlight the continuing importance of clinical experience to Irish students and the differences between male and female students' experiences. Irish medical schools were largely 'exporting schools' in the nineteenth and twentieth centuries.[71] This chapter explores the personal consequences of emigration during this period.

---

66 For a detailed account of the history of the first Irish women doctors, see Laura Kelly, *Irish women in medicine, c.1880s–1920s: origins, education and careers* (Manchester: Manchester University Press, 2012).

67 Alessandro Portelli, 'What makes oral history different', in Robert Perks and Alistair Thomson (eds), *The oral history reader* (London and New York: Routledge, 2003), p. 67.

68 Lynn Abrams, *Oral history theory* (London: Routledge, 2010), p. 96.

69 Portelli, 'What makes oral history different', p. 69.

70 Portelli, 'What makes oral history different', p. 67.

71 See Greta Jones, '"A mysterious discrimination": Irish medical emigration to the United States in the 1950s', *Social History of Medicine* 25(1) (2011): 139–56 and Greta

This book aims to provide an insight into what it was like to be a medical student in Ireland in the past through an exploration of Irish medical students' experiences of education and their day-to-day lives in the nineteenth and twentieth centuries. It will also further develop our understanding of commonalities in the experiences of medical students internationally. Moreover, through an examination of the history of medical education, the book builds on our understanding of the Irish medical profession while also contributing to the wider scholarship of student life and culture.[72]

Jones, '"Strike out boldly for the prizes that are available to you": medical emigration from Ireland, 1860–1905', *Medical History* 54(1) (2010).

72 See, for example, Andrew Warwick, *Masters of theory: Cambridge and the rise of mathematical physics* (Chicago: University of Chicago Press, 2003), which charts the experiences of mathematical physics students at Cambridge in the nineteenth and twentieth centuries; Carol Dyhouse, *Students: a gendered history* (London: Routledge, 2005), a gendered social history of students at British universities in the twentieth century; Paul R. Deslandes, *Oxbridge men: British masculinity and the undergraduate experience, 1850–1920* (Bloomington: Indiana University Press, 2005), a gendered history of student experience at Oxford and Cambridge universities; and Helen Lefkowitz Horowitz, *Campus life: undergraduate cultures from the end of the eighteenth century to the present* (Chicago: University of Chicago Press, 1988), which investigates the experiences of students at American universities.

1

The Medical School Marketplace, *c*.1850–1900

The early nineteenth century has been frequently hailed as the 'golden age of Irish medicine' as a result of the work of physicians Robert Graves and William Stokes, whose emphasis on bedside teaching earned fame for the Meath Hospital where they were based. However, by the 1850s, Irish medical education had fallen into ill repute. This condition was to prevail for most of the remainder of the nineteenth century. In an address to students in Cork in 1853, a young medical graduate, Thomas Holland, outlined the deficiencies of Irish medical education. In his view, the Irish School of Medicine was living on past glories, and although its system of clinical instruction as derived from German medical schools had been successfully introduced, Irish schools had been less successful in introducing aspects of the 'highly scientific and truth-searching character of the German mind'.[1] In Holland's view, the Irish School of Medicine had reached its 'culminating point, and must of necessity decline, if we continue basking in the sunlight of our teachers' names'. Moreover, he argued that 'Irish medicine must assume a new character; a truly scientific spirit must be reinstilled into our school, if we desire that it shall keep pace with the advance of science'.[2]

Irish medical schools from the mid- to late nineteenth century suffered from economic difficulties which resulted in the emergence of irregularities which were distinctive to Irish institutions, such as the sham certificate system, night lectures and 'grinding'. Students also had a choice with regard to the type of qualification they aimed at, meaning that there was

---

1 Thomas S. Holland, 'The Irish School of Medicine as it is and as it ought to be; an address: introductory to a course at pathological anatomy and histology in relation to the practice of medicine and surgery delivered at the Royal Cork Institution by Thomas S. Holland MD' (Cork: George Purcell & Co., 1853), p. 8.
2 Holland, 'The Irish School of Medicine', p. 9.

a different type of qualification to suit every pocket. Much attention has been given to the medical marketplace of the eighteenth and nineteenth centuries whereby practitioners competed for patients.[3] In this chapter, I wish to apply the concept to Irish medical schools, suggesting that for the second half of the nineteenth century, owing to intense competition between the different institutions, medical students wielded a great amount of power as consumers. The chapter will also focus on several case studies of student protest and what these tell us about students' concerns in the period. Moreover, students' involvement in these disputes and their mobilisation over educational concerns, suggests that they were beginning to view themselves as active members of the Irish medical profession with an entitlement to contribute to professional issues.

'The Irish system is open to grave abuses'

By the mid-1850s, students had several options for medical study in Ireland. These included Trinity College Dublin (founded in 1592), the Royal College of Surgeons (1784), the three Queen's Colleges (1845), the Catholic University School of Medicine (1854) or one of several private medical schools which were primarily located in Dublin. Numbers of medical graduates were high and supply exceeded demand. In the five-year period from 1876 to 1880, for instance, there were 517 men who graduated with MB and MD degrees from Irish institutions, compared with 402 men in England and 1,536 in Scotland. The Irish figure would actually have been higher than 517 as it did not take into account the numbers of graduates with MB degrees from the Queen's Colleges.[4] Despite the fact that Irish medical education was governed and regulated by the General Medical Council, established under the Medical Act of 1858, differences between standards of education in Britain and Ireland were frequently referred to in the contemporary medical press. Moreover, Irish students, in contrast with their counterparts at English and Scottish schools, had more freedom

---

3 See, for instance, Roy Porter, 'Before the fringe: "quackery" and the eighteenth-century medical market', in Roger Cooter (ed.), *Studies in the history of alternative medicine* (Basingstoke: Macmillan, 1988), pp. 1–25 and, for Ireland, see Catherine Cox, 'The medical marketplace and medical tradition in nineteenth-century Ireland', in Ronnie Moore and Stuart McClean (eds), *Folk healing and health care practices in Britain and Ireland: stethoscopes, wands and crystals* (New York: Berghahn Books, 2010), pp. 55–79.

4 See 'Number of graduates in medicine admitted during the five years, 1876–1880 in England, Scotland, and Ireland, taken from the Reports of the Royal Commission', Table 1 in Walter Rivington, '"The medical profession of the United Kingdom", being the essay to which was awarded the First Carmichael Prize by the Council of the Royal College of Surgeons in Ireland, 1887' (Dublin: Fannin & Co., 1888), p. 257.

in terms of their educational choices. In 1879, in their 'Students' Number' the *Medical Press and Circular* referred to the fact that in England medical students were encouraged to enter at a particular school and hospital and that they would take their whole education there, a path that the majority of students followed.[5] This had its advantages in that it meant that students were placed 'under the absolute control' of their teachers and supervised to a much greater extent than elsewhere. In Ireland, however, there was much more freedom. Students could go to any school or hospital they wished and enter their name for any number of lectures. Indeed, out of cities in the British dominions, Dublin was only surpassed by London in terms of institutional diversity.[6] According to the article, if a student 'does not like his school or hospital, he most probably migrates to a rival institution on the first opportunity'. Critically, the article remarked:

> The Irish system is open to grave abuses, which need not be dwelt on at present; but it has certainly the great merit of rendering the student perfectly independent, and forcing schools to compete energetically for a continuance of his patronage. It will be obvious, however, that the system which enables the student to pay a lump sum, and thus relieve himself of the trouble of entering for lectures, and paying fees in detail, is a convenient one, especially for the beginner, who is altogether ignorant of the system, and therefore the requirement which is provided for in England by the dean of the school, is met in Ireland by individual teachers or 'apprentice' holders.[7]

Evidently, Irish medical schools were in extreme competition with each other for student fees. Moreover, the article drew attention to the fact that students could pay for lectures but that there was no pressure on them to attend. This was a particular problem in the Irish system of medical education in the nineteenth century and was often referred to in the medical press as the 'sham certificate' system, whereby students produced certificates with the signatures of their teachers which merely indicated that they had paid for the lectures but not that they had attended them. This meant that students could potentially put themselves forward for an examination without having attended the prescribed classes. Attendance on lectures does not appear to have been rigorously enforced. The *Medical Press and Circular* reported in 1879 that the average student in Dublin was

---

5 'Students' Number', *Medical Press and Circular*, 24 September 1879, p. 266.
6 David Dickson, *Dublin: the making of a capital city* (London: Profile Books, 2014), p. 314.
7 'Students' Number', *Medical Press and Circular*, p. 266.

supposed to attend twelve courses of lectures, six of these extending over six months and six extending over three months, which totalled 52 months of lecturing. Students were also expected to dissect simultaneously and to attend demonstrations for a period of an hour and a half daily for eighteen months and to attend hospitals for at least two hours a day for 27 months, as well as spending three months in a chemical laboratory. This meant that a student typically could qualify in about five years, if they followed this timetable. At Trinity College, students were required to attend three-quarters of the prescribed lectures, but the journal remarked that the other Irish licensing bodies accepted as 'diligent' attendance the presence of the student at all, a few, or none of the lectures which the student had paid for. Condemning this system, the *Medical Press and Circular* remarked, 'the average student thinks himself exemplary if he works his hospital, dissections, demonstrations, physiology, lectures, and grind, and drops in occasionally to the other courses'.[8]

Matters do not seem to have improved moving into the 1880s. Writing in his account of the medical profession in Britain and Ireland in 1888, Walter Rivington accused Irish medical schools of systematically discouraging the registration of their medical students and denounced them for ignoring the recommendations of the General Medical Council. He claimed that this meant that students could commence their medical studies at any point in the academic year and were credited with attendance at the whole session regardless of when they started. For example, students who ought to have commenced their studies in October could be accepted as late as the following March or April, and, allegedly, could count three weeks' attendance as six months of professional study which meant that these individuals could complete their education in a shorter time period than their counterparts elsewhere in Britain.[9] Indeed, a study conducted by the Statistical Committee of the General Medical Council found that of medical students in the five-year period from 1871 to 1875, Irish students on average qualified after just over four and a half years compared with English and Scottish students who qualified after five years.[10] Irish students also had a higher failure rate than English and Scottish students. Of students registered in 1871, for instance, 27.55 per cent from the English medical students had not registered any qualification, compared with 29.82 per cent in Scotland and 34.5 per cent in Ireland.[11] Students could drop out of a medical course for a variety of reasons such as academic failure, illness,

8 'Students' Number', *Medical Press and Circular*, p. 267.
9 Rivington, '"The medical profession of the United Kingdom"', p. 650.
10 Rivington, '"The medical profession of the United Kingdom"', Appendix E, p. 1030.
11 Rivington, '"The medical profession of the United Kingdom"', Appendix E, p. 1021.

family commitments, lack of financial support or a change of heart about medicine as a profession.

From 1883, measures were introduced by medical schools to try and do away with the sham certificate system. At the Royal College of Surgeons, teachers were now required to specify on students' certificates the exact number of lectures delivered by the teacher and attended by the student, in contrast with the old system where professors merely reported whether the student had 'diligently' attended lectures. Although this was an improvement on the previous system, the *Dublin Medical Press* advised that there was still potential for 'sham certifying ... by the less scrupulous teachers'. Students could still sign for other students in the hospital signature book and others who signed their names at 9 a.m. returned to their day jobs by 9.30 a.m. Likewise, because attendance on lectures was ascertained by roll-call, this meant that students could answer for each other.[12]

Competition also drove some of Dublin's medical schools to exaggerate the number of pupils in their classes in their returns to the Anatomical Committee with the dual purpose of appearing successful and also securing a larger number of cadavers. Although schools had to pay £1. 1s. for every student for "subject money" (the cost of cadavers), some of this money could be withdrawn at the end of the session if so large a supply of subjects was not required.[13] The *Dublin Medical Press* condemned the practice in 1883, and although they did not name the guilty schools, the number of students listed for the Ledwich School (228), one of the smaller private colleges which had been established by George Hayden in 1836, suggests that it was guilty of including in its returns 'all sorts of sham pupils and dead-heads ... a crowd of perpetuals and chronics who have long since disappeared from the study of the profession, and a large number of night lecturers'.[14]

The most controversial aspect of the Irish medical education system in the late nineteenth century, however, was the practice of night lectures. This system appears to have been distinctive to Irish medical schools and again stemmed from competition and the monetary benefits to be gained by medical schools from having a larger number of students on their books. Although the practice gained widespread condemnation in the 1880s, it had a longer history. In 1845, the *Dublin Medical Press* reported that some of the private schools in Dublin, in order to attract pupils, had been keeping their

---

12 'Retrospect of the year 1883: Ireland', *Dublin Medical Press*, 25 December 1883, pp. 548–9.
13 'The Dublin student class', *Dublin Medical Press*, 19 December 1883, pp. 539–40.
14 'The Dublin student class', pp. 539–40. For more on the private Dublin medical schools, see Sir Charles A. Cameron, *History of the Royal College of Surgeons in Ireland and of the Irish Schools of Medicine including numerous biographical sketches; also a medical bibliography* (Dublin: Fannin & Co., 1886), pp. 513–40.

dissecting rooms open at night, 'and have them lighted up with gas, which has led to great evils and irregularities'.[15] Over forty years later, in 1889, the *Lancet* estimated that 10 per cent to 15 per cent of Irish medical students pursued their course of study through attendance at night lectures provided by some of the medical schools. According to the article, 'they stick to their business or desk during the day and become medical students at night, with such accommodation as some schools in Dublin provide for them'. The *Lancet* criticised this, suggesting that such a system was not 'one of true medical education'.[16] Similarly, Walter Rivington remarked in 1888 that 'there is no objection to evening lectures, but there would be great objection to admitting candidates to the examinations who have neither dissected properly nor paid sufficient attention to work in the hospital wards as dressers and clinical clerks'.[17] The *British Medical Journal* was more sympathetic, suggesting that night lectures allowed men working in offices, pharmacies and counting houses a means of entry to the profession and that this class often comprised 'the most hard-working and intelligent men, and many of them have become excellent and successful practitioners'.[18] The two main schools in the 1880s which were operating a system of night lectures were the Ledwich School and the Carmichael College in Dublin, which were smaller private medical schools. Both schools were criticised by Thomas Laffan in 1883 for having teaching staffs which were far in excess of requirements.[19]

The condemnation of the practice of night lectures stems from three main issues. First, members of the larger medical schools were quick to denounce the practice because of competition from the private medical schools. Secondly, it was argued that training attained through night lectures meant that students were not attaining a proper means of education. However, another possible reason was that night lectures allowed men of a lower class a means of entry to the profession. Irish medical students in the second-half of the nineteenth century were predominantly drawn from the middle classes. John William Moore, Fellow and Registrar of the KQCPI, Physician to the Meath Hospital and lecturer in the practice of medicine, Carmichael College, defended the Dublin system of night classes in 1888, arguing that it provided a means 'for a deserving class of students' to undertake medical education. He claimed that the 'evening students' had 'more than their share of prizes in our schools

---

15 'An appeal to students on behalf of students', *Dublin Medical Press*, 29 October 1845, p. 285.
16 'Nocturnal medical education', *Lancet*, 30 March 1889, p. 644.
17 Rivington, '"The medical profession of the United Kingdom"', p. 748.
18 'Night lectures', *British Medical Journal*, 9 April 1887, p. 794.
19 Thomas Laffan, '"The medical profession in the three kingdoms in 1887", the essay to which was awarded the Carmichael Prize of £100 by the Council of the Royal College of Surgeons, Ireland, 1887' (Dublin: Fannin & Co., 1888), pp. 194–5.

and hospitals', that these students were, to his knowledge, diligent in the hospital setting and had passed their examinations 'on excellent, sometimes on brilliant, answering' and, finally, 'that the justice of affording facilities to men, who in the face of the greatest difficulties exhibit untiring energy in their efforts to enter the profession of Medicine' had been conceded by some of the leading members of the Irish medical profession.[20] However, one constant theme throughout the history of the medical profession 'has been the effort to define who is a member and who is not'.[21] The objections towards night classes are revealing, and they suggest narrowing definitions of what it meant to be a member of the medical profession. As John Harley Warner's work has shown in the American context, professional identity was at a turning point in the period from the 1860s to the 1880s.[22] It was redefined and there was a shift 'from behaviour towards knowledge as the base of professional legitimacy'.[23] Professional identity now meant expertise in scientific matters and the possession and application of specialised knowledge.[24] From the late nineteenth century, as attendance at medical school became even more important to the development of a corporate and professional identity, night classes came to be viewed as an inadequate means of aiming at becoming a fully indoctrinated member of the medical profession. However, they were not the only means for less-well-off students to find a way to qualify as a physician. As will be shown later in this chapter, Irish medical students could aim at a variety of qualifications depending on their economic position and how much time they were willing to spend on medical study.

The Royal College of Surgeons ceased to accept certificates of attendance at night lectures from 1883.[25] Although the Royal University passed a motion declaring that they would follow suit in 1887, they revoked this and allowed certificates from students who had 'advanced in their studies'.[26] The Board of Trinity College agreed not to accept certificates of attendance at night lectures under any circumstances; however, there appear to have been no

20 'Medical education and examinations in 1887' by John William Moore, Fellow and Registrar of the KQCPI, Physician to the Meath Hospital and Lecturer in the Practice of Medicine, Carmichael College, *Dublin Journal of Medical Science*, 2 January 1888, p. 45.
21 Toby Gelfand, 'The history of the medical profession', in Roy Porter and W.F. Bynum (eds), *Companion encyclopedia of the history of medicine*, vol.2 (London: Routledge, 1993), p. 1119.
22 John Harley Warner, *The therapeutic perspective: medical practice, knowledge and identity in America, 1820–1885* (Princeton, NJ: Princeton University Press, 1997), pp. 258–64.
23 Warner, *The therapeutic perspective*, p. 263.
24 Warner, *The therapeutic perspective*, p. 262.
25 'Night lectures', *British Medical Journal*, 23 December 1882, p. 1272.
26 'The Royal University and night lectures', *British Medical Journal*, 28 May 1887, p. 1190.

objections from Royal College of Physicians until the 1890s.[27] By 1894, the system of night lectures had been abolished in Dublin, with one commentator remarking that this may have contributed to a decline in numbers of medical students. In Ireland in 1862, 352 students were registered, while in 1892 the number had fallen to 175. This was in contrast with increases in Scotland from 324 to 578 and in England from 676 to 1,007 in the same period. Dublin surgeon John McArdle, writing in 1894, attributed the decrease in numbers of students to the decline of prosperity in the country, the employment of many educated men in the Civil Service Departments, the extension of the time of study and the abolition of night lectures. Adding to this, he specified local causes such as frequent changes of regulations, the constant addition of new subjects and uncertainty of examinations.[28] William Stoker, in an address to students at the Royal College of Surgeons in the same year, argued that the falling off in numbers of students studying medicine in Dublin did not imply a 'material decadence'. In his view, it was due to two main factors: the opening up of medical schools in Belfast, Galway and Cork, and the fact that many Irish students, though educated at Irish schools, went to England or Scotland for their diplomas.[29]

'Grinding' was also a significant and distinctive aspect of the Irish medical student's educational experience from the 1840s, if not earlier, up until the mid-twentieth century. Grinding was a system of private tuition conducted in classes by private tutors with the aim of helping students to pass their examinations.[30] According to James Duncan, speaking to students in 1864, grinding was essentially a form of cramming where pupils were 'taught a certain number of answers to appropriate questions, which they afterwards repeat with little more intelligence than a parrot'.[31] At British medical schools, students would sometimes go to a 'coach' if they had failed an examination and wished to prevent another failure. However, at Irish schools, attendance on a grinder appears to have been more common, and students often attended one before examinations.[32] Davis Coakley, in his recent study of the medical

27 Rivington, '"The medical profession of the United Kingdom"', p. 748.
28 J.S. McArdle, 'Medical education as it is and as it should be', *Dublin Journal of Medical Science* 98 (1894), p. 395.
29 William T. Stoker, 'Some lessons on life', *Irish Journal of Medical Science* 98 (1894), p. 468.
30 The practice of 'grinding' is mentioned in the *Dublin Medical Press* on 18 October 1843 ('The approaching medical session', p. 254).
31 Introductory lecture delivered in the Adelaide Hospital, Dublin at the commencement of the clinical course, 31 October 1864, by James F. Duncan, AM, MD, TCD (Dublin: Alexander Thom, 1864), p. 18 in Annual Reports of Adelaide Hospital, 1858–65 [Trinity College Manuscripts, IE TCD MS 11270/11/1/1].
32 Colonel Robert J. Blackham, *Scalpel, sword and stretcher: forty years of work and play* (London: Sampson Low, Marston & Co. Ltd., 1931), p. 30.

school at Trinity College Dublin, has suggested that 'the primary source of knowledge for Trinity medical students and for students in the other schools was not their formal lectures but the private tuition they received from their grinders'.[33] Robert Blackham, who studied at the Ledwich School, believed that the 'grinder' took the place of the master of the 'apprenticeship days of surgery which were still within the experience of many then living'.[34] The practice appears to have been condoned by the medical schools and many of the tutors who conducted these classes were associated with the different medical schools. In 1900, the Catholic University medical faculty referred in a report to the 'want of common rooms for professors, students and grinders', suggesting that grinders at that institution were viewed as part of the establishment.[35]

Grinders advertised openly in the press and in student newspapers.[36] Students occasionally also advertised requests for grinders.[37] An advertisement which appeared in the *Irish Times* in 1890 stated that 'a firm of medical grinders are forming classes in Anatomy, Physiology and Histology, Chemistry and Physics, and Botany and Zoology'. The price for one month was two guineas, with special rates being offered for longer periods.[38] By 1907, it was estimated that grinding fees were usually about £3. 3s.[39] Thomas Garry blamed the system of teaching in Dublin medical schools for the booming business of grinding, believing that because students were left to their own devices they were forced to place themselves under the guidance of a 'grind', as he himself did. He condemned grinding as 'a most pernicious form of cramming. It deprives the student of all initiative and reasoning

---

33 Davis Coakley, *Medicine in Trinity College Dublin: an illustrated history* (Dublin: Trinity College Dublin, 2014), p. 176.
34 Blackham, *Scalpel, sword and stretcher*, p. 30.
35 25 May 1900, in Catholic University School of Medicine Governing Body Minute Book, 1892–1911 [UCD Archives, CU/14].
36 See, for instance, classified advertisement for medical student grinds 'in chemistry, physics, *materia medica* and therapeutics for pre-registration and professional examinations' (*Irish Times*, 6 February 1924, p. 1); classified advertisement seeking students for grinds (*Irish Times*, 23 October 1913, p. 2 and p. 1; advertisement by Mr T.A. Robb for grinds in *materia medica* (with specimens) at Lisburn Road, Belfast, *Q.C.B.* 8(4) (1907): 15; advertisement for Dr Bronte's grinds in pathology and physiology for College of Surgeons, Dublin University and NUI examinations, in *R.C.S.I. Students' Quarterly* 1(1) (1917), Kirkpatrick collection: Clubs and Associations [RCPI Heritage Centre, TPCK/6/7/12].
37 Classified advertisement, *Irish Times*, 16 January 1917, p. 1, advertisement of student seeking grind in anatomy for the second professional examination in April of that year.
38 Classified advertisements, *Irish Times*, 5 February 1890, p. 1.
39 Ella G.A. Ovenden, MD, 'Medicine', in *Open doors for Irishwomen: a guide to the professions open to educated women in Ireland*, ed. Myrrha Bradshaw, Issued by the Irish Central Bureau for the Employment of Women (Dublin, 1907), p. 36.

power as well as self-confidence, the most essential trait in the character of a medical practitioner'.[40] Contemporary medical journals such as the *Medical Press and Circular* suggested that the lecture load for students was very heavy and that to fulfil the nominal requirements of a medical education students would need to work nearly nine hours daily. As a result, attendance was lax, and students instead resorted to grinds for their tuition and were thought by professors to be more inclined to attend grinds than lectures.[41]

Occasionally, issues arose with the practice of grinds. In 1898, the committee of the Senate of the Royal University of Ireland charged two Dublin examiners with holding grinds immediately before the final examinations and accused that one of the examiners had discussed the exact questions set on the paper.[42] In February 1901, an extraordinary case came before the Commission Court in Dublin where a man called Joseph Haddock was accused of impersonating two medical students, Robert F. Cooper and Alexander Fyffe, and taking some of their preliminary examinations for the Royal College of Surgeons for them. This was an act which Sergeant Dodd, stating the case, called an offence which 'struck at the very root of a most important element of society'. Fyffe, in court, said that he had been receiving grinds with Haddock and had arranged to pay him £5 if he passed the examination. Haddock dyed his hair a light shade and shaved off his moustache in order to pass for the two students. Haddock was found guilty in court of impersonating Cooper and Fyffe and the case was adjourned until the next commission meeting in April.[43] Fundamentally, the practice of grinding was a distinctly Irish phenomenon and highlights the inadequacies with Irish medical education in the period. Moreover, the business of grinding and the fact that medical schools appear to have been complicit in this, with many of the grinders being informally associated with certain medical schools, highlights potential conflicts of interest. However, ultimately, the economic benefits to be gained from this practice overrode potential ethical concerns.

40   Thomas Garry, *African doctor* (London: John Gifford, 1939), p. 11.
41   W. Battersby, '"Medical education", an address delivered in the dining hall of Trinity College at the opening meeting of the second session of the Dublin University Medico-Chirurgical Society, November 27th, 1868 by the auditor W.E. Battersby, B.A. Med. Sch.' (Dublin: M. & S. Eaton, 1868), p. 26 and 'Students' Number', *Medical Press and Circular*, 24 September 1879, p. 267.
42   'General meeting of the BMSA held in the McMordie Hall on Friday, 4th of November 1898, Secretaries' report of year 1897–98', Belfast Medical Students' Association Minute Book, November 1898–November 1907 [QUB Special Collections].
43   'Medical examination scandal: extraordinary evidence', *Irish Times*, 16 February 1901, p. 18.

Choosing a qualification

Students had two choices with regard to the type of primary qualifications they could attain in the period – medical degrees and licences. Degrees could only be conferred by a university and allowed students to sign the letters MB BCh BAO after their names. Licences, on the other hand, allowed students to practise medicine after they passed the examinations of one of the corporate bodies, these being the Royal College of Physicians, the Royal College of Surgeons, or the Apothecaries Hall.[44] The difference between the two was that degrees took longer to gain but were held in higher esteem by the profession. The degree of the Royal University, for instance, involved students passing a matriculation examination, before devoting one year to the study of Arts, and then commencing medical studies, while in order to begin the course of study required for a medical licence, students were only required to pass a simple preliminary examination.[45] Students could also later aim at the higher MD degree.

Choice of primary qualification also depended on the student's financial circumstances. A guide for Irish medical students published in 1872 stated that if the student intended to 'make a fortune and enlighten his generation as a metropolitan practitioner, and if money and education are plenty', he should take the option of the university degree. However, 'if the attainment of good professional rank on moderate terms be desired, the College of Surgeons and College of Physicians will serve every purpose'.[46] University degrees required a longer period in college, with students having to undertake prolonged studies in classics and science in addition to their medical studies. However, if the expense and labour involved were accepted, the graduate 'will enter the Profession with all the prestige of an educated gentleman'.[47] Nonetheless, the guide noted that the licence of the Colleges of Physicians and Surgeons would 'stand well beside any in the United Kingdom' and 'as they do not require either residence or anything more than a single Arts examination, they continue to be the licensing bodies for the rank and file of the Profession in Ireland', and would be suitable for a student considering provincial, dispensary, army or navy practice.[48]

44 *Guide for medical students, more especially for those about to commence their medical studies, by the registrar of the Catholic University School of Medicine* (Dublin: Browne & Nolan, 1892), pp. 8–9.
45 *Guide for medical students, more especially for those about to commence their medical studies*, p. 9.
46 *The Irish medical student's guide: an epitome of medical education in Ireland and the public medical services* (Dublin: Office of the Medical Press and Circular, 1872), p. 28.
47 *The Irish medical student's guide*, p. 29.
48 *The Irish medical student's guide*, p. 29.

Medical degrees were seen as being more prestigious than licences, with the author of one university guide mentioning anecdotally of knowing many men who had qualified with a licence and who regretted not having attained the degree, and who had retraced their steps and begun their studies again in order to obtain a medical degree.[49] The degree was viewed as having a 'higher value in the professional scale than a licence and tells favourably in seeking appointments'.[50] Indeed, Emily Winifred Dickson initially graduated with a medical licence from the Royal College of Surgeons in 1891, but recollected: 'finding to my surprise I was apparently capable of passing examinations easily (I had the knack) I regretted not aiming at a proper degree and so matriculated at Royal University Dublin', qualifying with a medical degree in 1893.[51]

Students who had the financial means and more time to spend on studying were therefore encouraged to read for the medical degree. The cost of the qualification also had to be taken into consideration, with degrees evidently costing more than licences. Students who had previous training in Arts were also encouraged to go for the option of the medical degree, while those who had defective training in Arts were urged to aim for the licence.[52] Patrick McCartan, who started his medical studies in 1905, decided to take the course of the Royal University 'though it is the harder but by far the better degree'. In McCartan's view, the course offered by the College of Surgeons 'only gives one a licence to practise medicine ... the time is the same at both places but the examinations are harder in the Royal University. However, I hope with good application to be able to get through in the five years though I find a great many don't.'[53] However, five years later, McCartan had changed his course. Writing again to his friend Joseph McGarrity, he decided to aim for the licence examination of the College of Surgeons and Physicians because he wanted to be qualified by October 'in order to get into hospital as House Surgeon for the winter' as he would not be ready for the June Royal University degree examinations.[54] He believed that once qualified in the College of Surgeons he would

> have a free hand and can go up for the degree in the National or in Belfast at any time ... If I went up for the final in the National in Oct

49 *Guide for medical students, more especially for those about to commence their medical studies*, p. 10.
50 *Guide for medical students*, p. 10.
51 Typed memoirs of Emily Winifred Dickson (RCSI Heritage Collections, RCSI/IP/Dickson/4/1/1).
52 *Guide for medical students*, p. 11.
53 Letter from Patrick McCartan to Joseph McGarrity, dated 19 October 1905 [National Library of Ireland, Manuscripts Department, MS 17,457/23(1)].
54 Letter from McCartan to McGarrity, dated 7 May 1910 [National Library of Ireland, Manuscripts Department, MS 17,457/97].

they could pluck me if they liked no matter how I knew my work and thus keep me back six months when they could pluck me again. When I could have the Diploma of the Surgeons however I might not care so much.[55]

McCartan's testimony highlights how choice of qualification hinged on individual students' finances.

Students who were interested in gaining distinctions during their medical studies which would be useful for their future careers were also encouraged to aim for medical degrees. Licensing bodies awarded no honours or distinctions, while the Royal University offered several exhibitions in each year of the course, in addition to scholarships and studentships at the end of it.[56] Finally, the question of ability was also important. Students who were well above the average intelligence were encouraged to read for the degree but those who were below average were encouraged to aim at the licence. In order to obtain a university degree, students were required to pass every subject, and failure to do this meant losing the whole examination. However, for the licence, students could get credit for any subject, and thus could take their subjects one by one until they passed. There were also thought to be differences between the standard of the various qualifications. According to the Catholic University guide, the licence of the Conjoint Colleges of Physicians and Surgeons was viewed as being superior, while that of the Apothecaries Hall was believed to be 'cheaper and easier'.[57] Charles Bell Keetley, who published a guide for medical students in 1878, explained that a medical degree from Trinity College was of higher value than those of other Irish medical schools:

In the eyes of the profession in England, Scotch and Irish university medical degrees, excepting those of Edinburgh and Trinity College, are regarded as being very much on a level with ordinary legal qualifications to practise; because it is believed that the examinations necessary to obtain most of them are not more difficult. The MD of Trinity College Dublin has to graduate in Arts, and gets credit for that in the profession.[58]

Furthermore, in the nineteenth century, it was also common for Irish students to conduct their studies in Ireland and then take the examinations

---

55 Letter from McCartan to McGarrity, dated May 27, 1910 [National Library of Ireland, Manuscripts Department, MS 17,457/98(1)].
56 *Guide for medical students*, pp. 11–12.
57 *Guide for medical students*, p. 12.
58 Charles Bell Keetley, FRCS, *The student's guide to the medical profession* (Macmillan and Co., London, 1878), p. 15.

of a Scottish or English medical corporation. It is unclear why such students decided to take their qualifications in England or Scotland. According to William Stoker, it was not necessarily due to the diplomas in England and Scotland being cheaper. In England, the cost of the diploma examinations was the same as in Ireland and in Scotland; the difference was so small that he felt it was unlikely to have influenced students' decisions. Stoker instead believed it may have been because the charges for re-examination for the Scottish diplomas were less and also because there may have been a sense that the Scottish examinations were easier to pass, and thus he commended the Irish schools for not entering into 'an unworthy downward competition' and instead having 'in the best interests of the public good maintained a proper standard of professional fitness and refused to flood the market with practitioners of inferior merit'.[59]

According to Thomas Garry, who trained in Galway and Dublin in the late 1880s, in the late nineteenth century, 'the Scotch diploma was not considered of much account. But it granted the recipient full legal rights to experiment with the health and lives of the community and in the opinion of some students, what else mattered?'[60] Writing about the exodus of Irish students to Scotland for examinations, he recalled:

> The periodic departure of students from Dublin to Edinburgh was always observed as a great event. Crowds of us would go to the North Wall to give them a cheerful send off, and also to offer them a parting drink which we knew perfectly well they would refuse, as they were in strict training for the forthcoming entrance tests. But they had no objection to borrowing a quid which they promised to repay out of their first fees, for they were all perfectly certain to pass and I cannot recall a single failure.[61]

This quote suggests that there was a sense among the students themselves that the Scottish examinations were difficult to fail. Following this exodus, the medical students returned a few weeks later 'in tall hats and frock coats, now fully fledged "doctors". They generally passed us without a sign of recognition. When they did condescend to speak, their manner was most patronising and they were even said to speak sometimes with a strong Scotch accent'.[62] Students who qualified in Scotland were occasionally mentioned in the Irish press. One article in the *Irish Times* in 1894, for instance,

59 Stoker, 'Some lessons of life', p. 468.
60 Garry, *African doctor*, p. 16.
61 Garry, *African doctor*, p. 17.
62 Garry, *African doctor*, p. 17.

listed the names of students who had passed the 'triple' qualifications of the Royal College of Physicians, Edinburgh, Royal College of Surgeons, Edinburgh and the Faculty of Physicians and Surgeons, Glasgow. Amongst the forty-eight students who passed the final examination were eleven Irish students including John Jamison Wallace from Belfast, John Gardner from Downpatrick, and John Meade from Kilmallock, Limerick.[63]

Allegations persisted in the nineteenth century that Scottish qualifications were not up to the same standard as English and Irish ones. Evidence presented to a Select Committee established in 1879 to consider amendments to the Medical Act revealed English anxieties surrounding the standards of Scottish qualifications and allegations were put forward that Scottish examinations were less rigorous.[64] Andrew Wood, representing the Royal College of Surgeons in Edinburgh, was confronted by the contention that failed Irish students always headed for Scotland to take their examinations there.[65] When asked why persons from England and Ireland went to Scotland to take their examinations, he replied, first, that it was because the standard of education 'is very high indeed'. However, the main reason he attributed to Irish and English students taking the Scottish qualifications was because students could attain a 'double' qualification after one examination. Quoting from a student he had met, he explained:

[O]ne of the chief reasons (and I think that ought to be explained) why we have so many English and Irish students coming for licences to Scotland, is this; it is owing to the colleges of physicians and surgeons not forming combinations similar to ours. Just the other day a student came to me and said, 'I am come to Scotland to get your double licence' I said, 'Why do you come here; why not go to the English body?' and he said, 'Because if I want a double qualification, in England I must go through two separate examinations by two separate bodies, and it is the same in Ireland; whereas if I come here, by one series of examinations, I get the double qualification'.[66]

Samuel Haughton, representative of Trinity College on the General Medical Council, also gave evidence to the committee. He remarked on the pattern of Ulster students migrating to Scotland to attain qualifications, stating 'As a matter of fact, the Irish do go to Scotland, but I should be sorry to

63 'Irish medical students in Scotland', *Irish Times*, 23 April 1894, p. 3.
64 James Bradley, Anne Crowther and Marguerite Dupree, 'Mobility and selection in Scottish university medical education, 1858–1886', *Medical History* 40 (1996), p. 3.
65 Bradley, Crowther and Dupree, 'Mobility and selection', p. 4.
66 Special Report from the Select Committee on the Medical Act (1858), Amendment (no.3) Bill [Lords], 1878–9 (320), Q. 4030, p. 287.

say that they go there because they can get a lower standard. It is, perhaps, rather because, as you are aware, the province of Ulster is virtually part of Scotland, though it is really in Ireland; they do not believe in bishops in that part of Ireland'.[67] Irish students from the north of Ireland not only went to the Scottish institutions for qualifications, but a significant number left Ireland to study in Glasgow and Edinburgh in the nineteenth century.[68]

Dr A.H. Jacob, in evidence before the Royal Commission on the Medical Acts in 1882, produced a table illustrating the place of study and subsequent qualifications of Irish medical students registered in the ten-year period 1865 to 1874. The table highlighted a pattern of Irish students obtaining diplomas from the Scottish colleges, with 232 surgical diplomas granted by the Edinburgh College to Irish students, 151 of these coming from the Queen's Colleges. In Jacob's view, the reason for students aiming at Scottish qualifications was economic. He stated that

> a student attending in a Queen's College may obtain all the lectures necessary for a Queen's University degree, or a Scotch double diploma in two years, not more than two courses of lectures being required in any subject. That student, if he were to come to Dublin, would be obliged to put in a third year, to attend a third course of lectures, pay for his maintenance in Dublin, and maybe his fees. Consequently, he does not come to Dublin; but when he seeks a diploma outside his own university, he goes direct to the Faculty at Glasgow, or to the Colleges of Physicians and Surgeons at Edinburgh.[69]

The perception that the Scottish examinations were easier to pass again became apparent in this particular commission. Mr Gamgee of Birmingham testified that his students had told him, 'We know very well that the Scotch colleges give the easiest examination. If a man is plucked here, he can go there, and, to use a student's expression, bring his ticket back'.[70] Similarly, Christopher Heath, professor at University College London, remarked similarly of this practice, stating, 'A man was plucked the third or fourth

67 Special Report from the Select Committee on the Medical Act (1858), Amendment (no.3) Bill [Lords], together with the proceedings of the committee, minutes of evidence and appendix, 1878–9 (320), Q. 3665, p. 255.
68 Laura Kelly, 'Migration and medical education: Irish medical students at the University of Glasgow, 1859–1900', *Irish Economic and Social History* 39(1) (2012): 39–55.
69 Medical Acts Commission, Report of the royal commissioners appointed to inquire into the medical acts, with minutes of evidence, appendices, and index, 1882 [C.3259-I], Q. 1374, p. 69.
70 Medical Acts Commission, Report of the royal commissioners appointed to inquire into the medical acts, with minutes of evidence, appendices, and index, 1882 [C.3259-I], Q. 3229, p. 173.

time at the premary [*sic*] examination at the College of Surgeons in anatomy and physiology. He afterwards, at my recommendation, went to Glasgow, and came back with a double qualification'.[71] Heath was asked if he knew of any students who had gone to Ireland and passed under similar circumstances, to which he said that he had known 'one or two' and that these cases had been of an extreme kind.[72] As this section has shown, Scottish examinations provided students of lesser means with a surer way of qualifying as a member of the medical profession in the nineteenth century. Evidently, Irish students had a remarkable amount of choice, not only with regard to options for medical schools, but also with regard to their qualifications.

The power of medical students as consumers

Thomas Holland, writing in 1853, remarked that Irish students were not conscious of the moral power they possessed, arguing that if students put this power into action, it would be 'productive of most important results'. In his view, 'students alone can judge the competency of their teachers; the long winter session forms, as it were, one vast arena for the display of the professor's abilities; his audience ought to be his judges here as they are elsewhere'. If the professor was seen to be lacking, Holland felt that students had the right to write a 'memorial', or petition, to the professor 'to improve the character of his instruction'. If improvements were not made following a respectful request, Holland felt that an appeal to replace the professor in question was justified.[73] He warned that student appeals 'should meet with the best attention of the authorities, and if not, the public journals are ever open to the aggrieved', drawing attention to the example of the Queen's Colleges where students were invited to lay any complaints before the visitors at the triennial visitations that took place there.[74]

As will be discussed in the next chapter, from the mid-nineteenth century, the medical student was 'reformed' and became more respectable. Much scholarly attention has been paid to how medical students were improved as the nineteenth century progressed. Reports of badly behaved medical students became less common moving into the late nineteenth

71 Medical Acts Commission, Report of the royal commissioners appointed to inquire into the medical acts, with minutes of evidence, appendices, and index, 1882 [C.3259-I], Q. 3998, p. 205.
72 Medical Acts Commission, Report of the royal commissioners appointed to inquire into the medical acts, with minutes of evidence, appendices, and index, 1882 [C.3259-I], Q. 4024–5, p. 206.
73 Holland, 'The Irish School of Medicine', pp. 11–12.
74 Holland, 'The Irish School of Medicine', p. 12.

century, although it was suggested by one commentator, Thomas Laffan, who was at one point an anatomist at the Catholic University and later surgeon at Cashel Infirmary in 1887, that 'school managers too often wink at the misconduct of their students under the pressure of the too keen competition for recruits'.[75] Although it has been claimed that the Irish student of the late nineteenth century was 'generally speaking, contented and conformist' and 'did not want to set the world to rights or change "'the system"',[76] there is evidence to suggest that medical students began to take a more active role in shaping their education and making demands for improvements in standards. These demands could often take the form of riots and protests. Such protests enabled students to invert the traditional norm of deference to their professors and to have a real voice in academic matters. Less attention has been paid to students' involvement in professional matters; however, an analysis of some of these complaints indicates that students were aware of their power as consumers in nineteenth-century Ireland.

Student protests were often concerned with appointments to hospital or university staff with which students did not agree. For instance, in 1874, students at the Catholic University in Dublin voiced their disagreement with the appointment of a Dr Gunn to the office of demonstrator. Gunn had studied at Queen's College Cork and the Carmichael Medical School in Dublin, but students complained that he had 'barely finished his studies' and that his appointment would be regarded by the public as 'a triumph for the Queen's Colleges, and as a self condemnation of the Catholic University'.[77] Similarly, in 1880, the *Freeman's Journal* reported 'serious disturbances' in Dr Steevens' Hospital, Dublin. The students there resented that their lecturer in anatomy, Dr Warren, had been overlooked in the board's recent elections. The medical students, it was asserted, 'resented the rejection of Dr Warren, the lecturer in anatomy, so warmly that they were guilty of 'very outrageous conduct" towards Drs Speedy and Hayes, the gentlemen whom the Board of Governors had elected'.[78] Often these protests were sectarian in nature. Students appear to have rejected appointees who did not come from the feeder medical school, and thus, potentially did not share their political or religious allegiances, or sense of institutional identity. In 1883, students at the Catholic University School of Medicine complained to the Medical Board of the Mater Misericordiae Hospital over the appointment of an assistant-surgeon. Although they acknowledged that the appointed man was accomplished, well-educated and in the possession of 'very

75 Laffan, '"The medical profession in the three kingdoms in 1887"', pp. 206–7.
76 McDowell and Webb, *Trinity College Dublin*, p. 332.
77 *Irish Times*, 23 October 1874, p. 2.
78 *Freeman's Journal*, 27 February 1880, p. 4.

distinguished abilities', they pointed out that previous to the appointment 'he had no connection with the hospital, or with the Catholic University Medical School'. Pertinently, they also mentioned that 'for some time past he has held a position as Anatomical Demonstrator in an institution in the city of all others most opposed to the Catholic University', beating two gentlemen who had qualified through the Catholic University School of Medicine. The memorial further remarked, 'We are all students of the Catholic University, and we came there, in the first place, because we are Catholics and wished ... to uphold a Catholic Institution; secondly, we were told that the University Medical School was founded for the education of Catholic Medical Students, and that wherever Catholic influence prevailed, and a vacancy as medical officer existed, these students, when qualified, would get the preference'. Christopher Nixon, secretary of the Medical Board of the Mater Hospital, replied that the Medical Board could not discuss the appointment with the students.[79]

Such protests by medical students were not confined to the Catholic University student body. Members of the Medical Students' Association at Queen's College Cork wrote to the College Council in 1896 to state that with regard to appointments being made by the Council or coming before the Council for its sanction, 'the interests of our College would be best consulted by giving those appointments to gentlemen, who, other things being equal, shall have read their course at, and shall have gained Honours for this institution'.[80] Likewise, in 1901, students from Queen's College Belfast expressed their indignation at the appointment of a non-Queen's graduate as resident surgeon to the Royal Victoria Hospital in Belfast. According to the editorial in *Q.C.B.*, the student magazine, 'not only is the local man, trained in the hospital, rejected by the very men who taught him, but the man who is pointed out by the staff as a man of the very highest qualifications, and a credit to the teaching of the Belfast school, comes in with fewer votes than the Dublin man'.[81] At a meeting of the committee of the Belfast Medical Students' Association and the Medical Committee of the Students' Representative Council, students made it clear that they felt that preference for such appointments should be given to men trained in Belfast. They argued that because these men had been educated in Belfast and worked as resident pupils in the Royal Victoria Hospital, their qualifications were of the same standing as 'any outsider' and that 'to appoint an outsider

79 'The Catholic University School of Medicine and the Mater Misericordiae Hospital', *Irish Times*, 19 November 1878, p. 2.
80 Letter dated 16 December 1896, from QCC Medical Students' Association to College Council [UCC University Archives, UC/COUNCIL/19/296].
81 Editorial, 'House surgeons in the Royal Victoria Hospital', *Q.C.B.* 2(7) (20 May 1901), p. 1.

would cast a slur on the teaching of this School, and discourage the students attending it'.[82]

Squabbles over appointments were not always centred around institutional loyalties. In 1896, a group of students of the Royal College of Surgeons met to protest against a reply received to a memorial they had sent to the College Council expressing their dissatisfaction at the appointment of a woman as Senior Examiner in Midwifery and requesting that a gentleman be appointed instead. A student, Mr L. Geraty, suggested that they had two options: 'to boycott the College and take out their lectures elsewhere' or to form a students' union to use to defend themselves in future. Geraty believed that the former option would be 'cowardly' and that he would be in favour of them forming an association. The Chairman at the meeting, Henry T. Conyngham, added

> that one of the ways by which they could effect their object was to take away as much money as they could from the College. That had worked well before. The College, he regretted to think, was always doing unpopular things. When the students sent in a petition on a former occasion they were told the fare to Edinburgh was so much, and they could go. That was not, he took leave to think, a dignified way of meeting their request.[83]

Geraty's and Conyngham's statements are revealing in that they exhibit an awareness of the importance of fees to the Royal College of Surgeons and the fact that this was viewed as an effective, albeit, in Geraty's eyes, cowardly, means of addressing their concerns. Ultimately, these examples highlight that Irish medical students had a strong sense of loyalty to their schools and that a corporate identity was fostered so much so that it led students to reject those whom they perceived to be 'outsiders' being employed in these schools.

Student complaints could also take the form of personal attacks on individual professors. Bonner has suggested that in the early nineteenth century, students across Europe and the United States were often critical of their teachers and the way that their studies were conducted, usually valuing those teachers who could prepare them the best for their future careers.[84] Criticisms were not merely oral or in written form, but occasionally could take the form of riotous action. Thomas Garry recalled students attacking and breaking all of the windows of the private residence of a German

82 'Appointment of a Resident Surgeon to the Royal Victoria Hospital', *Q.C.B.* 2(7) (20 May 1901), p. 15.

83 'Royal College of Surgeons: meeting of students', *Irish Times*, 1 July 1896, p. 6.

84 Thomas Neville Bonner, *Becoming a physician: medical education in Britain, France, Germany and the United States, 1750–1945* (Oxford: Oxford University Press, 1995), pp. 80–1.

professor of French at Queen's College Galway in the 1880s, after 'some insulting remarks about the hopelessness of teaching French to the Irish' that he had made earlier that day. According to Garry, 'We would have done more but for the interference of the police. He took his revenge later, however, by ploughing us unmercifully in the examinations'.[85] In 1890, a group of 100 students from the Royal College of Surgeons marched out of the institution following an address from a professor whose 'demeanour' they disagreed with. The students formed a procession, beginning at Stephen's Green and marching down Grafton Street, Westmoreland Street, and up Sackville Street, carrying two small flags. Upon reaching the top of Sackville Street, some of the students marched to Mecklenburgh Street and 'seized a number of brooms, which they flung at the windows of the houses as they passed along'. The students allegedly jostled several people as they walked by 'and behaved generally in so rough and rowdy a manner as to cause the interference of the police'. Seven of the students were brought before the Southern Divisional Police Court and each fined 20 shillings.[86] In March 1894, a petition was drawn up by students from the Royal University, Royal College of Surgeons and Catholic University Medical School, who had formed an association. A meeting was held by students of the Catholic University Medical School with students of the other schools to discuss the petition, who unanimously adopted the resolution: 'That we, the medical students of the several Dublin schools, pledge ourselves to stand by each other in the upholding of our common rights'.[87] In the same month, students complained about the teaching of one of the professors at the Royal College of Science in Dublin. According to the *Dublin Medical Press*, 'the Council appear to have shelved the memorial and the anger of the students thereat took the form of remarks of a very emphatic sort made within the College and in the presence of the students and teachers' with the student who made the remarks being suspended and fined £10.[88]

Students also went through official means in order to have their demands met. For example, at the Queen's Colleges in Galway, Cork and Belfast, students' complaints sometimes resulted in visitations whereby a group of senior members of the medical profession would visit the college in question and conduct an inspection and investigation into standards of teaching. In 1869, for example, Mr Andrew Smith Melville, a student at Queen's College Galway, wrote to the *Lancet* medical journal to complain about the standards of teaching at his university. Melville was the son of Alexander Melville,

85 Garry, *African doctor*, p. 9.
86 '"Procession" of medical students', *Irish Times*, 24 March 1890, p. 5.
87 'Medical students' petition', *Lancet*, 10 March 1894, p. 645.
88 'The Dublin Students', *Dublin Medical Press*, 21 March 1894, p. 316.

professor of natural history at the college. Andrew Melville made a formal complaint about the clinical tuition against Professor Richard Doherty, the professor of midwifery, and his clinical tutor. Following a special meeting of the Academic Council about the complaints, Melville was informed that he had been suspended for three years for bringing the university into disrepute. What followed was a series of exchanges in the *Lancet* between members of the Academic Council, professors of medicine, Melville and his fellow students. This public airing of grievances meant that Melville was granted an Extraordinary Visitation as he wished. This was convened in Dublin Castle over two days at the end of March 1870.[89] In a letter to the council, Melville stated that the Academic Council believed he had violated all discipline. He said, 'I deny this, and assert that a student has every right to complain of an act of a Professor or of the Council; the fact of his being a student does not make him any the less a free British subject, and no law can or will compel him quietly to put up with injustice or tyranny'.[90] Not only had Melville irritated the medical teaching staff by writing to the *Lancet*, he had also been impudent while a student. Dr Browne, during the course of the visitation, alleged that Melville had been:

> extremely rude. He looked at me in the face, laughed at me, and was impertinent in his manner. One day driving up against my carriage with an old jaunting car, I asked him not to drive against my carriage; he did not take the slightest notice of me, but stared me in the face. When he entered the hospital, his conduct was of a piece with the rest. I did put him out. On that day, the whole of the students did go round, and I had an operation ... When I addressed him, his manner was disrespectful. He never attempted to acknowledge me, or do as students do. As every gentleman is aware, in the hospitals they show the surgeons a little respect. The very contrary was the case with him. With an air of very great impertinence he walked through the hospital by me.[91]

The Presidents of the Royal College of Physicians and the Royal College of Surgeons were requested to write a report on the conditions of clinical teaching in Galway and found it to be satisfactory.[92] Richard Doherty,

---

89 Timothy Collins, 'Dodos and discord: a biographical note on A.G. Melville of Queen's College Galway', *Journal of the Galway Archaeological and Historical Society* 50 (1998), p. 101.

90 *Queen's College Galway Report of an Extraordinary Visitation of Queen's College Galway held in Dublin Castle on 30th and 31st March 1870* (Dublin: Alexander Thom, 1870), p. 4.

91 *Queen's College Galway Report*, p. 24.

92 *Queen's College Galway Report*, pp. 50–1.

professor of midwifery, responding to criticisms about clinical teaching at Galway, argued that his teaching was 'a truly practical mode of teaching, one calculated to direct the student aright and facilitate the acquisition of knowledge at the bedside'.[93] Melville's suspension from the college was reduced to one year, and he was provided with his certificate of hospital attendance which he had been previously refused, but since he had chosen to pursue his studies at Edinburgh, the former was of little bearing. Dr John Banks, president of the Royal College of Physicians, had the final say, telling Melville that when a few years had passed over his head, he would 'greatly regret' the expressions he had used.[94] Unfortunately, Melville died suddenly in Edinburgh before he completed his medical studies.[95]

University authorities appear to have taken particular issue with students like Melville who addressed issues in the press. In 1884, a visitation took place at Queen's College Cork in response to the appeal of certain seven medical students against the decision of the College Council to suspend one and fine the others for various breaches of discipline. These breaches of discipline included the students meeting on two occasions in the Barrack Street Band Room publicly to criticise the constitution and management of the college; the sending of letters and reports to public newspapers on the same subject; and the conduct of the students before the College Council.[96]

Similarly, 15 years later, in 1899, a visitation occurred at Queen's College Cork. The inquiry took place in the Examination Hall, at which students were reported to have behaved in a disorderly manner and frequently interrupted proceedings. The students, represented by a solicitor, had a few requests, such as that the dissecting room should be kept open from 10 a.m. to 6 p.m., the establishment of a bone room in the medical school as well as a recreation ground, and that their fees for the summer session should be reduced. The visitors recommended that the dissecting room should be kept open from 9 a.m. to 5 p.m. but the students' other requests were not met.[97] Following the visitation and the refusal to meet their demands, 120 medical students conducted a demonstration in the college grounds. The students first destroyed most of the furniture in the Examination Hall, before taking possession of the fire appliances and going to the President's House where they turned on the hose in the window of the dining room, 'some of the persons in the room coming in for an unwelcome shower-bath'. After this, the students

---

93 'Statement laid before the visitors by Doctor Doherty respecting the nature and scope of his clinical lectures', *Queen's College Galway Report*, p. 3.
94 *Queen's College Galway Report*, p. 50.
95 Collins, 'Dodos and discord', p. 102.
96 Handwritten report of the Extraordinary Visitation of QCC, 15–16 May 1884 [UCC University Archives, UC/PRESIDENT/5/10(1)].
97 'Visitation at Queen's College Cork', *Irish Times*, 28 November 1899, p. 7.

wandered around the grounds of the college, breaking glass and demolishing gas lamps before gathering portable implements such as wheelbarrows, shovels and garden tools and walking towards the Western Road, with one of the students carrying a banner. The students seized a passing prison van. However, the shafts and the front portion of the car parted company with the main body and the students made themselves scarce. The riots continued at the Palace Theatre, where a group of students 'diverted themselves during the entertainment to the amusement of a portion of the audience and to the extreme chagrin of another section'. At the end of the show, the students left the building in a procession, walking through the streets singing national songs, in the direction of the college. They were prevented from reaching the college by the police, who stopped them. They dispersed shortly afterwards, although 'a few of them who were singing loyalist songs got into difficulty with some parties who evidently entertained different political opinions'.[98]

There is some evidence to suggest that students' complaints were listened to by the Irish medical hierarchy. In 1883, 500 students of the Royal College of Surgeons composed a petition to complain about new regulations for acquiring the licence of that body. The College Council had implemented a new rule which meant that students needed to be registered for 45 months before they could present themselves for the Letters Testimonial of the College. In their petition, the students argued that 'many men joined the Royal College of Surgeons solely on the ground that they could get their degrees there more quickly than anywhere else'. There were two points to the petition, first, that students would now need to spend an extra twelve months to graduate, a fact which they had not been made aware of when they began their studies, and second, that 'men of more limited means' would be unable to meet the expense of an extra year of study and would be forced to terminate their studies, having lost out on the expense of three years of study. In the discussion that followed a meeting of the students, a Mr Kennedy suggested that if the students' petition was refused 'there were a great many courses open to them. They could, if they chose, cross the silver stream – (laughter) – and get just as good and better a degree across the water as they could get here, and for less money. (applause and laughter)'. A Dr Auchinleck, also present at the meeting, sided with the students, arguing that 'it was a most ill-advised proceeding on the part of the College of Surgeons, with such a power as that on their flank to render themselves unpopular to the students, upon whom they depended'.[99] In response to the petition, the Council of the Royal College of Surgeons withdrew the

---

98 'The College students' riotous conduct: prison van demolished', *Quarryman*, March 1931, p. 47.
99 'The College of Surgeons Council and students', *Irish Times*, 14 March 1883, p. 3.

retrospective clause in their regulations so that only students matriculating after 1882 would qualify in the time that they had expected to. The *Irish Times*, reporting on this, stated that the college had 'acted with equity and a promptness which establishes that their desire was throughout not to inflict damage upon any one, and to improve medical training so as to increase the confidence felt in the profession in this country'.[100]

Likewise, in 1894, a deputation of students at the Royal College of Surgeons had a meeting with members of the College Council to complain about students being charged to take out another course of lectures after having failed their examinations and about the fees that were being charged for examination and re-examination. The President applauded the students for adopting 'a very proper course in memorialising the council on subjects to which they wished to call the attention of that body. It was a far better plan than that of breaking glass and general rowdy conduct, a means which students were only too fond of availing themselves of'. Similarly, Dr Carte sided with the students, with the *Irish Times* reporting that he felt that 'already the pockets of their parents were deeply dipped into and further calls were unjustifiable'. With regard to the issue of examination and re-examination fees, the deputation was less sympathetic, with Dr Thomas Myles stating that students had entered the college knowing what the fees were and, if they wanted to, they could get a return ticket to London for 30s. or to Edinburgh for 17s., while Dr Swanzy was more sympathetic and felt that the students were justified in asking for a reduction in fees. After discussion by the committee, it was decided that students would only have to take out another course of lectures after having failed their examination in cases where they displayed gross ignorance, while the matter relating to the reduction in the examination fees was passed on to the conjoint board for discussion.[101] Disappointed by this outcome, a declaration was signed by a large group of students binding themselves to take the summer courses of Trinity College or of the Catholic University pending the reply of the council to their memorial.[102] In April, 300 candidates for the conjoint examinations of the Royal College of Surgeons and the Royal College of Physicians in Ireland compiled a memorial which was presented to the President of the Royal College of Physicians and the President of the Royal College of Surgeons requesting a reduction of the fees for examination and a reduction of the fee for re-examination from 3 guineas to 1 guinea, adding, 'may we respectfully remind you that a re-examination fee was established to cover the cost to the Colleges of that examination, and not as a source of revenue'.[103]

100 Untitled article, *Irish Times*, 16 March 1883, p. 4.
101 'Medical students' petition', *Irish Times*, 20 March 1894, p. 6.
102 'Medical students' petition', p. 6.
103 'Medical students' agitation', *Lancet*, 7 April 1894, p. 906.

Archibald H Jacob, secretary of the Council of the Royal College of Surgeons replied to the students stating that a reduction in examination fees could only be processed with the consent of both the college and the Royal College of Physicians but that a scheme of reduction would be submitted to the Fellows of the RCPI for consideration. With regard to the question of re-examination fees, the College agreed that this could be modified considerably 'in the direction suggested by the memorialists'. Adding to this, the College agreed to consult with an architect with regard to the provision of a luncheon room, as requested by the students.[104]

Conclusion

This chapter has attempted to highlight some of the problems at Irish medical schools in the mid- to late nineteenth century. It is clear that although Irish medical schools were regulated under the General Medical Council there were a variety of distinctive issues such as the sham certificate system and economic difficulties which meant that Irish institutions were in competition with each other for students. However, in spite of student complaints, as Chapter 4 will demonstrate, it is evident that in many Irish medical schools poor standards persisted throughout the nineteenth and early twentieth centuries.

As a result of the geographical proximity to Great Britain, Irish medical students had a variety of options which meant that if they were not happy with educational standards or the price of qualifications in their own medical schools, they could educate themselves elsewhere. As a consequence, it is clear that Irish medical students held the upper hand as consumers in the period. An examination of student protests at the time illustrates not only that medical students were beginning to take an interest in professional affairs, thus mimicking their more senior counterparts, but also that they were to an extent aware of the power they had as consumers.

In recognising this, it appears that in some cases, such as in the instance of the Royal College of Surgeons, the hierarchies of Irish medical schools were willing to listen to students' complaints about educational standards. However, this was undoubtedly so long as students went about their complaints in the appropriate manner. In other instances, such as the case of Andrew Melville at Queen's College Galway, or in the riots at Queen's College Cork and where grievances were aired publicly in medical journals and newspapers, it is evident that examples were made of students who behaved badly.

104 'The students in the Royal College of Surgeons', *Irish Times*, 9 April 1894, p. 6.

2

'Entering upon an Honourable
and Important Profession':
Irish Medical Student Image and
Representation in the Age of Medical Reform,
c.1850–1900

A rriving at the Catholic University Medical School at Cecilia Street in 1905, a first-year medical student gave the following account of his registration:

> On the opening day of the winter term I first presented myself and standing in the draughty hall, allowed myself to be patronised by some of the men, all the time essaying to show an acquaintance with the place which I was far from feeling. My first awakening was rude and sudden, occasioning much laughter to such of the men as were congregated in the porch at the time, and leaving your humble servant utterly crushed and abashed.[1]

This description was typical for many students on the first day at university and highlights the anxiety that this student felt at his new surroundings while also drawing attention to the male-dominated sphere of medical school life. Other students recalled the difficulties in finding digs, or accommodation for their time at university. Leaving their home place and moving to study medicine was for many an important turning point in their lives. James Little, a student at the Royal College of Surgeons in the 1850s, remarked that being 'a country lad, and a country lad who had been kept by himself and in

---

1 'First impressions', *St. Stephen's: A Record of University Life* 2(9) (December 1905), p. 195.

seclusion', he felt 'rather afraid' at his digs and among the medical students initially, worrying that he did 'awkward things without being aware of it'.[2] Upon arrival and registration at a medical school in the nineteenth century, students attended introductory lectures given by their professors in which they were first initiated in the doctrines of the 'honourable and important profession' that they had now entered.[3]

There has, as yet, been little work done on the image that Irish doctors were trying to promote in the late nineteenth century and beyond. In recent years, historians of the United States and Britain have paid more attention to the different ways that doctors constructed, 'performed' and articulated their professional identity.[4] Michael Sappol has shown effectively how American doctors in the first half of the nineteenth century embraced narratives concerning anatomy in order to forge a sense of collective identity.[5] Delia Gavrus has also explored how neurosurgeons in the United States in the first half of the twentieth century articulated their professional identity through the use of narrative, paying close attention to the arguments, the language and the stories employed by neurologists and neurosurgeons.[6] Ludmilla Jordanova has shown how medical practitioners in the late eighteenth and early nineteenth centuries promoted a collective image of themselves as reliable, dependable and 'politely manly' through the medium of portraiture.[7] In many ways, as Christopher Lawrence has argued, doctors can be accommodated into the category of the 'forgotten middle class', when considered in terms of their promotion 'of respectability and intellectuality, their professional organisation, their praise of meritocracy and their apparent aloofness from the struggle of income'.[8]

This chapter is divided into three sections. The first explores representations of Irish medical students in the press from the mid- to late nineteenth century and how members of the medical profession attempted

2   Diary of James Little, p. 5 [RCPI Heritage Centre, TPCK/6/5/10].
3   William Stokes, 'An address delivered to the class of the Meath Hospital and County of Dublin Infirmary, session 1858–1859' (Dublin: Browne & Nolan, 1858), p. 12.
4   See, for instance, Michael Brown, *Performing medicine: medical culture and identity in provincial England, c.1760–1850* (Manchester: Manchester University Press, 2011).
5   Michael Sappol, 'The odd case of Charles Knowlton: anatomical performance, medical narrative, and identity in antebellum America', *Bulletin of the History of Medicine* 83(3) (2009): 460–98.
6   Delia Gavrus, 'Men of dreams and men of action: neurologists, neurosurgeons and the performance of professional identity, 1920–1950', *Bulletin of the History of Medicine* 85(1) (2011), p. 60.
7   Ludmilla Jordanova, 'Medical men 1780–1820', in Joanna Woodall (ed.), *Portraiture: facing the subject* (Manchester: Manchester University Press, 1997), p. 102.
8   Christopher Lawrence, 'Incommunicable knowledge: science, technology and the clinical art in Britain 1850–1914', *Journal of Contemporary History* 20(4) (1985), p. 503.

to play down reports of bad behaviour in the newspapers. The second section examines the practical advice given to Irish medical students in the period and aims to explore the traits and ideals expected of medical students. It will assess what was considered to be a 'good' medical student and how these ideals developed from the mid- to late nineteenth century. The third section will examine the importance of honour and heroism as traits in the medical profession. The link between education and professional identity will be discussed in more detail in subsequent chapters. This chapter will draw primarily on professors' introductory addresses to medical students. These constitute an important source for analysing the professional concerns of the Irish medical profession and what was expected of medical students commencing their studies in the period. As will become clear, the traits of nobility and heroism became important facets of professors' addresses in the period.

Representations of medical students

Although historians have argued that the debauched image of the medical student had significantly improved by the late nineteenth century, there were still occasionally reports of bad behaviour by medical students in the Irish press. In and around the mid–nineteenth century, as a result of the unregulated nature of Irish medical education, students had the freedom to spend their time indulging in less than gentlemanly activities. Although the period 1850 to 1900 was a crucial one for medical reform in Britain, Irish medical schools appear to have been slower to standardise, and medical education in this period was fragmented in nature. Students could attend a number of medical schools with little cohesiveness between them. Dublin remained the centre of medical education in Ireland, with a number of institutions there, and it was also the home of two important licensing bodies, the King and Queen's College of Physicians in Ireland and the Royal College of Surgeons. In Ireland, students followed a prescribed curriculum as set out by the General Medical Council and received certificates to show that they had attended their lectures; however, they could essentially pick and choose where they attended their various courses. From the late nineteenth century, however, as education became more regulated, student behaviour generally improved.

Accounts of student misconduct and pranks were rife in the Irish press around the middle of the nineteenth century. In 1853, the *Freeman's Journal* reported on the discovery of a human skeleton by a man lowering the ground floor of a back kitchen in a house at Gloucester Place, Dublin. The incident was reported to the police and an investigation was conducted by the police detectives and the city coroner, Dr Kirwan, with the police looking into former inhabitants of the house. Kirwan examined the bones and 'having investigated the matter as far as possible, and considered all the information that could be obtained, he and the various other gentlemen present were led to suppose that the bones had been deposited in the kitchen by some medical or anatomical student some twelve or fifteen years since, judging by their appearance'. Kirwan believed that an inquest was unnecessary, condemning the prank which he believed 'was calculated to excite groundless suspicions, and in years afterwards to cause considerable annoyance to the inhabitants of the house and neighbourhood'.[9] Knocker-wrenching appears to have been a popular prank for medical students in Dublin. For instance, in 1879, Robert Henry Moore, a medical student at Trinity College, aged 21, was charged with having wrenched the knockers off the hall-doors of numbers 20, 45 and 17 York Street and with the illegal possession of four other knockers. He was also charged with having assaulted the police constable who arrested him. When the judge remarked 'the entire affair is very bad', Moore responded that he had not known who the constable was and that 'he was not in a condition that he could be held accountable for his actions'.[10] Similarly, in 1884, Mr Sidney Herbert was accused in court of stealing three billiard balls, the property of the Kapp Brothers tobacco shop on Grafton Street. A witness in the case stated that the defendant had recently passed his 'half' examination and 'went about enjoying himself afterwards'. The defendant claimed that he had taken the balls after a drunken spree.[11] Herbert's testimony indicates the potential for such activities negatively to affect his future career. He requested that he would not be sent to prison because if he was 'his whole career would be blasted, and he never could go on with his profession'. He was sentenced to a fine of £5 or two months' imprisonment.[12] These are just a few examples, but, needless to say, in the Irish public's mind, the medical student was rowdy and badly behaved, an image which persisted late into the nineteenth century.

The changing system of medical education was often to blame for students' bad behaviour. In particular, it was felt that the demise of the apprenticeship system, whereby a student was apprenticed to a master for his years of medical training, had negative consequences. In 1843, the *Dublin Medical Press* lamented that since the petering out of the apprenticeship system 'inexperienced boys are now merely put on top of a coach, and sent

---

9 'Discovery of a human skeleton', *Freeman's Journal*, 7 April 1853, p. 3.
10 'Knocker wrenching', *Freeman's Journal*, 26 November 1879, p. 3.
11 'Charge against a medical student', *Belfast News-letter*, 6 September 1886, p. 3.
12 'Charge against a medical student', p. 3.

to grope their way to professional eminence through the dangerous paths before them in a large city, and exposed to temptation and imposition, left to follow their own vagaries as to the course of education to be pursued without counsel or constraint'.[13] Similarly, William Henry Porter, in an introductory address to students at the Meath Hospital in 1861, painted the following picture of the medical student coming up from the country to study in Dublin:

> Dropped at the railway station alone, and without a friend to meet him, or perhaps, as is more likely, consigned to some friend or acquaintance as ignorant and inexperienced in medical matters as he is himself, much of that young man's future welfare depends on the hands into which he may first chance to fall. Open and unsuspicious as youth generally is, at an age when impressions for good or evil are most easily received, and, as too frequently happens, proud of his recently acquired independence, and confident in his strength, he falls, or is easily led into difficulties and dangers that impart an unhappy tinge to the whole character of his future life.[14]

This quote from Porter is revealing as it provides an insight into contemporary fears about the dangers and corrupting influence of the city on the youth.[15] The city has been described by historians as being 'associated with sexual danger and disorder from the late eighteenth century onwards', and constructed as a site of particular danger for women and the youth.[16] Given the relatively young age that many students began their medical studies, it was inevitable that medical students would become targets for wider social anxieties. As Waddington has shown for the nineteenth century, the city was presented as 'a dangerous and polluting environment'. The behaviour of medical students, he argues, mirrored fears of the urban and 'not only seemed to embody the corrupting influence of the city; it was made worse by the fact that it ran counter to an emerging middle-class culture that was trying to escape the corruption associated with urbanisation and the coarseness of the

13 'The approaching medical session', *Dublin Medical Press*, 18 October 1843, p. 254.
14 William Henry Porter, quoted in Lambert Ormsby, *Medical history of the Meath Hospital and County Dublin Infirmary from its foundation in 1753 down to the present time; including biographical sketches of the surgeons and physicians who served on its staff; with the names of apprentices, resident pupils, clinical clerks, and prizemen; also all students who studied at the hospital from the year 1838*, 2nd edn (Dublin: Fannin & Co., 1892), p. 31.
15 John Demos and Virginia Demos, 'Adolescence in historical perspective', *Journal of Marriage and Family* 31(4) (1969), p. 639.
16 Matt Houlbrook, 'Cities', in H.G. Cocks and Matt Houlbrook (eds), *Palgrave advances in the modern history of sexuality* (Basingstoke: Palgrave Macmillan, 2006), p. 140.

proceeding century'.[17] In this way, medical students, and particularly those coming up to Dublin from the country, were painted as vulnerable figures, open to the temptations of the city and also as being susceptible to being led astray by others. Irish members of the medical profession particularly bemoaned the lack of collegiate residences which they believed meant that Irish medical schools lacked the discipline of their British counterparts. The *Dublin Medical Press* in 1845 doubted whether collegiate residences could ever be established in Dublin, because of the fact that the medical schools were broken up 'into so many insignificant sections, all jealous of collegiate control'.[18] This issue persisted as an area of concern late into the nineteenth century. William Henry Porter, writing in 1860, blamed the lack of enforcement of 'a strict discipline' at Irish institutions and also believed that because medical students spent so much time together it was inevitable that mischief would occur. He remarked that 'whenever young people are assembled together, the chances of mischief and the certainty of idleness are exactly in proportion to the numbers congregated for mutual encouragement'.[19] Similarly, Edward Dillon Mapother, professor of anatomy and physiology at the Royal College of Surgeons, wrote in 1868 that he believed that students were left 'desolate and friendless, without anyone to guide and control his studies', suggesting that Irish medical schools should adopt a system of collegiate residence and discipline, as was done in Bartholomew's Hospital, London, and to a limited extent at King's College London.[20] George Porter advised students in 1889 to avoid the company of 'idlers', and to 'cultivate the society of studious and industrious men, who are devoted to their profession'.[21] Thomas Garry, who studied in Galway and Dublin in the 1880s, believed that if there had been hostels attached to the hospitals in late nineteenth-century Dublin, 'many dismal tragedies' would have been avoided, remarking that owing to the lack of supervision of any kind it was 'not surprising that many young students made the worst possible use of their time'.[22] Some were more sympathetic to medical students. The *Irish Times* in 1875 drew attention to the difficult aspects of medical student experience:

17 Keir Waddington, 'Mayhem and medical students: image, conduct, and control in the Victorian and Edwardian London teaching hospital', *Social History of Medicine* 15(1), p. 49.
18 'An appeal to students on behalf of students', *Dublin Medical Press*, 29 October 1845, p. 285.
19 'Medical education' (address by Professor William Henry Porter at the opening of the session of the Meath Hospital, or County of Dublin Infirmary), *Irish Times*, 6 November 1860, p. 3.
20 E.D. Mapother, *First Carmichael Prize: the medical profession and its educational and licensing bodies* (Dublin: Fannin & Co., 1868), p. 114.
21 'A noble profession', *Weekly Irish Times*, 12 October 1889, p. 3.
22 Thomas Garry, *African doctor* (London: John Gifford, 1939), p. 15.

Anyone who may feel inclined to criticise very severely the conduct of a medical student should bear in mind the very peculiar character of his studies, and the singularly arduous nature of his duties. He is for hours daily in a dissecting room where he goes through the most repulsive course of training that it is possible to imagine; he is obliged to do work from which an ordinary man would shrink with the utmost horror. In the mornings at the hospitals he helps to alleviate every variety of human agony in the midst of loathsome diseases, contagion, and death.[23]

This suggests that pranks were seen as a rite of passage, and were excused as being a type of release for students. As a result, bad behaviour on the part of students both inside and outside the classroom was often excused or ignored by university professors and staff. For instance, Willie Stewart, a medical student at Queen's College Belfast in 1876, wrote the following account to his mother:

The latest tip in the classes is every one has a walking stick and the benches are ranged round like in a circus so they reach down with their sticks and give some one a tap on the head like the way Johnny fillips the ear. Lighted matches and fuses are pitched up in the air and fall down on some one amidst loud cheers and laughter. It is a prime ground where there are some warm boys. The porter stands quite unconcerned as if nothing unusual were going on. I have got into the way of working now and don't care a hair for nobody.[24]

Thomas Rawdon Macnamara, a former president of the Royal College of Surgeons, speaking in 1881, also took a compassionate perspective of bad behaviour, arguing: 'That some of these young gentlemen may be a little wild – that some of them may commit acts of which the more sober minded may not approve, is but to state that young shoulders do not carry old heads, and for my own part I am happy to think they do not do so'.[25]

Macnamara had not been immune to such acts of wildness himself. On 15 October 1842, at the age of 20, he was taken into custody by the Dublin police after they were made aware of a duel that was to take place the following day at six in the morning between Macnamara and another

23 'Dublin portraits: our medical students', *Irish Times*, 13 September 1875, p. 5.
24 Letter from Willie Stewart to his mother, dated 18 November 1876 [PRONI, D/953/3]. With kind thanks to Georgina Laragy for sending me this source.
25 Rawdon Macnamara, 'A lecture introductory to the session 1881–1882 delivered in the Royal College of Surgeons' (Dublin: J. Atkinson & Co., 1881), p. 11.

medical student called Robert Hussey. According to the newspaper report about the incident, the dispute had started after one party had said to the other, 'You are no gentleman', at the Royal College of Surgeons. The pair was discharged from custody after finding security of £100 and two sureties of £50 to preserve the peace.[26] Speaking with the wisdom of age, Macnamara offered students three pieces of advice: first, that they should honour God, secondly, never to taste intoxicating liquors before dinner and, finally, 'never descend to jealous-minded rivalry with your compeers, never seek by detraction to gain at their expense honors [sic] or distinctions'.[27]

However, it was felt by some members of the profession that medical students did not deserve the bad reputation they received. In 1867, Dr Robert Temple Wright (1843–1902), a scholar at King's College London who later worked for the Indian Medical Service, was so aggrieved by the bad press that medical students were receiving that he wrote a pamphlet defending them. In this, he claimed that defendants often called themselves medical students, when they were in fact 'some office-clerk who has had wit enough left to call himself a medical student, being aware of the general prejudice against us'.[28] Similarly, one year later, the Irish professor Edward Mapother claimed that the behaviour of medical students was no more 'frivolous or dissipated than that of any other class of youths exposed to the temptations of a great city', remarking on his belief that many 'police-office roués' dubbed themselves medical students when they were in fact not medical students at all. From Mapother's experience of several hundred medical students, he believed that they were 'imbued with a love of their profession, a full sense of its responsibilities, and an ardent but discriminating admiration for its teachers', commenting that, particularly in recent years, there had been 'great amelioration in students' conduct and industry'.[29] In 1884, Dr Rawdon Macnamara, in an address to students at the Meath Hospital, remarked that

> any midnight brawler, when he gets into the hands of the police, if only he wears a decent coat, can call himself a medical student, and the hardened street scamp thus induces, many a time, a good-natured magistrate to treat him as if he were a mere, wild, thoughtless boy just free from the trammels of school, erring through ignorance and

26 'Affair of honour', *Freeman's Journal*, 15 October 1842, p. 2.
27 Macnamara, 'A lecture introductory to the session 1881–1882', p. 18.
28 R. Temple Wright, MD, late scholar of King's College, London, 'Medical students of the period: a few words in defence of those much maligned people, with digressions on various topics of public interest connected with medical science' (Edinburgh and London: William Blackwood and Sons, 1867), p. 8.
29 Mapother, *First Carmichael Prize*, p. 116.

exuberance of those animal spirits which are expended in most unwise fashion.[30]

It is difficult to determine how many of the crimes reported as having been committed by medical students in the period were actually attributable to medics and not offenders pretending to be students.[31] By the 1880s, a Register of Medical Students was established by the Branch Medical Council for Ireland. The Irish police had access to this register and this enabled them to discover whether those claiming to be medical students were in fact self-decorated.[32] It appears that after this there was a decline in the Irish press of reports relating to medical students. However, the behaviour of medical students still remained an area of concern well into the twentieth century.

Advice to students

Medical students received guidance from a range of figures from the beginning of their studies while a number of student guides were published starting in the 1870s. These guides, generally aimed at the parents of prospective students, outlined the various options for medical study and the career paths afterwards.[33] Student guides sometimes summarised the qualities necessary for a student considering pursuing medical education. Charles Bell Keetley's guide, published in 1878, suggested that students should have 'a tolerably good memory for dry facts to get him through his examinations, and a fair judgement to use them when he becomes a doctor', as well as common sense.[34] A guide published by the Catholic University in 1892 suggested that anyone with average intelligence and who had obtained

---

30 Untitled article, *Irish Times*, 4 November 1884, p. 4.
31 Wright, 'Medical students of the period', p. 8.
32 Rawdon Macnamara, 'An address, introductory to the session 1884–1885, delivered in the theatre of the Meath Hospital and County of Dublin Infirmary' (Dublin: J. Atkinson & Co., 1884), p. 9.
33 See, for instance, 'The Irish medical student's guide: an epitome of medical education in Ireland and the public medical services' (Dublin: Office of the Medical Press and Circular, 1872); William Hemming, 'The medical student's guide: or, plain instructions as to the best course to be pursued by those entering the medical profession', reprinted from the *Student's Journal and Hospital Gazette* (London: Bailliere, Tindall, & Cox, 1876); Charles Bell Keetley, FRCS, *The student's guide to the medical profession* (London: Macmillan and Co., 1878); *Guide for medical students, more especially for those about to commence their medical studies, by the registrar of the Catholic University School of Medicine* (Dublin: Browne & Nolan, 1892).
34 Keetley, *The student's guide to the medical profession*, p. 8.

a fair pass in his Junior Grade intermediate examinations in English, Latin, French (or Greek), Arithmetic, Algebra, Euclid and Natural Philosophy would be suited for medical study.[35] Guides generally proposed that students should have a good general education, and, if possible, to have studied Arts for one year or attained an Arts degree (an Arts degree was an essential qualification for those studying medicine at Trinity College Dublin).

Although professors' addresses and medical student guides were generally directed at male students and did not contain specific advice directed at female students, early women doctors arguably took contemporary advice on behaviour on board, and in their writings emphasised the importance of traits such as industry and determination to budding young doctors. Elizabeth Garrett Anderson, one of the first female English medical graduates, advised in a medical student guide in 1878 that prospective women doctors should possess 'tenacity of purpose, natural good sense, and unwearying industry; and if these can be found in conjunction with good health, fair intellect, and sound preliminary education, their possessor probably is rather an exceptional woman, though she may not think so herself'.[36] In 1899, Emily Winifred Dickson, an early female graduate of the Royal College of Surgeons, suggested that 'a love for her work' was the most important quality. According to Dickson, 'If a girl naturally takes in hand any of the occasional invalids of her family, if she is active and cool and cheery with the sick folk, and finds pleasure in tending them, it is certain that she has in her the elements of either a nurse or a doctor'. Dickson also put forward the importance of good health and 'good spirits' for prospective women doctors.[37] Echoing Dickson and Garrett Anderson in 1907, Ella Ovenden, who had graduated with a medical degree in 1904 after study at the Catholic University, stated that love of the work was the most important personal qualification for prospective women doctors, and that 'This love must be for the actual work itself, not for the vision of a position of influence, or a comfortable consulting-room'. She also suggested that 'a girl should have fairly good health, she should be diligent, steady, and endowed, with a rich spring of humour and hope'.[38]

Before starting at a medical school, some students recalled meeting with the registrar as a turning point. Oliver St John Gogarty and his mother

---

35 *Guide for medical students, more especially for those about to commence their medical studies*, p. 5.

36 'A special chapter for ladies who propose to study medicine by Mrs. Garret Anderson, MD', in Keetley, *The student's guide to the medical profession*, pp. 43–4.

37 E. Winifred Dickson, 'Medicine as a profession for women', *Alexandra College Magazine* 14 (1899), pp. 368–9.

38 Ella G.A. Ovenden, MD, 'Medicine', in Myrrha Bradshaw (ed.), *Open doors for Irishwomen: a guide to the professions open to educated women in Ireland* (Dublin: Irish Central Bureau for the Employment of Women, 1907), p. 35.

initially met with Dr Birmingham, the registrar of the Catholic University Medical School. However, on finding that Birmingham had an evident 'want of manners', Gogarty was driven to Trinity College to be entered in the medical school there.[39] According to Gogarty, his mother agreed to send him to Trinity because of the gentlemanly nature of the registrar there, Dr Anthony Traill, who not only offered his mother a seat, but also remembered her deceased husband, Henry Gogarty.[40] J. Johnston Abraham, who studied at Trinity, also recalled in his memoirs his meeting with Dr Traill. Arriving in Dublin at the age of 18 from the 'black North' in 1885, he recalled passing by College Green and feeling 'thrilled to think that presently I might soon be as privileged as the black-gowned figures I could see passing in and out of the front gate'.[41] The following morning, feeling 'shy and self-conscious', he met with Traill and recalled the following exchange:

'Ha, you want to be a doctor, do you?' he barked, looking me up and down fiercely.
'Yes, sir' I murmured meekly.
'Well, it's five years' hard work to get qualified, and you've got to take your degree in Arts as well before you get your degree in Medicine. D'ye understand that?'
'Yes, sir' I replied, more meekly.
'All right, come to breakfast in Hall tomorrow at nine a.m. and you'll learn the arrangements then.'[42]

For all students, the first day was usually marked by attendance at an introductory lecture. Writing about his first day, Patrick McCartan, a student at University College Dublin in 1905, remarked, 'I attended my first lecture at the University to-day and enjoyed it. Of course it is not very important as the real work only begins on Nov 2nd.'[43] These introductory lectures were commonplace and represented a means of attempting to instil students with the ideals of the profession. As John Harley Warner has outlined, introductory lectures at medical schools, like presidential addresses to medical society meetings and medical theses, were responsible for setting exemplars for the medical profession and outlining the traits

---

39 Oliver St John Gogarty, *It isn't this time of year at all! An unpremeditated autobiography* (London: Sphere Books, 1983), p. 25.
40 Oliver St John Gogarty, *Tumbling in the hay* (London: Sphere Books, 1982), p. 14.
41 J. Johnston Abraham, *Surgeon's journey: the autobiography of J. Johnston Abraham* (London: Heinemann, 1957), p. 39.
42 Abraham, *Surgeon's journey*, p. 40.
43 Letter from Patrick McCartan to Joseph McGarrity, dated 19 October 1905 [National Library of Ireland MS 17,457/23(1)].

that were desirable for physicians to possess.[44] In the nineteenth century, practical knowledge, morality and interaction with patients were believed to be essential to professional identity, but 'a sense of responsibility, duty, judgement, piety, intellectual achievement, patience, industry, Christian faith and citizenship' were also viewed as important characteristics.[45] Introductory lectures were an important social occasion for Irish doctors and were usually attended by members of the medical profession, friends of the professor, as well as medical students who were now seen as being part of this medical community. Such lectures generally took the form of advice from a senior member of the profession to students. In particular, they often referred to the necessity of proper study habits, the importance of a good preliminary education, and student conduct. Addresses often drew attention to important medical issues of the day, while also sometimes outlining the course of study that was to follow.[46] The role of the lecturer in shaping student decorum was important with some lecturers, such as Robert Graves, the eminent Irish physician, quoted in an address by William Stokes in 1858, referring to medical students as being 'instruments of good or evil', with the teacher having an enormous responsibility in helping to dictate which path the student chose.[47]

Medical schools, as well as licensing societies and medical journals, were important vehicles through which the beliefs and values of the profession could be codified and transmitted.[48] Lecturers' addresses are a useful way of interrogating the behavioural traits that were expected of medical students in the period. Conscious of the importance of regulating students' behaviour, medical students were often advised by professors to be wary of the temptations that might lead them to pursue the wrong path. Charles Benson, in a lecture to students at the City of Dublin Hospital in 1859, suggested that students should write home once a week to their parents, believing that this would 'act as a valuable check upon your conduct in the intervals'.[49] Dr Power, speaking at the City of Dublin Hospital, Baggot Street, in 1860, believed that 'Many temptations beset the young student leaving home for

44 John Harley Warner, *The therapeutic perspective: medical practice, knowledge and identity in America, 1820–1885* (Princeton, NJ: Princeton University Press, 1997), p. 15.
45 Warner, *The therapeutic perspective*, p. 15.
46 Such lectures might be described as a ritual of admission and entering. Kathleen Manning, *Rituals, ceremonies and cultural meaning in higher education* (Westport, Conn.: Bergin & Garvey, 2000), p. 8.
47 Robert Graves, speaking in 1838, cited in William Stokes, 'An address delivered to the class of the Meath Hospital and County of Dublin Infirmary, session 1858–1859' (Dublin: Browne & Nolan, 1858), p. 12.
48 Warner, *The therapeutic perspective*, p. 16.
49 Charles Benson, 'Address delivered to the students in the City of Dublin Hospital on Tuesday, November 8th, 1859 (Dublin: Fannin and Co., 1859), p. 19.

the first time, freed from parental control, and finding himself his own master but these temptations should be sedulously resisted'.[50] Similarly, William Stokes, speaking to students at Trinity College in 1864 remarked: 'A young man, often little more than a boy, is sent from his parent's roof, and plunged into a medical school in a large city. As to discipline, there is none for him; as for example, has that of his fellows. There are none to care for him. He may degrade himself to the last extreme'.[51]

Poor behaviour and conduct during student days was thought to result in reduced opportunities for medical students in their future careers. In 1860, Robert Adams, in his introductory lecture to students at the Meath Hospital, warned students that from the moment they entered into education their character was before the public. He remarked on how poor conduct during student days could result in severe consequences for a student's future career:

> But there cannot be a greater error: even now, when you believe that no one heeds you, many eyes are upon you, whether you are diligent in your studies, striving to your utmost to obtain a knowledge of your profession – honorable in your dealings with others – conducting yourselves as gentlemen; or whether you are idle and inattentive, wasting the precious hours which should be devoted to study, in frivolous pursuits – all these things are noted to your advantage or disadvantage, and ultimately you will find that it is not on accidental circumstances, but on the character which you have made as students, that your success as practitioners depends.[52]

Likewise, four years later, Alfred Hudson, physician to the Meath Hospital, explained to students:

> If, unhappily, there should be those among you who, careless of their own reputation, care not for that of the hospital, and will throw discredit upon it by idleness, dissipation, and neglected opportunities, they will assuredly meet the same fate in their onward career that many like them have experienced – it may be summed up in three words – disappointment, disgrace, death.[53]

50 'City of Dublin Hospital, Baggot-Street', *Freeman's Journal*, 9 November 1860, p. 3.
51 William Stokes, 'Medical education in the University of Dublin, a discourse delivered at the opening of the School of Physic in Ireland session 1864–65' (Dublin: Printed at the University Press by M.H. Gill, 1864), pp. 13–14.
52 Robert Adams, 'Richmond, Whitworth and Hardwicke Hospitals: introductory lecture delivered on Thursday, November 1st, 1860' (Dublin: J.M. O'Toole, 1860), p. 14.
53 Alfred Hudson, '"The study of clinical medicine": a lecture delivered in the Meath Hospital at the opening of the session 1864–5' (Dublin: William McGee, 1864), p. 29.

One's reputation before the public was seen as very important. Arthur Wynne Foot, speaking to students in 1883, stated that students should possess 'the habits, manners, and feelings of gentlemen. A fair character is a more lucrative thing than people are generally aware of'.[54] Likewise, Walter Rivington, writing in 1888, argued that bad conduct on the part of students was a severe blunder which damaged the reputation of the student and meant that he would be passed over for hospital appointments.[55] Students were therefore encouraged to be well behaved, with the warning that failure to be so would result in their future careers being tainted. Such beliefs persisted into the late nineteenth century. In 1893, James Craig remarked:

> The character which is formed in your student days will not readily leave you. Strive, then, to keep fresh and green the innocence in which most of you have left the pure atmosphere of home. The antidote to the many temptations which surround you will be found in work, in healthful recreation, and in the charm that some outside hobby will yield you. Idleness is the vice which will lead you into many traps, work is the potion with which you will drug the monster of temptation and win your Golden Fleece.[56]

Craig encouraged students to use their recreational time valuably, in particular suggesting that students should involve themselves in sport. On the other hand, students who proved themselves during their student days could gain the approval of their seniors, and attain testimonials that were crucial for attaining posts. These testimonials provide a further insight into the qualities and traits expected of junior medical practitioners. For example, William Henry Porter, surgeon to the Meath Hospital, noted in his testimonial for Robert Jones that Jones had been a diligent student at the Meath Hospital and that this and his attention 'merited the approbation of his teachers as well as his general conduct their respect'.[57] Similarly, the testimonials of Dr Thomas Mulhall Corbet (d.1918) pay testament to his good behaviour and conduct. George Porter, surgeon to the Meath Hospital,

---

54 Arthur Wynne Foot, 'An address delivered in the theatre of the Royal College of Surgeons in Ireland at the opening of the session, October 29, 1883' (Dublin: John Falconer, 1883), p. 23.
55 Walter Rivington, '"The medical profession of the United Kingdom", being the essay to which was awarded the First Carmichael Prize by the Council of the Royal College of Surgeons in Ireland, 1887' (Dublin: Fannin & Co., 1888), p. 700.
56 James Craig, 'Introductory address delivered at the opening of the session of 1893–4 in the theatre of the Meath Hospital' (Dublin: John Falconer, 1893), p. 13.
57 Testimonial for Robert Jones by William Henry Porter, dated 11 January 1840 [Wellcome Library].

wrote that Corbet had been 'a most diligent pupil. His conduct at all times was steady and gentlemanlike'.[58] Edwin Lapper, a lecturer in chemistry at the Ledwich School of Medicine, remarked that he was 'an able, courteous, and well-qualified gentleman', while Thomas P. Mason, physician to the Mercer's Hospital and lecturer in anatomy at the Ledwich School, commented that Corbet had been 'an earnest, steady, industrious and intelligent student', whom he would recommend as being 'pre-eminently suited to take charge of any Institution which may require the services of a skilful and courteous Medical Officer'.[59] At the Theatre of Anatomy and School of Surgery at Peter Street, Dublin, students who had paid 'unremitting attention to their studies' would have the words 'diligently' or 'with exemplary diligence' added to their certificates from the school. Any student who disturbed the class would be excluded from the next lecture, while a repetition of the offence would result in exclusion for one week, and 'perseverance in any riotous irregularity' was punishable by exclusion for one month.[60]

Poor behaviour on the part of students while undertaking clinical experience in hospital could reflect badly on them, with Robert Graves lamenting in 1848 that some students 'come, not to listen but to speak; they consider the hospital a place of amusement rather than of instruction'.[61] In response to this address, the *Dublin Medical Press* suggested that the sooner the medical student 'ceases to be the boy and commences to be the man the better'. It acknowledged that although the 'tricks and practical jokes of the school-room may be borne in the dissecting-room or the lecture theatre ... no such displays of puerile mind is to be tolerated for a moment where the sick are congregated'. Students were advised to conduct themselves 'with as much masculine gravity' as possible in the hospital.[62] Students were warned by Edward Hamilton in 1885 that the hospital was

> ill-suited to the ribald jest, the merry jibe, or the ill-timed practical joke. The character which you make here, be it good or evil, will follow you further than you think. The weak and helpless occupant of the hospital bed may in your future be a tower of strength, a sincere

58 Testimonial for Dr Thomas Mulhall Corbet by George H. Porter, dated 22 January 1887 [RCSI Heritage Collections].
59 Testimonial for Thomas Mulhall Corbet by Edwin Lapper, dated 25 January 1887, and by Thomas P. Mason, dated 24 January 1887 [RCSI Heritage Collections].
60 John Kirby, *Theatre of anatomy and school of surgery, Peter-Street, Dublin, established in the year, 1810* (Dublin: Hodges and McArthur, 1827), p. 6 [RCSI Heritage Collections].
61 Robert J. Graves, *Clinical lectures on the practice of medicine*, 2nd edn, ed. J. Moore Neligan, MD MRIA, vol.1 (Dublin: Fannin & Co., 1848), pp. 2–3.
62 'Address to students on medical education', *Dublin Medical Press*, 1 November 1848, p. 282.

and valuable friend, or an equally determined and dangerous enemy, sowing the tares of detraction among the growing wheat of your practice; a chilling frost which nips the tender leaves of your hope.[63]

From the late nineteenth century, student discipline began to be more rigorously enforced. Punishments, when issued, were generally mild, such as small fines or written apologies, reflecting a certain amount of tolerance. In 1875, for example, two pupils at the Adelaide Hospital were reprimanded and forced to write an 'ample apology' after letting off a cracker outside the room in which the General Committee was meeting.[64] At Queen's College Belfast in the 1880s, students could be fined 2s. 6d. by their professors for any breach of discipline in class, while signature of certificates could be withheld if a student behaved badly.[65] Clinical and resident students at hospitals were expected to adhere strictly to the duties expected of them and were often provided with a set of rules governing their duties and their behaviour.[66] William A. Seymour, resident surgeon pupil at the Meath Hospital, was brought before the Medical Board in February 1889 after having reportedly remained out of the hospital on the night of 26 February without leave and not returning until 27 February at 5 p.m. Seymour was 'seriously reprimanded by the Chairman' and warned that if there was the 'slightest repetition of such conduct during his term of office he would be dismissed without further notice'.[67] The following month, the honorary secretary of the Medical Board, Mr Ormsby, reported that in the discharge of his duty as surgeon on duty he had suspended Seymour for misconduct. This action was approved by the board and Seymour was called up to resign his position.[68] In 1897, the professor of zoology at Queen's College Cork fined two students sixpence each for their disorderly conduct at a lecture.[69] At the Catholic University Medical School, the Dean of Residence, Father Darlington, complained to the faculty on the matter of student discipline in 1904. It was decided that students found to be gravely neglecting their studies would be reported by the Registrar to

---

63 Edward Hamilton, 'Royal College of Surgeons inaugural address, session 1885–86' (Dublin: Gunn & Cameron, 1885), pp. 15–16.
64 '17 September 1875', Adelaide Hospital Medical Board Minute Book, 17 September 1875–8 May 1880 [Trinity College Manuscripts, IE TCD MS 11270/2/3/3/2].
65 Rivington, '"The medical profession of the United Kingdom"', p. 699.
66 See, for instance, *Rules and regulations of the City of Dublin Hospital* (Dublin: Browne & Nolan, 1896) [National Archives of Ireland]. The minute books of the Adelaide and Meath Hospitals also regularly refer to the rules and regulations of these hospitals.
67 'Meeting of the Medical Board held on Thursday March 28th, 1889, Meath Hospital Medical Board Minute Book, June 1879–1899', p. 329 [National Archives of Ireland].
68 'Meeting of the Medical Board held on Thursday March 28th, 1889.
69 Letter: Professor of Zoology, QCC, 9 March 1897 [UCC University Archives, UC/COUNCIL/19/364].

Darlington who was to 'call at the student's lodgings and if necessary bring home influences to bear upon him'. If the student failed his examination more than once, the matter was to be brought before his parents. The faculty, in another attempt to improve behaviour, also decided that a sodality for the medical students should be formed.[70]

Students did not always accept these punishments nor were they rigorously enforced. In 1880, when a group of students at the Adelaide Hospital broke the glass of their sitting room door, they were ordered to pay for its replacement. However, several months later the Managing Committee reported that the glass had not been replaced.[71] Rules for resident students were usually quite strict in nature. At the City of Dublin Hospital, resident students were required to visit the wards daily before 9 a.m. on weekdays and no later than 9.30 a.m. on Sundays. They were not permitted to have visitors after 10.30 p.m., or staying overnight, and were required to ask for special permission from the Medical Officer on duty if they were to be absent from the hospital after 10.30 p.m.

In addition to good conduct, the maintenance of good health was also seen as important. For a young student in the nineteenth century, the study of medicine had the potential to damage one's health. Although mortality rates for adult males in Britain were improving in the mid-nineteenth century, the life expectancy of a medical man was significantly lower than the national average in 1870 and was also lower than that for the other professions. Tuberculosis, enteric fever, pneumonia, accident and suicide were common causes of early death among young practitioners. The death rate of doctors between the ages of 20 and 25 was not as high as that of doctors aged between 25 and 30; however, this group still had a 5.5 per cent chance of reaching death before reaching the next age band.[72] The eminent Irish doctors, Stokes and Cusack, had drawn attention in the 1840s to the risks facing Irish doctors in the nineteenth century.[73] They attested that doctors working in Ireland faced a high risk of death as a result of the constant existence of fever in the country and the frequent epidemics of the disease and its highly contagious nature. They also attributed high

---

70 'October 20, 1904', Catholic University School of Medicine Governing Body Minute Book, 1892–1911 [UCD University Archives, CU/14]. Sodalities were Catholic confraternities which enjoyed a revival in the early twentieth century. For more, see Colm Lennon (ed.), *Confraternities and sodalities in Ireland: charity, church and sociability* (Dublin: Columba Press, 2013).

71 'Medical board meeting, October 11, 1880', Adelaide Hospital Medical Board Minute Book, 5 May 1880–7 June 1900, p. 24 [TCD Manuscripts, IE TCD MS 11270/2/3/3/3].

72 Crowther and Dupree, *Medical lives*, pp. 45–6.

73 'Drs Cusack and Stokes on the Mortality of Irish Medical Practitioners', *Dublin Journal of Medical Science* 4(7) (1847), pp. 134–45.

mortality rates to the want of ventilation and cleanliness in the houses of the poor as well as 'the moral and physical depression which the repetition of these influences is sure to produce on the practitioner, particularly when he reflects on his frequent inability to relieve the victims of want and disease by whom he is surrounded'.[74] Medical students were open to the risk of infection as a result of their clinical experiences in hospitals, and through entering the homes of the sick poor for obstetrical experience.[75] Moreover, some students would have served as dressers or clerks in the infirmaries or might have worked assisting a GP during their summer breaks.[76] Students occasionally picked up diseases in the dissecting room. J.H. Corbett, professor of anatomy, wrote to the Council of Queen's College Cork in 1862 to complain that several students had been 'seriously attacked by diarrhoea and all the symptoms of poisoning by impure exhalations', while he and the anatomy demonstrator had also taken sick with fever and similar symptoms. Corbett argued that if improvements were not made to the dissecting room that the College would have to answer 'for the death of some of the students of the Practical Anatomy Class from fever of the typhoid form as the weather becomes warmer in February, March and April'.[77] Contrarily, some members of the medical profession argued that medical study actually benefited the constitution of 'delicate youths', and that the majority of illnesses attributed to the dissecting room actually had different causes.[78] John T. Banks, in an address to students at the Richmond, Whitworth and Hardwicke Hospital in 1883, warned students not to 'shun the wards of the Hardwicke [fever] Hospital, as I have known some Students to do, fearing Infection.' He stated that if there were any students who feared 'to brave danger in every form it may present itself, there is no place for him in the Brotherhood of Physic'.[79]

Good health was thought to be maintained by undertaking regular exercise. Dr Charles Benson (1797–1886), professor of medicine at the Royal College of Surgeons, encouraged students to take exercise each day, as well as to eat 'good wholesome meals at regular hours' and advocated the importance of rising early.[80] He also encouraged students to avoid the

74 'Drs Cusack and Stokes on the Mortality of Irish Medical Practitioners', p. 140.
75 Crowther and Dupree, *Medical lives*, p. 46.
76 Crowther and Dupree, *Medical lives*, p. 46.
77 Letter from J.H. Corbett, Professor of Anatomy, to the Council of Queen's College Cork, dated 16 December 1862 [UCC Archives, UC/COUNCIL/6/109(i)].
78 Keetley, *The student's guide to the medical profession*, p. 9.
79 John T. Banks, 'Introductory address delivered on the opening of the medical session, 1st November 1883 at the Richmond, Whitworth and Hardwicke Government Hospitals' (Dublin: Gunn & Cameron, 1883), p. 28.
80 Charles Benson, 'Address delivered to the students in the City of Dublin Hospital on Tuesday, November 8th, 1859' (Dublin: Fannin & Co., 1859), p. 19.

company of students who smoked as 'you will certainly learn from him the same disgusting habit, and with it you will be led into sundry gross indulgences, and, perhaps, become idle, besotted, and immoral'.[81] In an earlier address, he gave the same advice, and also warned students against the dangers of snuff-taking, 'a filthy thing', which would not only make their breath offensive, derange their stomach and alter their complexion, but would also impair sight, hearing and smell.[82] He also encouraged students to take great care of their health, suggesting that 'if sickness of any kind should attack you, do not hesitate at once to consult a medical friend. If you are not better acquainted with, or have not either confidence in, any other, tell one of us, and you will find us willing to give you our best advice and treat you with kindness and consideration'.[83] Similarly, J.H. Wharton, in an address to students at the Ledwich School of Medicine in 1860, encouraged students to partake in regular exercise, not just for health's sake but so that they might maintain the 'integrity of the vital and organic functions' and so that they might ensure they adhered 'the more resolutely and the more cheerfully' to their avocations. He suggested visits to museums, Schools of Designs, art exhibitions, zoological and botanical gardens, as well as 'the pursuit of photography ... the enjoyment of music, of books, the acquisition of languages, conversation &c.' as valuable modes of recreation.[84] Members of the medical profession were conscious of the potentially damaging aspects of intense study. Edward Hamilton, in 1885, encouraged students to devote a set period of time every Saturday to undertaking a hobby or some form of amusement in order to help renew and refresh the mind.[85] Speaking to students in 1893, James Craig encouraged them to take up sport to prevent illness, suggesting that 'a broken collar bone or a sprained ankle are better companions than indigestion or consumption'.[86] As will be discussed in Chapter 5, from the late nineteenth century, sport became increasingly important for the maintenance of good health and fashioning doctors who were robust and well-rounded.

Above all, Irish medical students were encouraged to behave as gentlemen. From the mid- to late nineteenth century, medical men began

81 Benson, 'Address delivered to the students in the City of Dublin Hospital on Tuesday, November 8th, 1859', p. 19.
82 Charles Benson, 'A lecture introductory to the course of clinical instruction in the City of Dublin Hospital, for the session 1844–45' (Dublin: Medical Press Office, undated), p. 22.
83 Benson, 'A lecture introductory', p. 24.
84 J.H. Wharton, 'Introductory address to students at the Ledwich School of Medicine' (Dublin: 1860), pp. 13–14.
85 Edward Hamilton, 'Royal College of Surgeons inaugural address, session 1885–86' (Dublin: Gunn & Cameron, 1885), pp. 22–3.
86 Craig, 'Introductory address', p. 7.

to think of themselves more so as scientific professionals, and investment in 'scientific rationality and expert knowledge' became even more important in the 'social and cultural configuration of medical identity and authority'.[87] However, addresses to students suggest that gentlemanly qualities were still viewed as being important. Sympathy, kindness to patients and gentleness were often highlighted to budding doctors as important traits to cultivate.[88]

Honour and heroism

The two most important themes to emerge from professors' introductory lectures to first-year students were those of honour and heroism, which were often interlinked. Michael Brown's valuable work has highlighted the rhetoric of militarism and heroism that was an important part of physicians' writings in the nineteenth century.[89] He has shown how 'certain members of the medical profession invoked and elaborated visions of masculinity framed by war, heroism, and self-sacrifice'.[90] The introductory addresses given at Irish medical schools in the nineteenth century exemplify this. For instance, speaking to students at the Adelaide Hospital, Dublin, in 1889, Kendal Franks (1851–1920), senior surgeon, declared:

> The world expects that the medical man will not fail in the hour of need, and it is so accustomed to find that he can be relied upon, that any failure on his part is heavily visited. It expects that in sudden emergencies he will be calm; that when others have lost their heads, he at least will be cool and collected; that he not only will know what to do, but will be prepared to do it, whatever the risk to himself may be. When infection is rife, and friends and relatives have deserted the sufferers, the doctor must show no fear.[91]

Such images of the heroic doctor were commonplace in introductory addresses to medical students at Irish institutions in the nineteenth century in an attempt to encourage 'manly' ideals. Franks presents the doctor as

---

87 Brown, *Performing medicine*, p. 226.
88 Craig, 'Introductory address', p. 13 and Alfred H. McClintock, 'Introductory lecture delivered at the Lying-in Hospital, Rutland-Square, session 1857–8' (Dublin: Browne & Nolan, 1857), pp. 11–15.
89 Michael Brown, '"Like a devoted army": medicine, heroic masculinity and the military paradigm in Victorian Britain', *Journal of British Studies* 49(3) (2010): 592–622.
90 Brown, '"Like a devoted army"'.
91 Kendal Franks, 'Introductory address delivered at the opening of the session of 1889–90 at the Adelaide Hospital' (Dublin: John Falconer, 1889), p. 7.

the epitome of strength and composure, with the ability to make quick and rational decisions without trepidation. Students were required to possess 'steadiness, attention, propriety of conduct, good temper, and kindliness of disposition and manner in dealing with the sick'.[92] This is the type of doctor that medical schools were trying to promote in the period. It is a predominantly 'masculine' image, and from the late nineteenth century very few references were made to women doctors or the type of characteristics they should possess even though women had been admitted to take the licences of the King and Queen's College of Physicians in Ireland from 1877, and the degrees of Irish medical schools from the mid-1880s and early 1890s.[93] Female doctors, on the other hand, were thought by opponents of women to the medical profession to be lacking in these qualities.[94] Female doctors who had made arguably heroic contributions in the missionary field in the nineteenth century were not included as examples of heroic doctors in professors' introductory addresses. As Judith Rowbotham has argued more generally of the missionary field, 'modern heroic deeds, performed in dangerous surroundings, were shown to be a predominantly masculine preserve', while descriptions of the work of female missionaries were 'were heroic in ways that related to a more passive endurance of unpleasantness or hardship'.[95]

Medical students were described in one *Irish Times* article in 1875 as heroic, with the writer commenting that students would 'fearlessly penetrate into the darkest and most dangerous slums of the city, the abodes of desperate men and fallen women, they traverse bye places which the police themselves avoid when they can, they coolly and skilfully perform their functions in the cellars and garrets of the outcasts of society'.[96] This particular image of the Irish doctor as strong and heroic owes its roots to the pre-Famine period.[97] According to Geary, Irish doctors in that era

---

92 Dominic Corrigan, 'Introductory lecture, winter session 1858–9, Richmond, Whitworth and Hardwicke Hospitals' (Dublin: J.M. O'Toole, 1858), p. 10.

93 For more on the admission of women to Irish medical schools, see Laura Kelly, '"The turning point in the whole struggle": the admission of women to the King and Queen's College of Physicians in Ireland', *Women's History Review* 22(1) (2013): 97–125.

94 See, for instance, 'A lady on lady doctors', *Lancet*, 7 May 1870, p. 680, where women are described as lacking in the 'very coolness and strength of nerve' required by doctors.

95 Judith Rowbotham, '"Soldiers of Christ"? images of female missionaries in late nineteenth-century Britain issues of heroism and martyrdom', *Gender & History* 12(1) (2000), pp. 84–5.

96 'Dublin portraits: our medical students', *Irish Times*, 13 September 1875, p. 5.

97 The Irish Famine occurred between 1845 and 1852, resulting in a population decrease of about 2 million people who either emigrated or perished during the Famine (Peter Froggatt, 'The response of the medical profession to the Great Famine', in Margaret Crawford (ed.), *Famine: the Irish experience, 900–1900: subsistence crises and famines in Ireland* (Edinburgh: John Donald Publishers Ltd., 1989), p. 134).

characterised themselves in valiant terms, 'as a dedicated corps who, along with their families, were constantly exposed to the endemic poverty and epidemic diseases of Irish life'.[98] Similarly, in an address to students at the Meath Hospital in 1847, the worst year of the Famine, the Irish physician, William Stokes (1804–78), described the Irish medical profession as 'brave', 'learned', 'bountiful' and 'extremely hard working'.[99] In an 1848 survey of deaths of members of the medical profession during the Great Famine by Stokes and surgeon James William Cusack (1788–1861), Irish doctors were described as 'highly educated' and as members of the gentry who had brought 'the status, education and feelings of gentlemen' to the profession.[100] However, for much of the nineteenth century, the reputation of Irish doctors was plagued by accounts of nepotism, monopoly, favouritism, patronage and the sale of hospital appointments.[101] Dispensary doctors, in particular, did not hold the public's confidence and retained an image of being inept, inefficient, poorly qualified and occasionally as drunkards, who were more interested in establishing themselves professionally than in the welfare of their patients.[102]

The higher purpose of medical study and students' future duties to society were regularly referenced while fears about materialism were commonly articulated. Charles Benson, speaking to students in 1859, stressed the honourable and noble aspects of the medical profession, remarking that he wanted to impress students with a sense of the 'true dignity and usefulness' of Medicine so that they would 'study it with deep earnestness, and with a nobler and better aim than that of mere money-making'.[103] Students were encouraged not to think of earthly rewards and money-making and to ensure that they were entering into medical education for the 'right' reasons. This was an issue for the Irish medical

98 Laurence M. Geary, *Medicine and charity in Ireland: 1718–1851* (Dublin: University College Dublin Press, 2005), p. 7.

99 *Dublin Medical Press*, 17 November 1847, pp. 317–18, cited in Geary, *Medicine and charity in Ireland*, p. 150.

100 Cusack and Stokes, 'On the mortality of medical practitioners in Ireland', DQJMS 5 (1848): 115 cited in Geary, *Medicine and charity in Ireland*, p. 150. In the year 1847 alone, Cusack and Stokes estimated that of no more than 2,700 medical practitioners thought to be practising in Ireland, 178 had died, a proportion of 6.59 per cent (see 'The mortality of Irish medical practitioners', *Lancet*, 12 February 1848, p. 186).

101 Geary, *Medicine and charity in Ireland*, p. 128.

102 Geary, *Medicine and charity in Ireland*, pp. 137–8. For more on dispensary doctors, see Catherine Cox, 'Access and engagement: the medical dispensary service in post-Famine Ireland', in Catherine Cox and Maria Luddy (eds), *Cultures of care in Irish medical history, 1750–1970* (Basingstoke: Palgrave Macmillan, 2010).

103 Charles Benson, 'Address delivered to the students in the City of Dublin Hospital on Tuesday, November 8th, 1859' (Dublin: Fannin & Co., 1859), p. 9.

profession at the time, particularly as dispensary doctors, for example, were often criticised for being more interested in money and status than in patient welfare. The dispensary system also had 'a reputation for corruption and cronyism particularly in relation to appointments, which were sought for their relative security and entitlements'.[104] Honour and a particularly heroic vision of masculinity were intertwined. In an address to his fellow students at the Medico-Chirurgical Society of Trinity College, Dublin, in 1868, William Battersby, the auditor, suggested that medical education had a higher and more noble purpose than the reward of 'affluence, or of high name and station'. In his view, students' 'glorious ambition is neither to earn for ourselves a handsome fortune, or even world-wide reputation, but to lighten and lessen the pain and bitterness of disease, to alleviate the misery and sickness of mankind'.[105] In the nineteenth century, the various elements of medical professional identity hinged upon action and the idea of useful professional knowledge.[106] Battersby remarked that it was not simply the acquisition of knowledge and number of books read that made a good and successful physician, but 'far more the habits which our studies imperceptibly lead us into, the new powers with which we thence are gifted, the moral discipline which results in the production of those virtues and mental qualities which mark the true gentleman; these rather shall lead us to higher eminence and esteem among our fellowmen'.[107] Similarly, in 1869, William Stokes referred to students' duties to society, stating that they 'must be as soldiers in a field of battle – you must do good for God's sake, whether it be to the rich or to the poor, and not measure your needful exertions by the amount of any earthly reward'.[108]

Professors often emphasised the difficult path that medical students had chosen and the heavy responsibility that came with their career. First-year students were frequently warned by professors in introductory lectures of the difficulties that lay ahead of them. Some medical students appear

104 See Ruth Barrington, *Health, medicine and politics in Ireland 1900–1970* (Dublin: Institute of Public Administration, 1987), pp. 101 and 134, cited in Lindsey Earner-Byrne, 'Moral prescription: the Irish medical profession, the Roman Catholic Church and the prohibition of birth control in twentieth-century Ireland' (in Cox and Luddy, *Cultures of care*, p. 223).

105 W. Battersby, '"Medical education", an address delivered in the dining hall of Trinity College at the opening meeting of the second session of the Dublin University Medico-Chirurgical Society, November 27th, 1868 by the auditor W.E. Battersby, B.A. Med. Sch.' (Dublin: M. & S. Eaton, 1868), p. 29.

106 Warner, *The therapeutic perspective*, p. 16.

107 Battersby, '"Medical education"', p. 8.

108 William Stokes, '"Medical ethics": a discourse delivered in the theatre of the Meath Hospital, November 1, 1869' (Dublin: McGlashan and Gill, 1869), p. 11.

to have been aware of the challenging path they faced in their studies. Robert Murray, in an address to fellow students at a meeting of the Dublin University Medico-Chirurgical Society in 1850, remarked:

> Many a harrowing scene of affliction and woe we are destined to witness, many a piteous tale of suffering and want shall we hear, and in our fight with death, his triumph over our best directed efforts, shall often display the depths of despair, grief and anguish, which his presence so frequently produces. 'Tis true such trials as these beset our path, and that we become habituated to such scenes. But all is not thus dark and dreary; there are many glimpses of sunshine, which dispel this gloom, and shed a brighter light on our way.[109]

Similarly, William Battersby, speaking to students in 1868, argued that the path of medical education was 'a difficult and toilsome one; from the first step, our path is arduous and beset with dangers'.[110] However, with the aid of 'energy, industry and integrity', he believed that students would be equipped to overcome any obstacles they faced. Medical men were imbued with a sense of bravery and masculinity which were put forward to students as important attributes.[111]

Professors also reinforced these ideas using the analogy of a rugged path. John T. Banks (1816–1908), professor of medicine at Trinity College Dublin, told students in 1883: 'Do not suppose you are about to enter a profession in which you can enjoy ease and quiet; far from it; you can never call a moment your own; you are ever liable to be summoned at the call of suffering humanity; your path, so far from being smooth, is often rough and rugged'. In Banks' view, by following the path of relentless labour students could win their way to eminence and fame.[112] John Moore, speaking to students in 1905, advised them that they had 'started on a journey which lies along "no primrose way" but one beset by thorns. Hard work, self-denial and perchance disappointment in the end await you'.[113]

Industry, perseverance and earnestness were regularly put forward as important traits, in contrast with idleness which was viewed by one member

---

109 Robert Murray, 'An inaugural address delivered at the opening of the Dublin Students' Medico-Chirurgical Society, on Wednesday, January 9, 1850 by Robert Murray, President' (Dublin: Browne & Nolan, 1850), pp. 12–13.
110 Battersby, '"Medical education"', p. 29.
111 Brown, *Performing medicine*, pp. 6–7.
112 Banks, 'Introductory address', p. 25.
113 Sir John W. Moore, *'Clinical case-taking', reprinted from the Dublin Journal of Medical Science, November 1905* (Dublin: John Falconer, 1905), p. 4.

of the profession as being 'a moral syphilis, a swinish malady'.[114] Such traits were viewed as important more generally in the Victorian period. For instance, Samuel Smiles, a British reformer, who had originally started his career studying medicine at the University of Edinburgh, put forward his doctrine of 'self-help' in 1845, which placed emphasis on personal attributes such as perseverance, determination and diligence in attaining success.[115] It is clear that, as Waddington has argued, medical schools played a more central role in inculcating professional ideals of diligence and hard work than other historians have suggested.[116]

Henry Curran, speaking to students at the Carmichael School of Medicine in 1858, referred to the occasions 'of darkness, hesitation, or faintheartedness' that students would experience 'on the score of duty', but suggested that later on students would, 'like a conqueror on the battle field, survey the scenes of your early struggles, strewn with the remains of rebellious desires' and feel noble and proud for having gained victory over themselves.[117] Similarly, he referred to students as 'ministers of light and life – spirits of charity warring with pain'.[118] Likewise, Kendal Franks, speaking to students at the Adelaide Hospital in 1889 explained:

In the medical profession you are always on active service; you are on duty both by day and night; you have to contend against a foe not less real because unseen, and who never makes a treaty of peace. With your enemy it is war to the knife; victory means life, defeat is death; and in your daily struggle it is not your own life you defend, but the life of another, never knowing, never hesitating to think that your wily enemy may suddenly turn around and grapple you in his deadly embrace.[119]

Frederic Warren in 1883 advised students to avoid feeling discouraged at the thought that they could accomplish little individually, suggesting, 'Each of you resembles a link in a chain, a bee in a hive, a soldier in an army

114 Arthur Wynne Foot, 'An introductory address delivered at the Ledwich School of Medicine, November 1st, 1873' (Dublin: John Falconer, 1873), p. 17.
115 John D. Goldthorpe, *Social mobility and class structure in modern Britain*, 2nd edn (Oxford: Oxford University Press, 1987), pp. 3–4.
116 Waddington, 'Mayhem and medical students', p. 47.
117 Henry Curran, 'The introductory lecture of the winter session 1858–59 delivered in the Carmichael School of Medicine on Tuesday November 2nd, 1858' (Dublin: Browne & Nolan, 1858), p. 22.
118 Curran, 'The introductory lecture of the winter session 1858–59', p. 23.
119 Kendal Franks, 'Introductory address delivered at the opening of the session of 1889–90 at the Adelaide Hospital' (Dublin: John Falconer, 1889), p. 4.

– contributing a mite to the common good'.[120] Warren himself died at the age of 33, and was referred to in another address by Edward Hamilton, professor of surgery at the Royal College of Surgeons, as having nobly fallen at the post of duty, 'slain by the merciless typhoid'.[121]

In 1893, James Craig referred to the qualities of youth, hope and enthusiasm with which students commencing their studies were 'armed' as being 'splendid fighting gear' but also warned students to apply these virtues appropriately to their studies rather than to 'idle days' and 'much less important objects than daily work'.[122] Why did military rhetoric become so important in these addresses? As Brown's work has shown, some medical practitioners 'sought to capitalize on the imaginative appeal of war and empire to shape the cultures and values of medicine', while others, 'perceiving the army's popular ascendancy to come at some expense to themselves, articulated alternative discourses in which the humanitarian mission of medicine was presented as morally and politically superior to the baser qualities of martial valor'.[123] Arguably, such addresses also helped to preserve medicine as a predominantly masculine field of practice, particularly from the late nineteenth century when women were entering the medical field in Ireland in increasing numbers.

Doctors who had died as a result of their work were often held up as heroes by professors in their addresses. Stories of doctors who had died not only in literal battle but in the battle against disease were common tropes in the introductory addresses. Dominic Corrigan, speaking at the Richmond, Whitworth and Hardwicke Hospitals in 1858 stated that it was not uncommon for students to lose their lives in the course of their duty, remarking 'a year has seldom passed in which we have not had to deplore the death of some one or more of our most promising pupils', also noting numbers of graduates who had recently died at their posts in the Crimean War, 'the massacres of India'.[124] Similarly, in his 1860 address to students at the Meath Hospital, Professor William Henry Porter told the story of two past pupils of the hospital who had shown exceptional bravery during the Crimean War in 1855. On 16 August 1855, when the Russians were attacking the French and Sardinians posted on the river Tchernaya, these men crossed the fields, in spite of the cannon shots dropping around them,

120 Frederic W. Warren, 'Inaugural address delivered in the theatre of the Adelaide Hospital, introductory to the session 1883–84' (Dublin: George Healy, 1883), p. 27.
121 Edward Hamilton, 'Royal College of Surgeons inaugural address, session 1885–86' (Dublin: Gunn & Cameron, 1885), p. 24.
122 James Craig, 'Introductory address delivered at the opening of the session of 1893–4 in the theatre of the Meath Hospital' (Dublin: John Falconer, 1893), p. 7.
123 Brown, *Performing medicine*, p. 19.
124 Corrigan, 'Introductory lecture, winter session 1858–9, pp. 11–12.

to administer care to the wounded. According to Porter, 'they were not called on to perform any such service; yet there they were, unmindful of both fatigue and danger, and acting solely under the impulses of humanity, busily endeavouring to assuage the sufferings and preserve the lives of their deadliest enemies'. Upon meeting one of the men later, Porter asked him why he had 'so gratuitously thrust himself into danger'. The man replied, seemingly nonchalantly, 'I was riding about three miles off, and hearing the sustained pealing of the cannonade, I knew some mischief was going forward and hastened to the field in the hope of being of use'.[125]

It is evident that the possession of courage and self-sacrifice was seen as important. In his 1881 introductory lecture at the Royal College of Surgeons, Rawdon Macnamara referred to his two sons, both doctors. One of his sons had died in the discharge of duty while another had lost an eye. Macnamara argued that a career in medicine was not a profession but a mission, suggesting that such cases of bravery, which 'ennoble our calling', were not isolated and occurred 'daily, if not hourly'.[126] James Craig, in his address to students in 1893, referred to Thomas Heazle Parke (1857–93), who had recently died suddenly, noting that, 'in the memory of Thomas Heazle Parke all Irishmen possess an ideal of what a man should be'.[127] Parke was best-known for his bravery in his role as medical officer in charge of the Emin Pasha Relief Expedition (1886–9) with Henry Morton Stanley in Egypt, but had also worked in Egypt for some years previously, contributing several articles on health in Africa. Likewise, the *Irish Times* echoed these comments, remarking that 'no one was more gallant in action, more energetic in grappling with practical difficulties, more helpful and cheerful in times of disaster, more attentive, kind, and gentle to the sick and wounded, whether European or native, more generally respected and loved by all who came in contact with him, than Surgeon-Major Parke'.[128]

Conclusion

What can be said about the expectations of Irish medical students in the mid- to late nineteenth century? It is clear that the advice given to Irish medical students at the time was similar to that given to students in the

---

125 'Medical education', address by Professor William Henry Porter at the opening of the session of the Meath Hospital, or County of Dublin Infirmary', *Irish Times*, 6 November 1860, p. 3.
126 Rawdon Macnamara, 'A lecture introductory to the session 1881–1882 delivered in the Royal College of Surgeons' (Dublin: J. Atkinson & Co., 1881).
127 Craig, 'Introductory address', p. 13.
128 'Death of Surgeon-Major Parke', *Irish Times*, 13 September 1893, p. 5.

United States and Britain. Students were warned of the great responsibility that came with a medical career and of the importance of cultivating the traits of perseverance, diligence and hard work, and to avoid the company of idle students. Students were warned that bad behaviour in their student days would result in lessened opportunities following graduation, although by the mid-nineteenth century, reports of bad behaviour were beginning to decline. These addresses also reflect wider fears about the corruption of the youth, with professors being particularly concerned with young students who studied in Dublin. As the nineteenth century progressed, it is evident that the themes of honour and heroism became more prevalent in professors' addresses. This helped to reinforce ideals about medicine being a manly and noble profession, with concepts of manliness and masculinity becoming increasingly important as the twentieth century approached.

3

Beginnings: Medicine and Social Mobility, *c*.1850–1950

Medicine was a logical choice for me when I went to university. One could say that I had been initiated into it at the age of three when I first injured my ankle … My tuition had begun in the garden during my years of enforced inactivity, fortified by my visits to Dr. Minnitt's surgery. I was drawn by the humour of the various scenes I witnessed, rather than by a precocious interest in medicine but when the time came no other possibility entered my mind.[1]

Writing in his memoirs in 2007, Dr Louis Courtney recalled his enrolment in University College Dublin in 1912. Like many other students, Courtney was inspired by childhood experience of illness to pursue a medical education. Upon arriving in Dublin from Nenagh, Co. Tipperary, Courtney recalled finding digs and his immediate enrolment in the university sports clubs. Courtney was just one of thousands of medical students who have passed through Irish institutions since the nineteenth century. This chapter will explore the changing social and religious backgrounds of medical students at Irish universities in the period, as well as investigating students' varied reasons for studying medicine and the factors that impacted upon their choice of medical school over the period. As will become clear, the reasons why students entered into medical education were often personal and varied; however, students and their parents in both the nineteenth and the twentieth centuries were often driven by social mobility. An assessment of the social and religious backgrounds of students matriculating at Irish universities in the nineteenth and early twentieth centuries suggests that these varied from one institution to another.

---

1 Dr A.D. (Louis) Courtney, *…I go alone: memoirs of a rural Irish doctor 1878–1985* (Nenagh: Tipperary Manuscripts, 2007), p. 29.

Reasons for studying medicine and choosing a medical school

In their memoirs, Irish doctors often recalled the reasons why they decided to pursue medical study. Some students were very much aware of the opportunities that medical study could bring. Others, like J. Johnston Abraham, who studied at Trinity College Dublin in the late nineteenth century, recalled having simply wanted to be a doctor since their childhood.[2] Joyce Delaney, a student at Trinity College Dublin remarked that she was 'always filled with a sodden sense of shame' when she listened to her friends' 'laudable motives for taking up the practice of Medicine'. Delaney believed that she became a doctor because she 'couldn't think of anything else to do'.[3] Ken O'Flaherty decided to study medicine after his first year of study at University College Dublin in 1945 when he socialised with medical students in his digs and the rugby club. Having undertaken one year of Arts, he now felt imbued with the confidence to study medicine.[4] Others, like Louis Courtney, mentioned earlier, were inspired by personal experience. Emily Winifred Dickson, a student at the Royal College of Surgeons from the late 1880s, decided to study medicine after nursing her sick mother for a year.[5] Malachy Smyth, who studied at University College Dublin in the 1940s, injured his right knee one day when playing football, an incident he believed to be a catalyst for him becoming a doctor.[6] Others, like Anna Dengel, who studied at University College Cork in the 1910s, were inspired by a sense of vocation.[7] Michael Taaffe, who studied at Trinity College in the mid-1910s, began his studies because he felt the 'necessity of doing something useful during this uncomfortable period between the world of school and an adult life'. Believing that his reason for this choice was partly 'because it was one of the very few callings that constituted a generally accepted substitute for service in the armed forces', he was also affected by 'the romance of a doctor's life, powerfully evoked in me by the writings of Conan Doyle'.[8] John Lyburn, who started his studies at Trinity College in 1922, initially hoped to embark on an ecclesiastical career; however, after spending a year

2 J. Johnston Abraham, *Surgeon's journey: the autobiography of J. Johnston Abraham* (London: Heinemann, 1957), p. 39.
3 Joyce Delaney, *No starch in my coat: an Irish doctor's* progress (London: Cox & Wyman, 1971), p. 1.
4 Ken O'Flaherty, *From Slyne Head to Malin Head: a rural GP remembers* (Letterkenny: Browne Printers, 2003), p. 97.
5 Laura Kelly, *Irish women in medicine, c.1880s-1920s: origins, education and careers* (Manchester: Manchester University Press, 2012), p. 162.
6 Aubrey Malone, *A life in medicine: a biography of Malachy Smyth, MD, FACS, FRCS* (Baldoyle: Colour Books, 2005), p. 14.
7 Kelly, *Irish women in medicine*, pp. 52–3.
8 Michael Taaffe, *Those days are gone away* (London: Hutchinson, 1959), pp. 169–70.

in the Divinity School, he had a serious change of heart and decided that he 'could be of much more service to mankind as a doctor of medicine'.[9] A similar sense of vocation has also been reported by religious sisters in twentieth-century Ireland. Yvonne McKenna's work has shown how Irish women who entered into religious life were often imbued with a sense of sacrifice and believed in the importance of 'doing things for other people'.[10]

Many students were following family examples. In his autobiography, Oliver St John Gogarty remarked: 'Doctoring was in our family, so off to see Dr Bermingham [sic] [registrar of the Catholic University Medical School] my mother took me'.[11] A family history of doctors is reflected in the statistical evidence. Over 21 per cent of a sample of medical students matriculating at Trinity College Dublin between 1850 and 1913 had fathers in the medical profession, while 11.5 per cent of medical students matriculating at the Queen's Colleges in the later period of 1887 to 1917 came from medical backgrounds. Maureen, who studied at UCD between 1952 and 1958, felt that she was partly inspired by her father who had instilled in her the importance of women having independence, but also believed she had wanted to study medicine from an early age.[12] Sometimes students were inspired by friends who had studied medicine.[13] When asked for his reasons for deciding to study medicine, John, a student at the Royal College of Surgeons from 1947 to 1953, explained, 'It was ... A lot of my friends did it, you know, and it was contagious. I think that would be the answer. Catching, you know. There was something allegedly glamorous about white coats. Yes, even in the anatomy room.'[14]

Social mobility and a sense of middle-class respectability were often at the heart of the decisions of many to study medicine, as evidenced in the nineteenth-century records. Speaking to students in 1873, Arthur Wynne Foot, lecturer in medicine at the Ledwich School, stated that many students adopted the medical profession because it represented 'a means of procuring a livelihood as respectable as any other' or because of the unsuitability of other learned professions.[15] James Mullin, a student at Queen's College Galway in the late nineteenth century, felt that after four

---

9 John Lyburn, *The fighting Irish doctor (an autobiography)* (Dublin: Morris & Co., 1947), p. 48.
10 Yvonne McKenna, *Made holy: Irish women religious at home and abroad* (Dublin: Irish Academic Press, 2006), pp. 55–62.
11 Oliver St John Gogarty, *It isn't this time of year at all! An unpremeditated autobiography* (London: Sphere Books, 1983), p. 25.
12 Oral history interview with Maureen (UCD, 1952–8).
13 Arthur Wynne Foot, 'An introductory address delivered at the Ledwich School of Medicine, November 1st, 1873' (Dublin: John Falconer, 1873), p. 6.
14 Oral history interview with John (RCSI, 1947–53).
15 Foot, 'An introductory address', pp. 6–7.

years of medical study he would be 'confident of having an honourable and lucrative profession that would render me independent in any part of the world'.[16] Although a career in the Irish medical profession was not thought to be as remunerative as in England, medicine brought with it a certain prestige, with one guide for medical students in 1872 stating that 'Irish medical men pride themselves on holding a higher social position than the English general medical practitioner. They are entitled to meet the gentry of their locality on terms of equality, and it is not necessary or usual for them to endanger their prestige by the adoption of the trading or Christmas bill system which obtains elsewhere. In fact, what they lose in income they gain in rank.'[17] As Marguerite Dupree and Anne Crowther have argued, in their study of medical students in Glasgow and Edinburgh in the nineteenth century, 'for some families a medical career for their son was a considerable step forward, and sacrifices had to be made to achieve it'.[18] However, in the Scottish case, medical schools were now recruiting from higher social classes and students had often attended relatively expensive schools and studied classics before starting their medical education.[19] Irish medical students were predominantly drawn from the middle classes. In the period 1860 to 1880, Meenan has estimated that for an investment of £400 to £500, in addition to the cost of a high-quality intermediate education before this, a Catholic University medical student could gain a medical qualification.[20] They could then expect to earn a salary of at least £90 to £120 per annum, or a little more than this if they entered the Royal Army Medical Corps.[21] As Ciaran O'Neill has pointed out, this was a low return for their investment compared with the salary that could be earned from other professions, and 'the potential for a parsimonious lifestyle was surely a significant deterrent for those from elite backgrounds'.[22]

Students who attended university in mid- to late nineteenth-century Ireland were in the minority in the population, having had a secondary education. There were just over 22,000 children receiving secondary

16   James Mullin, *The story of a toiler's life* (Dublin and London: Maunsel & Roberts, 1921), p. 119.
17   'The Irish medical student's guide: an epitome of medical education in Ireland and the public medical services' (Dublin: Office of the Medical Press and Circular, 1872), p. 28.
18   Anne Crowther and Marguerite Dupree, *Medical lives in the age of surgical revolution* (Cambridge: Cambridge University Press, 2007), p. 35.
19   Crowther and Dupree, *Medical lives*, pp. 35–6.
20   F.O.C. Meenan, 'The Catholic University School of Medicine 1860–1880', *Studies: An Irish Quarterly Review* 66 (262–3) (1977), p. 140, cited in Ciaran O'Neill, *Catholics of consequence: transnational education, social mobility, and the Irish Catholic elite, 1850–1900* (Oxford: Oxford University Press, 2014), p. 119.
21   Meenan, cited in O'Neill, *Catholics of consequence*, p. 119.
22   O'Neill, *Catholics of consequence*, pp. 119–20.

schooling in Ireland in 1861, with the number rising to 35,000 by 1901 largely as a result of increasing numbers of Catholic students entering secondary education after the regularisation of partial state funding in 1878.[23] Additionally, as O'Neill's work has shown, there were also 1,500 to 2,000 Irish boys and an unknown but probably smaller number of girls from wealthy Protestant and Catholic elite families being educated outside of Ireland.[24] In Ireland, there were four socially exclusive boarding schools open to boys, these being Clongowes Wood College in Co. Kildare, St Stanislaus College in Co. Offaly (both run by the Jesuits), as well as Castleknock College in Dublin and Blackrock College, south of Dublin city. Catholic girls from elite families may have attended the Loreto Convent, Rathfarnham, the Sacred Convent at Mount Anville or Laurel Hill Convent in Limerick, or one of the other Ursuline, Loreto or Sacred Heart convents. Protestant girls, like their male siblings, were likely to have attended a school in England, and for those who remained in Ireland there was a limited choice outside of day-schools for girls in Dublin like Alexandra College.[25]

Medical students attending the Queen's Colleges in the mid-nineteenth century were likely to have attended local secondary schools: again, illustrating the middle- and lower middle-class status of many of these students. Catholic male students matriculating at Queen's College Cork between 1850 and 1924 were most likely to have attended local secondary schools: Christian Brothers College, Cork, the Presentation Brothers College, Cork or St Coleman's College, Fermoy while Protestant students were more likely to have received private tuition. Catholic women students, similarly, came from nearby convent schools such as St Angela's College, Cork and the South Presentation College, while Protestant women were also likely to have received private tuition. Galway students, matriculating in medicine between 1861 and 1944 were likely to have attended St Ignatius' College and later St Jarlath's College, Tuam or St Joseph's Seminary, while women students tended to come from convent schools such as Dominican College, Galway, St Louis' Convent in Kiltimagh or the Ursuline Convent, Sligo. Protestant students were educated at a range of schools, several of which were in the north of Ireland such as the Belfast Academy. As for Belfast students matriculating between 1850 and 1914, St Malachy's College, Belfast was a feeder school for many Catholic male medical students, while Protestant students were likely to have come from the Royal Belfast Academical Institution, Methodist College or have been privately educated.

23 O'Neill, *Catholics of consequence*, p. 9.
24 O'Neill, *Catholics of consequence*, p. 10.
25 O'Neill, *Catholics of consequence*, p. 12.

Victoria College, established by Margaret Byers, was an important feeder school for Protestant women students.

Following secondary education and having made the decision to undertake medical study, students now had to decide which institution to attend. As outlined earlier, students had a variety of options in the nineteenth century and a remarkable degree of freedom with regard to the path of study they could pursue. For students wishing to qualify with a licence or degree in the early nineteenth century in Ireland, there were four main options. Students could obtain a degree through the School of Physic at Trinity College Dublin, which had been in operation since the seventeenth century. Trinity was the only Irish institution that could award degrees until the establishment of the Queen's University of Ireland in 1850. Alternatively, students could obtain a medical licence through the Royal College of Surgeons (founded in 1784) or through the Royal College of Physicians (founded in 1692). The Apothecaries' Hall (founded in 1791) also offered licences for apothecaries. In the first half of the nineteenth century, students could also attend one of the private medical schools that existed in Dublin in the nineteenth century. Around 1830, there were at least ten of these in existence, but most were extinct by the mid-nineteenth century.[26] From 1845, students could also attend one of the Queen's Colleges at Galway, Cork or Belfast and from 1854 students could also attend the Catholic University Medical School at Cecilia Street. The Catholic University could not award degrees so students would usually take the examinations of another licensing body. Following study at one of the Queen's Colleges or the Catholic University, students would usually take the degree examinations of the Royal University of Ireland (later the National University of Ireland). As discussed in Chapter 1, Irish medical students had a great deal of autonomy with regard to their education. Students in Dublin, for instance, could attend classes at any of the medical schools so long as they produced certificates to show that they had

---

26 These included the Jervis Street Hospital School (1808–33), Kirby's School (1809–32), Medical School, House of Industry Hospitals (1812–26), the Theatre of Anatomy, subsequently the Anatomico Medical School, Moore Street (1820–37), the School of Anatomy and Surgery (subsequently termed the Theatre of Anatomy, Physiology, and Surgery), Lower Ormond Quay (1821–7), Park Street School (1824–49), the School of Anatomy, Medicine and Surgery, Richmond Hospital, later Carmichael College, the School of Anatomy, Physiology and Surgery, Bishop Street, School of Anatomy, Marlborough Street (1831–40), the Dublin School of Anatomy, Medicine and Surgery, 1832–57, the Theatre of Anatomy and School of Surgery, 27 Peter Street, 1832–41, School of Anatomy, Medicine and Surgery, Mark Street (1834–5), the Ledwich, formerly the 'Original' School, Peter Street (established 1836). Sir Charles A. Cameron, *History of the Royal College of Surgeons in Ireland and of the Irish Schools of Medicine including numerous biographical sketches; also a medical bibliography* (Dublin: Fannin & Co., 1886), pp. 513–33.

undertaken the prescribed curriculum for the qualification they were aiming at. According to Robert Blackham, who commenced his training in 1887,

> The student could select any school of medicine for any particular course of lectures or practical work. All the schools were recognised, even by the most conservative of institutions – Trinity College. If the student thought the course of lectures on *materia medica* – shall we say – was better at the Carmichael than at the College of Surgeons School, all he had to do was to give in his name to the lecturer and attend the course. He did not have to pay in advance, but only handed in his fee when he wanted a certificate for having attended the lectures.[27]

This meant that medical schools and hospitals were all actively competing with each other for students and that students were often swayed by the personalities of individual professors when choosing which course to follow.

Choice of medical school was inspired by a variety of factors. Charles Bell Keetley, in his 1878 guide for students considering the medical profession, summarised the choice of medical school as being guided by several factors: the student's father having attended the school before him; knowing or having had an introduction to members of the staff; or the reputation of the medical officers. The size of a hospital was also viewed as important, with both large and small hospitals conferring their own advantages. Large schools were thought to offer a 'greater choice of friends and acquaintances, a wider field for observation, and a much more perfect machinery for teaching the student the groundwork of his profession'.[28] Students were also thought to be influenced by more personal factors, such as a perception that the students at one school were more gentlemanly than another, better at football, or because the school was in a convenient or good part of town. Even in the 1940s, such factors appear to have been relevant. Ken O'Flaherty, who studied at University College Dublin from 1945, 'was delighted with the idea of going to U.C.D. mainly because it was the big centre for G.A.A. All-Ireland Finals and rugby and soccer internationals'.[29]

Fees were also a factor, although Keetley warned students to be aware of false economy when paying small fees.[30] Some students decided to obtain a licence through the Royal College of Physicians or the Royal College of

27 Colonel Robert J. Blackham, *Scalpel, sword and stretcher: forty years of work and play* (London: Sampson Low, Marston & Co. Ltd., 1931), p. 25.
28 Charles Bell Keetley, FRCS, *The student's guide to the medical profession* (London: Macmillan and Co., 1878), pp. 17–20.
29 Ken O'Flaherty, *From Slyne Head to Malin Head: a rural GP remembers* (Letterkenny: Browne Printers, 2003), p. 84.
30 Keetley, *The student's guide to the medical profession*, pp. 17–20.

Surgeons of Ireland because it was a cheaper option and meant that they could practise. *The Irish Medical Students' Guide* estimated in 1872 that the cost of obtaining a licence through the Royal College of Surgeons was a minimum of £83, including lecture fees, diploma fees and hospital teaching, but it was probably more likely to be between £114 to £140 if grinds were included.[31] Trinity College was the most expensive option but its degrees were thought to hold a certain prestige over those from the newer Queen's Colleges and Catholic University. In 1872, it was estimated that the total cost of a medical degree from Trinity would be £198. (This was £49. 12s. for lectures, £33. 12s. for hospital fees, £32 for the cost of the degree, and £83 for a degree in Arts, which was a necessary requirement for Trinity.) For a student at one of the Queen's Colleges, the guide estimated that the cost of education would be approximately £67.[32] Willie Stewart, a medical student at Queen's, wrote to his mother in 1876 that students sometimes took a year's break after completing one year of medical education in order to 'make some money and then return and complete their course'. Stewart also mentioned that he was able to economise by buying his books second hand, writing, 'they are not the latest editions, yet they will do'.[33] By 1892, the Catholic University guide for medical students gave the following costs for a medical education, including the cost of lectures, hospitals, special courses and examinations (i.e., all professional expenses with the exceptions of books, instruments and private coaching or 'grindings'): Royal University, £146; Conjoint Colleges of Physicians and Surgeons, £162; Conjoint College of Surgeons and Apothecaries Hall, £148.[34] There were also additional costs to be considered. According to Charles Keetley's guide for medical students, published in 1878, books would cost about £7 to £12, instruments about £2 and grinding up to £25, although it noted that 'an intelligent and industrious student requires little grinding in a school where the teaching is properly organised'.[35] Students who were unable to economise by living at home also had to consider the cost of digs. The *Lancet* reported in 1897 that rent in Dublin was almost the same as in London (£1 per week), while in Cork rent was usually not higher than 15s. (75p) a week, and in the Irish

---

31 'The Irish medical student's guide: an epitome of medical education in Ireland and the public medical services' (Dublin: Office of the Medical Press and Circular, 1872), p. 31.
32 'The Irish medical student's guide', p. 63.
33 Letter from Willie Stewart to his mother, dated 18 November 1876 [PRONI D/953/3]. With kind thanks to Georgina Laragy for sending me this source.
34 *Guide for medical students, more especially for those about to commence their medical studies, by the registrar of the Catholic University School of Medicine* (Dublin: Browne & Nolan, 1892), pp. 6–7.
35 Keetley, *The student's guide to the medical profession*, pp. 10–12.

provincial towns it was on average 5s. to 6s. (25p to 30p) a week.[36] By 1925, the cost of medical education had increased considerably, with the total cost being estimated at £1,000 before the First World War and up to £1,500 by 1925.[37] In 1947, the *Lancet* estimated that the cost of medical education in Britain was about £1,500 before the Second World War, but that allowances now had to be made for increased maintenance costs and increased tuition and examination fees at some universities.[38] By 1950, it was estimated by Dr Frank Kane, professor of physiology at University College Cork, that it cost an Irish medical student a minimum of £1,250 to qualify, with fees being cheaper than those in Britain (£300 in Dublin in comparison with £350 in London), but 'with the cost of his education and upkeep before starting the course, the minimum total cost was about £3,000'.[39]

Fees were therefore evidently an important consideration for parents of prospective medical students. However, Irish students often attended their local university as it meant that they could save money by living at home.[40] Writing to his friend Joseph McGarrity in 1910, for instance, Patrick McCartan, said that he had advised his friend Bulmer Hobson (who would become a leading member of the Irish Republican Brotherhood one year later) to start medicine as 'he could get through very cheaply in the new Belfast university. Being at home he would only have fees to pay'.[41] The Irish medical schools, with the exception of Trinity College Dublin, had more in common with the Scottish medical schools in that they lacked a 'resident corporate life' which was present in universities such as Oxford and Cambridge.[42] However, student 'corporate life' did not necessarily entail residence, and from the 1880s it developed strongly in Scotland, where students lived at home or in lodgings, while 'student unions, newspapers, political clubs, debating societies and athletics were all part of the Scottish model, and spread from there to the English civic universities'.[43] Like students in Glasgow and Edinburgh, students at Irish universities tended to live in digs or lodgings which were kept by landladies. Students were provided with a room and basic meals. Students at Trinity College, on the other hand, had more in common with students at Oxford and Cambridge and many of

---

36 'The cost of medical education', *Lancet*, 21 August 1897, pp. 437–8.
37 '2,796 new doctors', *Fermanagh Herald*, 12 September 1925, p. 6.
38 'The cost of medical education', *British Medical Journal*, 6 September 1947, p. 392.
39 'Overcrowding in universities', *Irish Press*, 15 April 1950, p. 7.
40 Kelly, *Irish women in medicine*, p. 58.
41 Letter from Patrick McCartan to Joseph McGarrity, dated 21 January 1910 [National Library of Ireland, Manuscripts Department, MS 17,457/92(4)].
42 Crowther and Dupree, *Medical lives*, p. 83.
43 Robert Anderson, *British universities past and present* (London: Hambledon Continuum, 2006), p. 111.

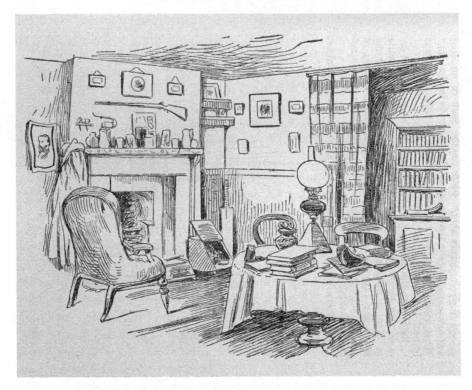

1   'A student's room', from: H.A. Hinkson, *Student life in
Trinity College, Dublin* (Dublin: J. Charles & Son, 1892).
Courtesy of the National Library of Ireland.

them were accommodated in College. According to H.A. Hinkson, writing
in 1892, 'to get a set of rooms to yourself, with an outer door for retreat,
and a dunscope for inspection of the casual visitor, is to enter at once into
one's kingdom of independence'.[44] The majority of students, however, found
lodgings in digs or shared lodgings with a fellow student.

Digs were essentially lodgings which comprised of a room and board in
a house. Thomas Garry, writing of digs in Dublin in the 1880s, commented
that they were 'cheerless', providing 'badly cooked food, not always cleanly
served'.[45] Sometimes, as in the case of Louis Courtney, who lived in digs on
Lower Baggot Street in Dublin in 1912, rent also covered one's own sitting-
room, which he used for studying.[46] Digs were a booming business in the

44   H.A. Hinkson, *Student life in Trinity College, Dublin* (Dublin: J. Charles & Son, 1892),
     p. 5.
45   Thomas Garry, *African doctor* (London: John Gifford, 1939), p. 15.
46   Courtney, *...I go alone*, p. 34.

university towns. In Dublin in the early years of the twentieth century, for instance, the cost of lodgings varied from 14s. to £1 a week.[47] Of students at University College Cork in the academic year 1943–4, 38.5 per cent of the men and 30.9 per cent of the women lived in digs, with about two-thirds of students living at home, with relatives or in religious houses or in hostels.[48]

Digs were often the subject of criticism in the student press. For example, one article in 1907 advised that the practice of living in digs was 'not only expensive, but entirely against the academic spirit', and as a result of a lack of information on the part of the university or Students' Representative Council about the standard of such accommodation decent digs were difficult to come by.[49] Students in Dublin were allegedly driven by the 'discomfort of digs' to the bar, the restaurant, the courts at Terenure and the National Library.[50] The *National Student* in 1919 drew attention to the problems facing students inexperienced in the art of digs hunting who arrived in Dublin from the country at the start of each academic year. The Catholic University provided a list of suitable lodgings to its students; however, this was greatly out of date.[51] By the 1940s, things had not changed much, with digs ranking as the fifth highest in a student questionnaire at University College Dublin in reply to the question: 'What do you dislike most about college?', with lectures, red tape, '86' (St Stephen's Green, where student 'hops' were held) and first-year women disliked more than digs.[52] Some student digs had a reputation for only taking medical students. For example, Thomas Hennessey, a student at University College Dublin in the 1950s, found lodging at a digs run by a landlady who informed him of the history of the digs' relationship with the UCD Medical School and who told him that she only took on medical students as she found them more reliable than other students, and because they stayed on longer due to the length of their course of studies.[53] The shared experience of living in digs had the effect of helping to cement social relationships between medical students. Ken O'Flaherty, a medical student at UCD from 1946, lived in digs in Ranelagh for his final year, along with his partner at the Coombe Hospital, Charlie Kehoe and his cousin James Lee, who was starting veterinary medicine. The three men studied together

47 Note of students' residences in Dublin (MS 17,457126(1), Letters of Dr Patrick McCartan to Joseph McGarrity, NLI).
48 'Our students', *Cork University Record* 1 (summer term 1944), p. 10.
49 'Student organisation: societies and clubs', *Hermes: an illustrated university literary quarterly* (February 1908), p. 111.
50 'The digs problem solved', *National Student* 33 vol.ix no.1 (June 1919), p. 9.
51 'The digs problem solved', p. 9.
52 'We ask you … College Questionnaire', *National Student*, new series, no.103 (May 1948), p. 19.
53 Thomas Hennessey, *My life as a surgeon: an autobiography* (Dublin: A. & A. Farmar, 2011), pp. 62–3.

at night in their digs and 'went for short walks around the block to revive our drooping spirits'.[54]

Ultimately, parents usually had the final say in choice of medical school. J. Johnston Abraham, from Coleraine, who began his studies at Trinity College Dublin in 1894, had the decision made for him by his mother. His uncle had been a graduate of the University of Edinburgh and Abraham's father wanted to send him there, but his mother had the final say. Impressed by the Trinity College team in the annual regatta, and the fact that the captain of the team carried 'his liquor like a gentleman', she said 'I like these Trinity boys. They have style, I think we'll send you there'. Abraham believed his mother may have been joking, and later learned that his headmaster's wife had suggested that Trinity would be the most suitable university given his love of the classics.[55]

Students' financial means had an impact on whether they could pursue medical studies and bright students were sometimes assisted by scholarships. James Mullin, the son of a widow, decided to attend Queen's College Galway because there the 'competition was not so keen' and he had a greater chance of obtaining a scholarship. Secondary reasons for choosing Galway were that 'living and lodging were cheaper, the place was quieter and the surroundings more salubrious and beautiful'. His mother was supportive of this decision, in spite of Mullin pointing out the difficulties which his absence would cause for her.[56] Similarly, Alexander Porter received a senior scholarship from Queen's College Belfast to help him to pursue his medical studies in the 1860s. In spite of this, it appears that Porter struggled financially, writing in April 1864, 'Money is really scarce and I am not getting on half so well this year as I did last'.[57] To his further dismay, later that month he received a letter informing him 'that I am to get only £25 for my Sch … it appears that it is an act of parliament. Fortune is fickle – so let us be content and make the best of our circumstances'.[58]

However, some students were pushed into medical study without being particularly suited for it. James Mullin observed that many students, particularly 'chronics' who failed to pass examinations, were

> the innocent victims of that parental vanity which flatters its possessors with the belief that their sons, merely because they are their sons, inherit enough talent to make them successful in any

54 O'Flaherty, *From Slyne Head*, p. 126.
55 Johnston Abraham, *Surgeon's journey*, pp. 38–9.
56 Mullin, *The story of a toiler's life*, p. 90.
57 Diary of Alexander Porter, 5 April 1864 [Harry Ransom Center].
58 Diary of Alexander Porter, 7 April 1864 [Harry Ransom Center].

profession, however difficult. And so, without measuring the capacity or consulting the tastes of their sons, they thrust them into the study of Medicine, the most difficult and probably the most disagreeable of all studies unless one is born with a natural talent, or at least aptitude for it.[59]

Similarly, a piece published in *Galway University College Magazine* in 1924–5, entitled 'Autobiography of a Medical Student' provides a revealing insight:

My parents were respectable, so I suppose I ought to be respectable too, but I'm not. People said I was clever also, but I have reason to doubt this now, because my examiners never seemed to think so. Now there is a tradition in the West of Ireland, which demands, that youths of such talent and such parentage as I possessed, shall confer the hall mark of respectability on their families by becoming either healers of souls or of bodies.[60]

Certainly, for much of the late nineteenth and early twentieth centuries, for Catholic families, having a 'priest in the family' brought prestige and was seen as a status symbol, and Irish mothers often desired for one of their sons to become a priest.[61] As Ferguson has outlined in his work on masculinity in late-modern Ireland, the priest became a role model for Irish masculinity and it was common for first-born sons to enter the priesthood.[62] As one 45-year-old priest, interviewed in 2001, put it, 'You really had it made in society in our country if you had a well in the yard, a bull in the field and a son a priest'.[63] Michael Flynn, born in 1917, the son of farmers, recalled

---

59 Mullin, *The story of a toiler's life*, pp. 124–5.
60 'The autobiography of a medical student', *Galway University College Magazine* 3(10) (1924–5), p. 39.
61 Harry Ferguson, 'Men and masculinities in late-modern Ireland', in Bob Pease and Keith Pringle (eds), *A man's world?: changing men's practices in a globalized world* (London: Zed, 2001), p. 120 and Tom Inglis, *Moral monopoly: the Catholic Church in modern Irish society* (Dublin: Gill & Macmillan, 1997), p. 200. Yvonne McKenna has also noted this in her book on religious sisters in twentieth-century Ireland, where the women she interviewed 'were aware that their vocation was not responded to as positively as a son's vocation for the priesthood might have been' (Yvonne McKenna, *Made holy: Irish women religious at home and abroad* (Dublin: Irish Academic Press, 2006), pp. 64–5).
62 Ferguson, 'Men and masculinities in late-modern Ireland', p. 120.
63 H. Ferguson and S. Reynolds, 'Gender and identity in the lives of Irish men', research report, Department of Social Policy and Social Work, University College Dublin (2001) cited in Ferguson, 'Men and masculinities in late-modern Ireland', p. 120.

his mother's hope that he would be the 'priest in the family', but at the age of 16 he decided that he would not be able to commit to a life of celibacy. Instead, his brother John, who was studying science at University College Dublin, advised Michael to study medicine. Although Michael recalled that he would have liked to have worked as a farmer like his father before him, 'in reality there was no prospect of this happening with my two older brothers already working the land, so medicine offered the best prospect for me'. Moreover, he felt that he 'already had a feeling for people', and so enrolled at UCD in 1934.[64] Without doubt, having a doctor in the family conferred a certain degree of prestige on late nineteenth- and early twentieth-century Irish families, in the same way as having a priest did. Certainly, doctors were thought to occupy a special place in Irish society, with Lambert Ormsby, then President of the Royal College of Surgeons, writing in 1903, that 'in many families the doctor is held in as great love and reverence as the priest'.[65] Undoubtedly, medical study could be converted into what Pierre Bourdieu has described as 'symbolic capital' for the families of medical students due to the status of the doctor in Irish society, in the same way that a vocation for the religious life could because of the status of Catholicism and of priests and religious sisters in Irish society.[66]

This was recognised by students themselves with articles in student newspapers occasionally referring to the link between medical study and social mobility. In a piece in *Q.C.C.* magazine in 1910, for instance, which addressed the overcrowding of the medical profession, the author argued that if medical schools continued to admit students at the current levels, the standards of the profession would be lowered and would become extremely competitive and mediocre, meaning that ambitious men might be dissuaded from entering. Moreover, the article described the genesis of the medical student as follows:

> At present the genesis of a doctor is very commonly something after this manner. A well-to-do farmer or prosperous business man has the universal and very laudable desire of raising the social position of his family. He cannot do it himself, so he decides his sons shall be fitted

---

64 Michael P. Flynn, *Medical doctor of many parts: memoirs of a public health practitioner and health manager, spanning sixty years of social change* (Dublin: Colourbooks, 2002), p. 2.

65 Sir Lambert Ormsby, President of the Royal College of Surgeons, 'An Address on the ideal physician: his early training and future prospects. Delivered to the Students of the Royal College of Surgeons in Ireland on November 2nd, on the opening of the medical session 1903-04', *Lancet* 162(4186) (1903), pp. 1413–16.

66 See Pierre Bourdieu, 'The forms of capital', in J. Richardson (ed.), *Handbook of theory and research for the sociology of education* (New York: Greenwood, 1986), pp. 241–58 and McKenna, *Made holy*, p. 65.

for a higher sphere. Therefore he makes Pat a priest, and there being nothing else left, Tim becomes a doctor. He takes an extra three years or so over his course, but his father can afford to pay for him. Then he drags through his final somehow, and buys a practice where he is known, not as old Jerry Buckley's son, but as young Dr. Buckley. The title of Doctor confers a certain social distinction, and a University education is supposed to be a certificate of many desirable attainments; so the old man's aim is achieved, and another undesirable is added to the roll of an honourable Profession. Now, this is not as it ought to be. The Profession deserves the best men, and it must get the best.[67]

The prospect of social mobility played an important part in students' decisions to undertake medical study in both the nineteenth and twentieth centuries. The professionalisation of British and Irish society began in the late eighteenth century, with the 100 years from 1750 to 1850 seen as a crucial period in the development of the modern professions.[68] During this period, the professions not only expanded numerically but also underwent important changes with regard to their organisation.[69] The ancient learned professions were those of divinity, law and medicine, while the military is often added to this grouping.[70] Although figures do not exist for Ireland, it is estimated that less than 3 per cent of the English and Welsh population were engaged in these professions between 1688 and 1851. From the second half of the nineteenth century, this percentage began to increase, eventually comprising 10 per cent of the overall population in the twentieth century.[71] The professions were an attractive option for the children of gentry families in decline or middle-class families in ascent.[72] They allowed these men and women to earn a steady salary while also granted a degree of respectability.[73] During the latter part of the nineteenth century, the 'new' professions were growing faster than the ancient three of 'divinity, physic and law'.[74] This was because as 'new and more varied businesses came into existence, the rise in the scale of business and government required more managers,

67 M.D., 'The overcrowding of the medical profession: being a guide for boards of studies and an awful warning to the young', *Q.C.C.* 4(3) (1910), p. 56.
68 O'Neill, *Catholics of consequence*, p. 113 and Marcus Ackroyd et al., *Advancing with the army: medicine, the professions and social mobility in the British Isles, 1790–1850* (Oxford: Oxford University Press, 2007), p. 1.
69 Ackroyd, et al., *Advancing with the army*, p. 1.
70 O'Neill, *Catholics of consequence*, p. 113.
71 O'Neill, *Catholics of consequence*, p. 114.
72 O'Neill, *Catholics of consequence*, p. 156
73 O'Neill, *Catholics of consequence*, pp. 156–7.
74 W.J. Reader, *Professional men: the rise of the professional classes in nineteenth-century England* (London: Cox & Wyman Ltd., 1966), p. 156.

administrators, office workers and supervisors, and the professions and would-be professions increased in size and numbers'.[75]

The comfortable middle classes, or 'the servant-keeping class', as described by Booth and Rowntree, stood below the rich and powerful and included taxpaying families with an income of between £160 (which was the income tax threshold in 1905) and £700 a year. According to Perkin, 'a few senior civil servants, clergymen, lawyers, doctors, local manufacturers and wholesalers, high-street shopkeepers, and so on, might rise to as much as £1,000 a year, but the average was perhaps a quarter of that figure'. At the lower end of the middle classes were the 'petty bourgeoisie', which included most shopkeepers, schoolteachers, clerks and white-collar workers who would have earned 'a good deal less than £160 a year but still stoutly claimed middle-class status'.[76]

Students from less-well-off backgrounds often worried about their finances. Alexander Porter, mentioned earlier, was born into a tenant farming family in County Down. Following the death of his father in 1856, Porter's family's circumstances changed drastically and he and his sister were reliant on the financial support of their two older brothers.[77] Porter regularly remarked in his student diary entries in the 1860s of his fears about his future career and earnings, particularly, it seems, since he had decided to study medicine as a result of a desire to make his brothers and sister financially comfortable. In January 1864, he wrote, 'I do not know what to turn to when I do get M.D., I don't feel at all sure of earning £100 a year. This time last year I thought that I might be pretty sure of earning £1000'.[78] He also frequently wrote in his diary about not feeling like he fitted in socially. For example, in April 1864, he wrote: 'No person likes me, I must have something repulsive about me. Why wasn't my father rich? Why was I not the son of a rich man? God forgive me for rebelling'.[79]

Fears about the lower middle-classes, like Alexander Porter, entering into the medical profession, were frequently expressed by members of the Irish medical profession. As early as 1844, Dr Jacob, delivering an introductory lecture at the Royal College of Surgeons, drew attention to the importance of young men being sufficiently educated to be members of the profession, stating,

---

75 Harold Perkin, *The rise of professional society: England since 1880* (London and New York: Routledge, 1989), p. 79.

76 Perkin, *The rise of professional society*, p. 78.

77 Christopher Shephard, '"I have a notion of going off to India": Colonel Alexander Porter and Irish recruitment to the Indian Medical Service, 1855–96', *Irish Economic and Social History* 41(1) (2014), p. 40.

78 Diary of Alexander Porter, 8 January 1864 [Harry Ransom Center].

79 Diary of Alexander Porter, 14 April 1864 [Harry Ransom Center].

If a person be so poor that he cannot educate his son as a professional man, he should not presume to foist him on the public for that which he is not; he should do what is much better for the boy, make a good shoemaker or tailor of him, by which he will be enabled to earn an honest and competent livelihood, instead of starving in the practice of disreputable arts and contrivances.[80]

Likewise, William Stokes, giving a lecture at the Meath Hospital in 1861, suggested that there had been an increase in young men 'of limited means' entering the medical profession because men had

a better chance of earning a livelihood at an early period of their career than at the Bar, and this is a reason why men of limited means are more tempted to enter Medicine than the other professions. The profession of Medicine, then, is more largely recruited from classes of society below those which value academic teaching, or that can well afford an extended education for their children. The *res angusta domi* is too often a cause of the neglect of the general, and the sole adoption of the special education.[81]

Concerns continued to be voiced throughout the nineteenth and twentieth centuries that those who were entering into medical study were not suitable for it or were entering medical schools for the wrong reasons. For instance, in 1919, an editorial in *T.C.D.: A College Miscellany* bemoaned the high numbers of students entering into Irish medical schools attracted by the false 'get-rich-quick allurements of the Medical School'.[82] By this point, the higher education had begun to be 'inspired by notions of humane, liberal culture, aiming to develop the whole personality, and feeding graduates into the professions and public services' as opposed to being a 'practical, examinable, market-driven, utilitarian affair'.[83]

However, many of these students would be forced to emigrate after graduation. As Greta Jones has shown, for each year between 1860 and 1875, there were over 1,000 medical students on average in Ireland, with the same number attending medical schools in the Republic of Ireland in the period

---

80 'The Introductory lecture delivered by Doctor Jacob at the Royal College of Surgeons for the session 1844–45' (Dublin: Medical Press Office, 1844), p. 8.
81 William Stokes, 'Medical education, a discourse delivered at the Meath Hospital' (Dublin: Hodges, Smith and Co., 1861), p. 11.
82 Editorial, *T.C.D.: A College Miscellany* 26(444) (3 December 1919), p. 33.
83 R.D. Anderson, *British universities past and present* (London: Hambledon Continuum, 2006), p. 111.

1938 to 1965.[84] This meant that parents who paid for a medical education for their sons and daughters were often aware that their children would have to emigrate following graduation.[85] Irish medical schools in this period were therefore 'exporting schools' and 'there was an expectation that opportunities for making a medical living outside Ireland would routinely be considered upon graduation or shortly after'.[86]

Noël Browne (1915–97), whose parents both died from tuberculosis in the 1920s, trained at Trinity College, beginning his studies in 1933, a decision he remarked was 'to be the first occasion on which, without any malicious intent, I ignored the dictat [sic] of the Archbishop of Dublin'.[87] Browne was given the opportunity to study there by the Chance family, who had sympathy for him because of his 'bleak future' and decided to fund his medical education. Lady Chance agreed that Browne could stay with them at their family home while he was undertaking his medical studies. Writing in his memoirs of this act of kindness:

> It was an extraordinary selfless decision to take. It was completely unexpected. I had never presumed to aspire to a university education, let alone become a doctor. It was difficult to assimilate the incredible news and all its implications at once, but I agreed gratefully to return to Dublin to begin a new life.[88]

Browne, who would later become Minister for Health, was not unique in being a Catholic studying medicine at Trinity College, Dublin. However, his quote gives an insight into how religious background could influence one's choice of medical school. This sets the Irish history of medical education apart from its European and American counterparts. For much of the nineteenth century, members of the Irish medical profession had been overwhelmingly Protestant. By the second quarter of the nineteenth century, Catholic medical practitioners began to expand in number, thus challenging the established medical order.[89] According to Laurence Geary, 'The Irish medical profession was racked by jealousy and suspicion and its members

84 Greta Jones, '"Strike out boldly for the prizes that are available to you": medical emigration from Ireland, 1860–1905', *Medical History* 54(1) (2010), p. 70.
85 Jones, 'Strike out boldly', p. 70.
86 Jones, 'Strike out boldly', p. 74. See also Greta Jones, '"A mysterious discrimination": Irish medical emigration to the United States in the 1950s', *Social History of Medicine* 25(1) (2011), pp. 139–56.
87 Noël Browne, *Against the tide* (Dublin: Gill & Macmillan, 1986), pp. 58–9.
88 Browne, *Against the tide*, p. 57.
89 Laurence Geary, *Medicine and charity in Ireland, 1718–1851* (Dublin: University College Dublin Press, 2005), p. 6.

were loath to see advantage and preferment conferred on their rivals, particularly if they differed from them in religion and politics'.[90] In one report in
the *Lancet* in 1869, it was claimed that 'Hospitals in Dublin are not only the
bought and sold property of their doctors, but they are also the appanages of
rival forms of religion'.[91] Writing in 1868, E.D. Mapother drew attention to
the sectarian considerations which influenced hospital elections in Dublin,
pointing out that of all the hospital officers in Dublin, 'over three-fourths
belong to one persuasion, which holds a still higher proportion among
the fellows of the Colleges of Physicians and Surgeons, a position usually
required to qualify for appointments'. He attributed the lower number of
Catholic doctors to the restrictions which had been placed in the way of
them in relation to university education, but also mentioned how directors
of hospitals were to blame for religious exclusion for hospital appointments.
He also mentioned that 'in at least four of the hospitals, appointments
are got by purchase' and that Catholics may not have been able to afford
these sums or would instead 'obtain greater bargains at hospitals where
those of their creed are readily accepted'.[92] Similarly, in the 1850s, with
the establishment of the dispensary service, there were allegations made
that these appointments depended on the candidate's religious and political
allegiances.[93] By 1871, just over three-quarters of the Irish population were
Catholic while 12 per cent were members of the Church of Ireland and a
further 9 per cent were Presbyterians. However, these statistics were not
reflected in the medical profession and it is estimated that only 34 per cent
of doctors were Catholic in 1870.[94] Numbers of Catholic doctors began to
rise moving later into the nineteenth century, with Catholics comprising
39 per cent of the medical profession in 1881 and 1891, and increasing to
43 per cent in 1901 and 48 per cent in 1911.[95]

The Queen's Colleges, founded in 1845 as an attempt at progressive
unionism, had the aim of educating non-Protestants who were barred from
attending Trinity College. These colleges faced a huge amount of backlash

90 Geary, *Medicine and charity in Ireland*, p. 6.
91 News cutting from the *Lancet*, 'The Irish Hospitals', 3 July 1869, p. 15 [RCPI Heritage
    Centre, TCPK/7/2/1–2].
92 E.D. Mapother, *First Carmichael Prize: the medical profession and its educational and
    licensing bodies* (Dublin: Fannin & Co., 1868), pp. 135–6.
93 Catherine Cox, 'Access and engagement: the medical dispensary service in post-Famine
    Ireland', in Catherine Cox and Maria Luddy (eds), *Cultures of care in Irish medical
    history, 1750–1950* (Basingstoke: Palgrave Macmillan, 2010), p. 62.
94 Cox, 'Access and engagement', p. 62.
95 John Hutchinson, 'Numbers of Roman Catholics in selected professions (1861–1911) and
    their percentage of the total', *The dynamics of cultural nationalism: the Gaelic revival
    and the creation of the Irish nation state* (London: Allen and Unwin, 1987), Table 8.2,
    p. 262. With thanks to Professor Greta Jones for alerting me to this source.

from the Irish Catholic bishops who viewed them as 'godless'. According to T.W. Moody, at Queen's College Belfast, the system of non-denominational education was a success so far as the Protestant churches were concerned, with Presbyterian, Anglican and Methodist students working 'harmoniously together as students'.[96]

Choice of medical school therefore was very much influenced by religious background. Between 1881 and 1901, at Trinity College, Catholics comprised between 4 per cent and 11 per cent of the students matriculating, or an average of six to ten men each year.[97] Catholic students who decided to attend Trinity College 'undoubtedly did so for both professional and social reasons'. A degree from Trinity was a 'valuable asset for young men intent on professional and bureaucratic careers', while Trinity also attracted the sons of leading Irish Protestant and Catholic families, so the potential for networking and cultivating useful connections was a distinct advantage of attending the university.[98] Similarly, as Kilbride has shown in his study of students from the southern states of the United States in Philadelphia in the nineteenth century, choice of medical school 'involved a judgment of social prestige and contacts as much as educational quality'.[99] In the Irish case, students would come into contact with their professors in both university and hospitals, and making a good impression would undoubtedly help them to secure a position following graduation.

Pressure for a state-funded Catholic university, or the 'Irish university question', was one of the most pressing political issues of the nineteenth century, capturing 'the attention of the Catholic church, British legislators and influential lay people, all of whom were aware of its potential impact on its beneficiaries, the future ruling class of Ireland'.[100] Charles O'Malley, writing to the *Lancet* in 1907, suggested that if a Dublin-based Catholic university with the ability to award degrees was to be established, then a non-denominational Ulster-based university should also be established 'where the students of Belfast, Galway and Cork could be examined for their medical degrees without the possibility of favouritism and in fair circumstances'.[101]

---

96 T.W. Moody, 'The Irish university question of the nineteenth century', *History* 43(148) (1958), p. 99.
97 Senia Pašeta, 'Trinity College, Dublin, and the Education of Irish Catholics, 1873–1908', *Studia Hibernica* 30 (1998–9), p. 11.
98 Pašeta, 'Trinity College, Dublin', p. 12.
99 Daniel Kilbride, 'Southern medical students in Philadelphia, 1800–1861: science and sociability in the "Republic of Medicine"', *Journal of Southern History* 65(4) (1999), p. 721.
100 Senia Pašeta, 'The Catholic hierarchy and the Irish university question, 1880–1908', *History* 85(278) (2000), p. 268.
101 C.D. O'Malley, 'Medical education and the university question in Ireland', *Lancet*, 4 May 1907, p. 1249.

Medical students were also actively engaged with this issue. At a General Meeting of the Belfast Medical Students' Association in 1899, students discussed the Irish university question and came to the conclusion that the present state of university education in Ireland was unsatisfactory; that the establishment of denominational universities would be detrimental to medical education in Ireland and, finally, that the Royal University of Ireland should be maintained, but that there should be adequate endowment for the various public colleges.[102] In the Secretaries' report for that year, it was stated that 'one of the largest and most important meetings of the year was that in which the University Question was discussed, several important resolutions were passed condemning Mr Balfour's scheme of a Catholic University'.[103] Similarly, at the Catholic University Medical School, the establishment of an association for medical students in 1904 had the main aim of agitating for 'a speedy and acceptable settlement of the University question'.[104] At a joint meeting of the Belfast Medical Students' Association and the Literary and Scientific Society of Queen's College Belfast in 1902, students debated the issue and aimed to find a resolution to the university question. Students discussed the merit of the creation of an Ulster University, with those in favour suggesting that mixed education was no longer possible and that an Ulster University 'could develop along its own lines'. Those opposing argued that if an Ulster University were established 'its degrees would be of very small value (a point which seemed to affect particularly the medical side of the house), and that there would not be enough students to support it'.[105] Religious rivalries between the medical schools persisted into the twentieth century. However, there is limited evidence to suggest that these impacted in a significant way on student experience, yet religious affiliation remained an important factor in choice of medical school and hospital.

102 Belfast Medical Students' Association Minute Book, November 1898–November 1907, letter pasted into Minute Book signed by W.A. Rice, BA (President), H.B. Steen, A.L. Black (Hon. Secs).
103 Session 1899–1900: Secretaries' report of previous year, 1898–9, Belfast Medical Students' Association Minute Book, November 1898–November 1907.
104 'Notes from the medical school', *St. Stephen's: A Record of University Life* 2(2) (1904), p. 32.
105 'Joint meeting of Literary and Scientific Society and the B.M.S.A.', *Q.C.B.* (February 1902), p. 96.

Social and religious backgrounds of students at
Trinity College Dublin and the Queen's Colleges

It is possible to provide an overview of the social backgrounds of medical students who matriculated at Irish universities in the nineteenth and early twentieth centuries through the use of matriculation registers. Matriculation registers have previously been utilised by Crowther and Dupree to provide an insight into the social and geographic backgrounds of students studying at the University of Glasgow and the University of Edinburgh in the nineteenth century. For this research, I examined the matriculation registers of the three Queen's Colleges and Trinity College Dublin.[106] Unfortunately, the registers of the Catholic University/University College Dublin were unavailable for consultation. These would undoubtedly have provided an interesting insight into the social backgrounds of Catholic students in the period. The registers of the Royal College of Surgeons do not provide information relating to father's occupation and religion. The matriculation registers of the other universities provide varying information: generally, they provide the student's name, date of entry to the university, home address, address while at university, father's name, religious persuasion and occasionally (from the 1880s) father's occupation. For students where no information was provided on father's occupation, it was possible to trace some of these students' fathers using the 1901 and 1911 censuses because of the other information provided, such as parents' address, age and father's name. Samples from each of the four medical schools were created by compiling the details of the tenth medical student matriculating in each year. In some cases at Queen's College Galway, where fewer than ten students matriculated each year, the details of the last student to matriculate that year were recorded. The information below, therefore, while incomplete, as it does not relate to students at the Catholic University or Royal College of Surgeons, provides an insight into the social backgrounds of students at the Queen's Colleges and Trinity College Dublin.

There are of course methodological issues when consulting student registers. As R.B. McDowell and D.A. Webb point out in their history of Trinity College, 'the aspiring student was often vague or misleading; one boy might describe his father as a cattle-dealer while two years later his younger

---

106   The matriculation registers of Trinity College from 1850 to 1913 were examined. Owing to the 100-year rule, it was not possible to look at later registers. The matriculation registers for 1850–1917 for Queen's College Cork and Queen's College Belfast and the matriculation registers for Queen's College Galway for the years 1861–1917 were consulted. Unfortunately, the matriculation registers for the earlier period for Queen's College Galway were unavailable.

Table 3.1 Social backgrounds of a sample of medical students matriculating at Trinity College Dublin, 1850–1913

Social background	Number of students	Percentage of traceable students
Medicine	79	21.6
Commercial and industrial	65	17.8
Land-related	52	14.2
Religious life	44	12.1
Law	39	10.7
New professions	37	10.1
Agriculture	19	5.2
Armed forces	14	3.8
Local/central government	8	2.2
Education	4	1.1
Skilled working class	3	0.8
Other	1	0.3
Totals	391	100
Deceased	5	–
Unknown/not given	21	–

Source: Trinity College Dublin Matriculation Registers, 1850–1913.

brother would say that he was the son of a landowner'.[107] Similarly, as Anne Crowther and Marguerite Dupree found in their study, students often provided vague descriptions of their fathers' occupations in their matriculation cards. The filling in of a university matriculation card in a university hall may have encouraged some students to inflate their family's socioeconomic position, while vague descriptions 'could disguise quite different backgrounds'.[108] Moreover, some of the registers provide incomplete information.

The matriculation registers of Trinity College provide detailed information, including father's name, father's occupation, religion (up until 1906, when the registers ceased to record this information), age and place of birth. Of a sample of 391 medical students studying at Trinity College Dublin from 1850 to 1913, the following information can be discerned. As Tables 3.1

107 R.B. McDowell and D.A. Webb, *Trinity College Dublin, 1592–1952, an academic history* (Cambridge: Cambridge University Press, 1982), pp. 506–7.
108 Crowther and Dupree, *Medical lives*, p. 27.

Table 3.2   Detailed social backgrounds of a sample of medical
students matriculating at Trinity College Dublin, 1850–1913

Father's occupation	Number of students	Percentage of traceable students
Commercial and industrial	65	17.8
Merchant	45	
Stockbroker	1	
Mill owner	1	
Grocer	1	
Bank manager	4	
Bank inspector	1	
Agent	7	
Auditor	1	
Railway official	2	
Stationmaster	1	
Hotel proprietor	1	
Agriculture	19	5.2
Farmer	19	
Medicine	78	21.4
Doctor	65	
Chemist	3	
Dentist	1	
Vet	2	
Surgeon Major/RAMC	7	
Religious life	44	12.1
Undefined clergyman	37	
Archdeacon	2	
Navy chaplain	1	
Minister	4	
Education	4	1.1
Teacher	1	
Headmaster	1	
Professor of elocution	1	
Fellow, TCD	1	
New professions	37	10.2
Engineer	11	
Clerk	21	

Father's occupation	Number of students	Percentage of traceable students
Secretary	2	
Accountant	1	
Architect	2	
Local/Central government	8	2.2
Civil servant	7	
Register of probate	1	
Armed Forces	14	3.8
Royal Irish Constabulary	1	
Navy Captain	2	
Army Officer	4	
Army Major	3	
Royal Marine	3	
Army Commander	1	
Land related	52	14.3
'Gentleman'	49	
Auctioneer	1	
Landowner	2	
Skilled working class	3	0.8
Builder/contractor	1	
Brewer	1	
Jeweller	1	
Law	39	10.7
Solicitor	22	
Barrister	11	
Justice of the Peace	1	
Magistrate	2	
Judge	3	
Other	1	0.3
Musician	1	
Totals	**364**	**100**
Deceased	5	–
Unknown/not given	21	–

Modelled on a table used in Crowther and Dupree, *Medical lives*, p. 28.
Source: Trinity College Dublin Matriculation Registers, 1850–1913.

and 3.2 illustrate, medical students at Trinity College in the period tended to come primarily from the upper middle classes. Notably, 21.6 per cent were the children of medical practitioners, with 17.8 per cent having fathers working in commerce and industry. Some 14.2 per cent of students were the sons of men in land-related positions – 49 of those traceable were the sons of 'gentlemen', which implied men of independent means who had not adopted a profession or trade.[109] Students at Trinity College Dublin, although much better off than their Catholic counterparts, were not as wealthy as their social equals attending the comparable institutions of Oxford and Cambridge in England.[110] According to W.J. Reader, 'Certainly the young men who went to Dublin virtually all expected to earn their own living, whereas a fair proportion at Oxford and Cambridge did not. For that reason, if for no other, Trinity College was even more professionally-minded, if that were possible, than the universities of Scotland'.[111]

As McDowell and Webb have noted, what becomes clear from a study of the social backgrounds of students at Trinity College in the nineteenth and twentieth centuries is that 'the professional class, although it was only in the second half of the nineteenth century that it constituted an actual majority, has always been the backbone of those who sent their children to Trinity'.[112] Certainly medical students at Trinity College were more likely to come from professional backgrounds with significant numbers of students having fathers working as physicians, clergymen, merchants or in law. John Stewart Swan is a typical example. Swan matriculated at Trinity College medical school in October 1886 at the age of 19. He listed his religion as Church of Ireland. His father was Robert Lafayette Swan (1843–1916), who worked as an orthopaedic surgeon at Dr Steevens' Hospital in Dublin. Swan's grandfather, John Wright Swan, had been a dispensary medical officer in Kilkenny.[113]

In contrast, as outlined in Tables 3.3 and 3.4, students attending the Queen's Colleges tended to come from middle-class backgrounds. The highest proportion of students from the sample of medical students matriculating at the Queen's Colleges had fathers working in the commercial and industrial sector (31.6 per cent) with 26.3 per cent of students coming from agricultural backgrounds. Some 11.5 per cent had fathers working in medicine, with 9.6 per cent coming from skilled working-class backgrounds, 6.7 per cent with

109 McDowell and Webb, *Trinity College Dublin*, p. 507.
110 Reader, *Professional men*, p. 134.
111 Reader, *Professional men*, p. 135.
112 Statistics relating to students. See McDowell and Webb, *Trinity College Dublin*, Appendix 2, p. 507.
113 'Obituary: Robert Lafayette Swan, F.R.C.S.I.', *British Medical Journal*, 18 November 1916, pp. 706–7.

Table 3.3   Social backgrounds of a sample of 281 medical students matriculating at the Queen's Colleges, 1887–1917

Social background	Number of students	Percentage of traceable students
Commercial and industrial	66	31.6
Agriculture	55	26.3
Medicine	24	11.5
Skilled working class	20	9.6
Education	14	6.7
New professions	10	4.8
Armed forces	6	2.9
Law	6	2.9
Religious life	5	2.4
Local/central government	3	1.4
Land-related	0	0
Other	0	0
Totals	209	100
Deceased	3	–
Unknown/not given	69	–

Source: Matriculation Registers of Queen's College Galway, Cork and Belfast.

fathers working in education and 4.8 per cent having fathers in the new professions (e.g., engineer, clerk, secretary, accountant, architect, journalist). The backgrounds of students at the Queen's Colleges contrast with those at Trinity College. For instance, at Trinity College, there were higher proportions of the sample that had fathers working in medicine, land-related, religious and legal professions, while students matriculating through the Queen's Colleges were more likely to come from commercial and industrial or farming backgrounds. Moreover, the percentage of students coming from skilled working-class backgrounds at the Queen's Colleges was 9.6 per cent for this sample, in contrast with 0.8 per cent for the sample of Trinity medical students, suggesting that for the students at the Queen's Colleges, the choice to study medicine may have had more to do with social mobility. Medical students at Trinity College had to spend extra time studying Arts, so the Queen's Colleges would have made more economic sense for middle-class families. John Stewart Weir, for instance, who enrolled at the Queen's College Belfast medical school in 1896 at the age of 18, was typical of the sample. From

Table 3.4   Detailed social backgrounds of a sample of 281 medical students matriculating at the Queen's Colleges, 1887–1917

Father's occupation	Number of students	Percentage of traceable students
Commercial and industrial	66	31.6
Merchant	27	
Shopkeeper	7	
Draper	8	
Grocer	2	
Publican	4	
Bank manager	1	
Bank agent	3	
Railway official	3	
Hotel proprietor	2	
Pawnbroker	1	
Commercial traveller	1	
Agent	1	
Manufacturer	3	
Manager	2	
Board of Trade surveyor	1	
Agriculture	55	26.3
Farmer	55	
Medicine	24	11.5
Doctor	19	
Chemist	3	
Indian Medical Service	1	
RAMC	1	
Religious life	5	2.4
Clergyman	5	
Education	14	6.7
Teacher	9	
Headmaster	2	
Schools inspector	1	
Art master	1	
Professor of theology	1	
New professions	10	4.8
Architect	1	
Clerk	3	
Secretary	3	

Father's occupation	Number of students	Percentage of traceable students
Accountant	1	
Journalist	2	
Local/central government	**3**	**1.4**
Superintendent, Board of Trade	1	
Collector of Customs and Excise	1	
Officer of Post Office	1	
Armed forces	**6**	**2.9**
Royal Irish Constabulary	4	
Navy Captain	1	
Army Officer	1	
Skilled working class	**20**	**9.6**
Builder/contractor	1	
Baker	1	
Bootmaker	2	
Butcher	2	
Clothier	2	
Cooper	1	
Decorator	1	
Engine driver	1	
Ironmonger	1	
Joiner/ carpenter	1	
Lard refiner	1	
Master coachbuilder	1	
Master plumber	1	
Tailor	1	
Victualler	2	
Vintner	1	
Law	**6**	**2.9**
Solicitor	3	
Justice of the Peace	1	
Councillor of Petty Sessions	2	
Totals	**209**	**100**
Deceased	3	
Unknown/not given	69	

Source: Matriculation Registers of Queen's College Galway, Queen's College Cork and Queen's College Belfast.

Derry, Weir was the son of a farmer and Presbyterian. Charles O'Connell, who enrolled at Queen's College Cork in the same year, was the Catholic son of a bank agent and from Dunmanaway in Cork. For these students, medicine offered a means of social mobility. However, most pertinently, the students came from backgrounds with parents who had the means to fund the five or six years of medical study necessary to qualify as a doctor.

Although students at the Queen's Colleges tended to be drawn from similar backgrounds, there were differences with regard to religious backgrounds, as Table 3.5 illustrates. Student registers were consulted for Queen's College Cork, Queen's College Belfast and Trinity College Dublin for the years 1850–1913 and for Queen's College Galway from 1861 to 1913. From 1906, Trinity College Dublin stopped recording students' religious affiliations. However, it was possible to trace many of these students in the 1901 and 1911 censuses.

Trinity was almost exclusively Anglican until the beginning of the twentieth century. According to statistics garnered by McDowell and Webb, 1902 was the first year when Anglican students did not comprise 75 per cent of the total.[114] As Table 3.6 illustrates, Protestants were overwhelmingly in the majority among medical students matriculating at Trinity College Dublin in the years 1873–93, with 68.7 per cent of the sample being a member of one of the Protestant churches. Some 12.5 per cent of students listed their religion as Presbyterian, with 15 per cent as Roman Catholic. As Senia Pašeta has shown, Catholics made up between 4 per cent and 11 per cent of Trinity College's annual intake between 1881 and 1901, with 4 per cent being the lowest figure, recorded in 1888, and between 6 per cent and 10 per cent being the average for each year.[115] The proportion of Catholic medical students appears to be higher than the percentage of Catholics in the student body overall. Numbers of Catholic students at Trinity College showed a steady increase from 1900, in spite of the hostility of the Catholic hierarchy.[116] This seems to have been the case in the medical faculty also, with a notable increase in the percentage of students listing 'Roman Catholic' as their religion after 1900. Catholic students comprised over 20 per cent of students at Trinity in the years from 1923 to 1930, but figures declined from the mid-1930s, with the proportion of Catholic students entering Trinity in the two years in the middle of the decade falling to as low as 8 per cent. From 1938, recovery began again, and continued, so that by 1950 the figure for Catholic students was 23 per cent.[117]

114 McDowell and Webb, *Trinity College Dublin*, p. 504.
115 Pašeta, 'Trinity College, Dublin', p. 11.
116 McDowell and Webb, cited in Pašeta, 'Trinity College, Dublin', p. 20.
117 McDowell and Webb, *Trinity College Dublin*, p. 504.

Table 3.5 Religious backgrounds of a sample of 549 medical students matriculating at the Queen's Colleges, 1850–1913 (1861–1913 in the case of Galway), and a sample of 391 Trinity College Dublin students matriculating 1850–1913

University	Protestant[a]	Roman Catholic	Presbyterian	Other Christian[b]	Not given	Jewish	Totals
Queen's College Belfast (sample of students 1850–1913)	49 (25.1%)	27 (13.8%)	109 (55.9%)	9 (4.6%)	1 (0.5%)	0	195
Queen's College Cork (sample of students 1850–1913)	75 (31.1%)	152 (63.1%)	8 (3.3%)	6 (2.5%)	0	0	241
Queen's College Galway (sample of students 1861–1913)	24 (21.2%)	58 (51.3%)	22 (19.5%)	8 (7.1%)	1 (0.9%)	0	113
Trinity College Dublin (sample of students 1850–1913)	262 (67.0%)	57 (14.6%)	36 (9.2%)	14 (3.6%)	2 (0.5%)	20 (5.1%)	391

[a] Including Protestant, Church of England, Established Church, Church of Ireland, Church of Scotland, Episcopalian.
[b] Including Society of Friends, Unitarian, Wesleyan, Plymouth Brethren, Methodist, Dutch Reformed Church, Dissenter, Baptist.
Source: Matriculation Registers of Queen's College Cork/ Queen's College Belfast, 1850–1913, Queen's College Galway 1850–1913, and Trinity College Dublin, 1850–1913.

Table 3.6 Religious backgrounds of samples of students matriculating, 1873–93 and 1893–1913

University Year	Protestant[a]		Roman Catholic		Presbyterian		Totals	
	1873–93	1893–1913	1873–93	1893–1913	1873–93	1893–1913	1873–93	1893–1913
Queen's College Belfast	26 (28.6%)	8 (13.1%)	3 (3.3%)	18 (29.5%)	52 (57.1%)	33 (54.1%)	91	61
Queen's College Cork	32 (28.8%)	10 (13.5%)	71 (64.0%)	59 (79.7%)	4 (3.6%)	3 (4.0%)	111	74
Queen's College Galway	6 (18.7%)	3 (15.0%)	19 (59.4%)	14 (70.0%)	5 (15.6%)	3 (15.0%)	32	20
Trinity College Dublin	110 (68.7%)	67 (53.6%)	24 (15.0%)	23 (18.4%)	20 (12.5%)	13 (10.4%)	160	125

University Year	Other Christian[b]		Jewish		Not given	
	1873–93	1893–1913	1873–93	1893–1913	1873–93	1893–1913
Queen's College Belfast	10 (11.0%)	1 (1.6%)	0	0	0	1 (1.6%)
Queen's College Cork	4 (3.6%)	2 (2.7%)	0	0	0	0
Queen's College Galway	2 (6.2%)	0	0	0	0	0
Trinity College Dublin	5 (3.1%)	8 (6.4%)	0	2 (1.6%)	1 (0.6%)	12 (9.6%)

[a] Including Protestant, Church of England, Established Church, Church of Ireland, Church of Scotland, Episcopalian.
[b] Including Society of Friends, Unitarian, Wesleyan, Plymouth Brethren, Methodist, Dutch Reformed Church, Dissenter, Baptist.
Source: Matriculation Registers of Queen's College Cork / Queen's College Belfast, 1850–1913, Queen's College Galway, 1850–1913 and Trinity College Dublin, 1850–1913.

A breakdown of the samples into two 20-year periods reveals an increase in Catholic students at both the Queen's Colleges and Trinity College Dublin from the late nineteenth century and a decline in the percentage of Protestant and other Christian students, while percentages of Presbyterian students remained more or less the same.

Conclusion

It is clear that members of the middle classes were predominant among entrants to medical schools from the mid-nineteenth to the early twentieth century. Although students' social backgrounds differed depending on institution, with students from Trinity College being more likely to have fathers in the medical or legal professions or the clergy, numbers of students with fathers in the commercial and industrial fields were significant. Students from the Queen's Colleges were more likely to have fathers in the middle or 'middling' classes. Although for the early nineteenth century members of the Protestant faith had been predominant in the medical profession, by the mid-nineteenth century, members of the Catholic middle-class were entering the profession in growing numbers. Students undertook medical education for a variety of reasons, sometimes personal, but often based around socioeconomic factors. Considering the expense involved in medical study, parents needed to be able to support their sons and daughters. Although statistics relating to students' social and religious backgrounds from the 1920s to 1950s are unavailable, it is clear that reasons for studying medicine remained consistent. Writing in 1954, William Collis, the Irish paediatrician commented that the first test for a student considering entering the medical profession was 'the financial position of their parents who must set aside a very substantial sum so as to be able to subsidise their sons or daughters for at least six years after having given them a secondary education'.[118] For the next generations of students in the first half of the twentieth century, class remained an important factor in deciding whether medical education could be pursued.

118 William Collis, 'The trend of medical education in Ireland', *Irish Journal of Medical Science*, 6th series, no.343 (July 1954), p. 316.

4

Educational Experiences
and Medical Student Life,
c.1880–1920

By the early twentieth century, some professors at Irish medical schools were promoting a sense of confidence about the achievements of Irish medical education and its 'scientific atmosphere'.[1] This transition had not been straightforward. As has already been suggested, Irish medical education was beset with many problems for much of the nineteenth century. From the 1880s, attempts were made by the General Medical Council to standardise medical education in Britain and Ireland. In 1886, under the Medical Amendment Act, medical education was extended to a recommended five-year programme. The subjects taken remained the same as in earlier years, but a clear demarcation was made between the pre-clinical subjects and the clinical subjects.[2] At Queen's College Galway in 1888, for instance, the medical curriculum was divided up into two periods, which were to take at least two years each. In the first period, students studied chemistry, practical chemistry, botany and zoology, anatomy and physiology, practical anatomy, comparative anatomy, practical physiology, *materia medica* and pharmacy. In the second period, they studied a second course of anatomy and physiology, a second course of practical anatomy, theory and practice of surgery, obstetrics and gynaecology, the theory and practice of medicine, state medicine (medical jurisprudence, hygiene, sanitary engineering) and pathology.[3] The other Irish medical schools followed a similar programme.

---

1 Newspaper cutting from the *Irish Times*, 'Dublin University Biological Association', 19 November 1908, TCD Biological Association Minute Book, March 1904–December 1908 (Minute Book 4) [TCD Manuscripts Department].
2 James P. Murray, *Galway: a medico-social history* (Galway: Kenny's Bookshop and Art Gallery, 2002), p. 123.
3 College calendar of Queen's College Galway, 1887–8, p. 20.

By 1909, the National University of Ireland (NUI) suggested that students should spend five years in medical study and that the subjects of physics, chemistry, biology (including botany and zoology) should be taken in the first year, with the option of anatomy and practical anatomy and practical chemistry. For the second year, students were required to study the optional subjects from the first year, as well as physiology, *materia medica* and hospital attendance. They also had the option of taking practical physiology and histology. In the third year, students studied anatomy, practical anatomy, practical physiology and histology and *materia medica* (if not taken in the second year), as well as physiology, practical pharmacy, hospital attendance and two of the following: medicine, surgery and midwifery. In the fourth and fifth years, students studied medicine, surgery, midwifery (if not taken in the third year), operative surgery, medical jurisprudence, pathology, ophthalmology and otology, sanitary science, mental diseases, practical midwifery, as well as continuing their hospital attendance. Students were required to attend a fever hospital as well as six post-mortem examinations and work for at least six months as clinical clerks and to have attended at least 20 labours, of which they were to have had personal charge, and to have undertaken a course in vaccination.[4] Hospital attendance was an important part of the curriculum and this is reflected in the fact that students were recommended to obtain this experience starting from their second year if they were aiming at the NUI examinations.

There has been limited research on the educational experiences of medical students at Irish institutions. This chapter aims to illuminate this theme through an examination of how the medical curriculum evolved between the late nineteenth and early twentieth centuries, in particular assessing the shifting importance of scientific subjects and clinical instruction to the identity of burgeoning new members of the Irish medical profession. Focusing on the various educational spheres – the lecture theatre, the laboratory, the dissecting room and the medical museum, this chapter will explore formative educational experiences as well as initiatives that students took on themselves in order to try and enhance their educational experiences. It is clear that certain rites of passage in medical education, such as one's first entry to the dissecting room, and clinical experience, were viewed as having particular importance for medical students. Additionally, medical study was often described as a transformative experience. Educational spaces such as the lecture theatre, dissecting room, laboratory and the hospital helped students to undergo the transformation from student to fully fledged practitioner, while also cementing a collective identity. The standard of education also varied from one institution to another, while choice of hospital was often

4 *NUI Calendar 1909*, pp. 146–58.

dependent on religious affiliation. The hospital, more so than any other sphere of education, was the most important educational setting for Irish medical students and, as will become evident, clinical education remained a crucial formative experience for Irish doctors well into the twentieth century.

The pre-clinical years

Upon entering first year of medical school, students generally had a core set of lectures in the basic sciences. Lectures remained an important part of the pedagogy at Irish medical schools throughout the nineteenth and twentieth centuries. Medical students themselves often condoned the fact that they had to study the more theoretical subjects which they viewed as less relevant to a career in the profession. Others, like J. Johnston Abraham, who studied at Trinity College Dublin in the 1890s, commented that once they began their hospital training they could see how these subjects were essential in providing a scientific foundation.[5] Botany and zoology, often referred to as 'bugs and weeds' in Trinity College from the late nineteenth century well into the twentieth century, faced the most criticism from students.[6] Professors of these subjects were not always treated in a respectful manner by students. In 1897, the professor of zoology at University College Cork, wrote to the College Council to complain about students' disorderly conduct at a zoology lecture.[7] At Trinity College Dublin, J. Johnston Abraham recalled the medical students referring to their professor of zoology as 'Tapes' behind his back, owing to his lecture on parasitic worms.[8] George Sigerson, who lectured at the Catholic University Medical School, taught Oliver St John Gogarty at the turn of the century, before Gogarty transferred to Trinity College. Gogarty recalled students putting parts of specimens that had been handed around in class in Sigerson's tall silk hat, which he would unknowingly then put on.[9] Similarly, Belfast students traditionally had a poor relationship with the professor of botany. On the first day of the second-year term, medical students in the 1920s traditionally attended the first-year lecture and caused

5   J. Johnston Abraham, *Surgeon's journey: the autobiography of J. Johnston Abraham* (London: Heinemann, 1957), p. 58.
6   'The Schools: I. The Medical School', *T.C.D.: A College Miscellany* 39(682) (23 February 1933): 114 and Oliver St John Gogarty, *Tumbling in the hay* (London: Sphere Books, 1982), p. 14.
7   Letter from Professor of Zoology to College Council, dated 9 March 1897 [UCC University Archives, UC/COUNCIL/19/364].
8   Abraham, *Surgeon's journey*, p. 41.
9   Oliver St John Gogarty, *It isn't this time of year at all! An unpremeditated autobiography* (London: Sphere Books,1983), p. 27.

disruption with missiles, setting 'the standards of behaviour for students of subsequent years', a practice that was still ongoing in the mid-1950s.[10] Florence Stewart, a student at Queen's in the late 1920s, commented that the professor of botany, Professor James Small (perhaps, understandably), 'did not like medical students' and recalled him addressing the class of students as 'ladies and gentlemen' (meaning the science students) 'and medical students'. This dislike of medical students she felt owed its roots to a 'Reception Rag' when he was appointed and the medical students had 'picked him up and left him in a flower bed in the Botanic Gardens'.[11]

Moving into the twentieth century, there were persistent pleas for the subjects of botany and zoology to be removed from the medical curriculum by both professors and students. A student writing in *Q.C.B.* in 1900 remarked, 'Both Zoology and Botany are dead and uninteresting, indeed cannot be learned, unless book-work go hand-in-hand with practical work in the Laboratory. It is a thousand pities that the most interesting subject in the preparatory curriculum should thus be made dry and lifeless to the average student'.[12] Henry Bewley, in a paper presented to the Dublin Biological Club in 1909, stated that he failed to see the relevance of botany and zoology to medical education.[13] Moreover, he commented that these subjects also presented a real challenge to students. In June 1909, 29 students out of 64 failed the botany and zoology examination at Trinity College, and at the October examination, 24 failed out of 33.[14] Similarly, Dr William Pearson, in a paper given to students at the Trinity College Biological Association in 1910, suggested that the 'less useful subjects' of botany and zoology should be cut from the medical curriculum as well as parts of *materia medica*, physiology and applied anatomy.[15] Others disagreed. Writing in the *Irish Journal of Medical Science*, in 1910, W. Thompson explained that botany had originally become part of the medical curriculum because a knowledge of plants was necessary for the understanding of the subject of *materia medica*, while zoology was important in helping students to understand human anatomy in relation to other animals. Thompson believed that if either of the subjects was to be removed from the medical curriculum the student would

10 Denis Biggart, *John Henry Biggart: pathologist, professor and Dean of Medical Faculty, Queen's University, Belfast* (Belfast: Ulster Historical Association, 2012), p. 23.
11 Florence Stewart Memoirs [PRONI D3612/3/1].
12 'The College from a student's standpoint – 1. Medical', *Q.C.B.*, vol.1, no.6 (21 May 1900), p. 7.
13 Henry T. Bewley, 'Medical education: a criticism and a scheme', a paper read before the Dublin Biological Club on 14 December 1909, printed in *Dublin Journal of Medical Science* (February 1910), p. 4. (RCPI).
14 Bewley, 'Medical education', p. 5.
15 24 February 1910, TCD Biological Association (Minute Book 5), January 1909–February 1914 [TCD Manuscripts].

lack the knowledge necessary for other subjects – for instance, 'the student on beginning physiology would lack a knowledge of what is meant by an animal or vegetable cell, and also the histological technique acquired in their study'.[16] Students often called for increased emphasis on the more practical elements of the curriculum and for the course content of subjects like botany to be revised or removed.[17] This suggests that the practical subjects were viewed as more important to students' sense of identity.

Lectures in botany and zoology were complemented by hands-on experience with specimens in the medical museum. As Jonathan Reinarz has noted, for nineteenth-century medical students, the medical museum 'was the site where theory first encountered practical learning, as ideas introduced in lectures were explained and illustrated with the help of preserved specimens'.[18] In spite of their importance to medical education in the period, with the exception of Reinarz's work, medical museums have received little attention from historians.[19]

All of the Irish medical schools appear to have possessed medical museums. The medical museum at the Royal College of Surgeons was open daily to matriculated students.[20] The museum contained four departments: an anatomical museum founded in 1841, a pathological museum containing over 5,000 specimens, a wax model collection containing 38 specimens, and the 'Butcher' museum which contained a series of surgical preparations collected by Richard G.H. Butcher, a former President of the College.[21] The College Museum was still advertised in the RCSI prospectus of 1938.[22] Similarly, at Queen's College Cork, there was a Natural History museum attached to the biological department which contained collections of native birds and animals as well as a 'Hortus Siccus', consisting of a general collection of about 60,00 named specimens and a native collection

16 W. Thompson, 'More about medical education', *Irish Journal of Medical Science*, 129 (March 1910), p. 183.

17 'Editorial Notes', *T.C.D.: A College Miscellany* 15(266) (10 November 1909): 133 and W. Battersby, '"Medical education", an address delivered in the dining hall of Trinity College at the opening meeting of the second session of the Dublin University Medico-Chirurgical Society, November 27th, 1868 by the auditor W.E. Battersby, B.A. Med. Sch.' (Dublin: M. & S. Eaton, 1868), p. 11.

18 Jonathan Reinarz, 'The age of museum medicine: the rise and fall of the medical museum at Birmingham's School of Medicine', *Social History of Medicine* 18(3) (2005), p. 420.

19 Reinarz, 'The age of museum medicine', p. 419.

20 *Royal College of Surgeons in Ireland Calendar, January 1886* (Dublin: Fannin & Co.), p. 80.

21 *Royal College of Surgeons in Ireland Calendar, January 1886*, pp. 115–16.

22 *Royal College of Surgeons in Ireland: Schools of Surgery Including Carmichael and Ledwich Schools* (Dublin: Ponsonby and Gibbs, 1938–9); Prospectus, Wellcome Library, p. 11.

containing a very large number of the British flora'.[23] Students were permitted to remove the specimens from their cases in order to examine and study them.[24] The Cork medical school also had a museum of *materia medica* containing 'specimens of crude and manufactured drugs, and of the plants, minerals &c., from which drugs are made'.[25] The Pathological Museum contained examples of ordinary morbid conditions as well as 'many rare cases of disease' while a large collection of surgical, gynaecological, obstetrical instruments and splints were available to students for consultation in the corridor of the Medical Building.[26] University College Galway also had a number of museums, such as a natural history museum, a *materia medica* museum, a collection of anatomical preparations and the Montgomery Museum which contained casts, models, and prepared specimens for instruction in obstetrics, as well as a selection of ancient and modern obstetric instruments.[27] However, as mentioned in a 1925 report on the teaching facilities at UCG, although the museum was seen as 'invaluable for teaching purposes', a lack of funds 'hamper[s] its complete development'.[28]

Certain Irish hospitals also possessed their own educational museums. For instance, Dr Steeven's Hospital provided a reading room and museum for students of the hospital in the late nineteenth century.[29] Although it is not possible to gauge the extent to which students themselves utilised these medical museums, some medical students appear to have recognised their educational potential. In 1896, members of the Cork Medical Students' Association wrote to the College Council asking that students should be provided with 'a proper anatomical museum and bone room to which they have free access', acknowledging that this would help students in preparing for the higher examinations in medicine and surgery.[30] Similarly, in 1899, students wrote again to the College Council requesting that recently

23 'The Cork School of Medicine: Queen's College, Cork and Associated Hospitals' (Cork: George Purcell & Co., undated), p. 5 [UCC University Archives, UC/COUNCIL/4/46(4)].

24 'The Cork School of Medicine', p. 5.

25 'The Cork School of Medicine', p. 7.

26 'The Cork School of Medicine', pp. 7–8.

27 *Calendar for University College, Galway, 1941*, pp. 66–73 and *Report on the Department of Midwifery and Gynaecology, 1924–25*; *Report on Medical School, University College Galway, 1925* (Galway: O'Gorman Printing House, 1925), p. 7.

28 *Report on the Department of Midwifery and Gynaecology, 1924–25*, p. 7.

29 E. Wooton, *A guide to the medical profession: a comprehensive manual conveying the means of entering the medical profession in the chief countries of the world* (London: L. Upcott Gill, 1883), p. 313.

30 Letter from Medical Students Association [UCC University Archives, UC/COUNCIL/21/32].

prepared dry specimens could be placed in the zoological museum and that specimens 'be placed in the Materia Medica Museum so as to bring it up the requirements of the British Pharmacopoeia (1898)'.[31] Professor J.J. Charles, the professor of anatomy at Queen's College Cork, in a letter to the College Council in 1896 remarked that he did not think it was necessary to keep the bone room open to students for consultation. On two occasions he had placed the bones of a skeleton in cases in the anatomical museum but, regrettably, these were stolen.[32] In 1897, the professor of zoology was commended by medical students at Trinity College Dublin for the new models he had introduced to the museum which illustrated the segmentation of the ovum and the early development of the embryo, providing students with 'ample opportunities' for 'studying this important branch of biology'.[33] Likewise, the committee of the Belfast Medical Students' Association wrote to the College Council in 1904 asking that the pathological specimens of the medical museum be rearranged and classified and a new catalogue created.[34]

Moving into the late nineteenth century, medical museums began to decline in importance with the rise of specialist medical institutions which meant that students could observe interesting cases directly by walking the wards.[35] J. Johnston Abraham remarked that the museum of comparative anatomy at Trinity College, which was curated by the professor of zoology, an unpopular figure amongst the medical students, 'was practically wasted. A few curious people came occasionally to see the huge skeleton of Cornelius McGraw [sic], the Irish giant, nearly eight feet high, but that was all'.[36]

Of more importance was the educational sphere of the dissecting room, with the first entrance to the dissecting room commonly described as one of the most important educational rites of passage.[37] The following poem, which appeared in the magazine of the Royal College of Surgeons in 1917, describes a medical student's first foray into the dissecting room:

31 Letter from QCCMSA, dated 18 January 1899, addressed to Alex Jack esq. [UCC University Archives, UC/COUNCIL/18/38(i)].
32 Letter to the Council of QCC, dated 20 March 1896 [UCC University Archives, UC/COUNCIL/19/165].
33 'News from "the schools": medical school by "Section X"', *T.C.D.: A College Miscellany* 3(38) (13 February 1897), p. 16.
34 Committee Meeting, Thursday, 11 February 1904, Belfast Medical Students' Association, Committee Minute Book, 1899–1925 [Royal Victoria Hospital Archives].
35 Reinarz, 'The age of museum medicine', p. 435.
36 Abraham, *Surgeon's journey*, p. 41. The correct name of the giant was Cornelius Magrath (1736–60).
37 Through the effective use of a range of photographs from American medical schools, John Harley Warner and James M. Edmonson have underlined the importance of dissection to professional identity. See Warner and Edmonson, *Dissection: photographs of a rite of passage in American medicine, 1880–1930* (New York: Blast Books, 2009).

When first the budding student goes
To the dissecting room, his nose
By odours strange is greeted:
And as he wears his new white clo'es
And stares at all around, his pose
Proclaims a mind unseated!
While round about on tables lie
The subjects on which bye and bye
His skill will be directed.
On them he casts a nervous eye,
And firmly he resolves to try
And keep his thoughts connected.[38]

As the verse suggests, a student's first experience of dissection usually engendered feelings of fear and trepidation.[39] William M. Hunter, who studied at Queen's College Belfast in the 1890s, recalled his first day in the dissecting room in the following way:

My first day in the Dissecting Room was pretty nerve racking. I will always remember the first time I saw so many dead bodies in different degrees of dissection. The first incision I made in the skin of a dead body was never forgotten.[40]

Irish medical students regularly reported needing reserves of courage to curb their feelings of anxiety. A student writing in St. Stephen's magazine in 1903 stated: 'A record day in the student's life will be his first visit, paid in fear and gruesomeness, to Peace's [medical porter] apartment', which he later described as 'the chamber of horrors'.[41] Others commented on the telling of ghoulish stories by other students prior to students entering the dissecting room.

Most doctors' memoirs recall the visceral nature of the dissecting room and its effect on their senses, particularly noting the smell. Robert Blackham, a student at the Ledwich School in Dublin in the late 1880s recalled the anatomy room as a 'long, ill kept apartment, cold and draughty in the winter and hot and stuffy in the summer session. The lighting was from flaring bats wing gas burners. The floors were dirty and the smell from the "subjects"

38 'The student's progress', R.C.S.I. Students' Quarterly 1(1) (February 1917), p. 5.
39 One poem published in 1917 remarked on the 'nervous eye' of the student upon entering the dissecting room ('The student's progress', p. 5).
40 William M. Hunter, 'Private life of a country medical practitioner', p. 7 (private memoir courtesy of the Hunter family).
41 'Medical notes', St. Stephen's: A Record of University Life 2(1) (December 1903), p. 18.

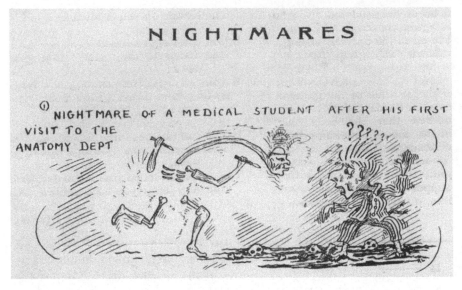

2   'Nightmare of a medical student after his first visit to the Anatomy Dept.'
From *Galway University College Magazine*, 2(9): 1922–3.
Courtesy of NUI Galway Archives and Special Collections.

was often overpowering'.[42] R.W.M. Strain, a student at Queen's University Belfast in the 1920s, wrote in his memoirs: 'When you go into the dissecting room with its unforgettable odours of formalin and strong carbolic soap you start a study that sets you apart from all the other Faculties. You get over the shock of the bodies'. For Strain, 'it was good to have the baptism over. It is quite a landmark'.[43] In G.M. Irvine's novel, *The Lion's Whelp*, the dissecting room at Queen's was described as 'a long, foul-smelling, ill-kept room, poorly equipped for the purpose of teaching anatomy. Along each side were arranged six tables, on each of which lay a dead body, or the remains – more or less scant – of a dead body with one or more of the limbs removed, or extensively mangled ... the whole place looked horrible, smelt horribly'.[44]

Owing to the Anatomy Act of 1832, which regulated the supply of cadavers to anatomy schools, subjects were in good supply. Under this legislation, the unclaimed bodies of persons who died in prisons or workhouses could

42 Colonel Robert J. Blackham, *Scalpel, sword and stretcher: forty years of work and play* (London: Sampson Low, Marston & Co. Ltd., 1931), p. 31.

43 R.W.M. Strain, *Les neiges d'antan. a two-part story: recollections of a medical student at the Queen's University of Belfast, 1924–30 and of a houseman, the Royal Victoria Hospital, Belfast, 1930–31* (Truro: R. Strain, 1982), p. 8.

44 G.M. Irvine, *The lion's whelp* (London: Simpkin, Marshall, Hamilton, Kent & Co. Ltd., 1910), p. 13.

be utilised as cadavers in the dissecting room.[45] In addition, members of the public could also agree to donate their bodies after death for the advancement of medical science. Robert Blackham recalled that many of the cadavers he saw as a medical student tended to be elderly or 'definitely deceased persons' but he recalled one occasion when the porter at the school called the students in to see the cadaver of a young girl. The experience affected Blackham and he wrote about the cadaver in a sexualised way: 'Her features were well nigh perfect and her long golden hair had not been removed – which was remarkable. We found no outward evidence of disease and it seemed amazing that there should be no one in the world to claim the exquisitely moulded body'.[46] Michael Taaffe, who trained at Trinity College from the mid-1910s, remarked that he felt an 'initial repugnance to sinking a scalpel' but that after eight months in the medical school he felt 'familiar enough with death as exemplified by the mummy-like subjects that had once been human beings'.[47] John Lyburn, a student at Trinity in the 1920s, remarked that his first entrance into the dissecting room 'was a bewildering, even nauseating sight ... for this was the first time I had ever seen a dead man without apparel, and now for the first time I gained an impression of the magnificent architecture of the animal and human body'.[48] Lyburn became fascinated with the 'craftsmanship of the human body', and he soon became 'full of fervour' for his work.[49] Although many students remarked on the fear they felt upon their first entrance into the dissecting room, it is evident that this space occupied a particular place in doctors' collective memory, as evident in their memoirs. As Chapter 5 will discuss in more depth, one's first encounter with the dissecting room was one rite of passage that had particularly masculine connotations.

The rise of the laboratory

By the mid-nineteenth century, medical classes across Europe generally consisted of a course of lectures and sometimes demonstrations in the newer sciences as well as traditional lectures in 'the institutes of medicine, surgery, medical practice, pharmacy, therapeutics and obstetrics and some

---

45 For more on the Anatomy Act, and on the history of dissection more generally, see Ruth Richardson, *Dissection, death and the destitute* (Chicago: University of Chicago Press, 2000).
46 Blackham, *Scalpel, sword and stretcher*, pp. 32–3.
47 Michael Taaffe, *Those days are gone away* (London: Hutchinson, 1959), p. 173.
48 John Lyburn, *The fighting Irish doctor (an autobiography)* (Dublin: Morris & Co., 1947), p. 52.
49 Lyburn, *The fighting Irish doctor*, p. 53.

provision for clinical or hospital instruction'.[50] As medical cosmologies shifted from hospital to laboratory medicine from the middle decades of the nineteenth century, the role of the practitioner transitioned from that of clinician to scientist with the perception of the sick man moving from that of case to cell complex.[51] Accordingly, from the 1870s, laboratory and scientific teaching came to play a more significant role in British and North American medical schools.[52] As Waddington has discussed in his work on St Bartholomew's Hospital in London, 'the growing acceptance of a limited definition of science in medical education saw the emergence of a more "modern" style of training. It forced the development of a new type of teaching space – the teaching laboratory – which provided a new discipline and mode of instruction'.[53]

The microscope became the new emblem of the laboratory. Writing in 1864, William Stokes, the famous Irish physician, hailed the rise of the microscope, which 'revolutionized the study of pathological anatomy'.[54] Likewise, Irish gynaecologist Henry Macnaughton Jones, speaking to students in Cork in 1877, encouraged each student 'to cultivate, early in his career, a familiarity with the microscopial appearances of diseased structures' and to invest in a microscope, which could be purchased for five or six guineas.[55] Indeed, some students themselves began to become aware of the increasing importance of the microscope. William Battersby, a student at Trinity College Dublin, in an address to his fellow students in 1868, accorded that research by British

---

50 Thomas Neville Bonner, *Becoming a physician: medical education in Britain, France, Germany and the United States, 1750–1945* (Oxford: Oxford University Press, 1995), pp. 217–18.

51 N.D. Jewson, 'The disappearance of the sick-man from medical cosmology, 1770–1870', *Sociology* 10(2) (1976): 225–44.

52 As Steve Sturdy has shown, from the 'mid-nineteenth century, the metropolitan licensing bodies and some of the elite universities began to set new standards for pre-clinical education by emphasising practical laboratory training, particularly in physiology and pathology'. Although some schools, such as the Sheffield Medical School, 'continued to adhere to an older model of pre-clinical education, which restricted practical experience to anatomical dissection, while physiology and pathology were taught entirely in the lecture theatre', medical schools were forced to introduce laboratory-based scientific instruction from the 1880s as ambitious students began to leave to attain their studies elsewhere (Steve Sturdy, 'The political economy of scientific medicine: science, education and the transformation of medical practice in Sheffield, 1890–1922', *Medical History* 36 (1992), p. 130).

53 Keir Waddington, *Medical education at St Bartholomew's Hospital, 1123–1995* (Woodbridge: Boydell Press, 2003), p. 116.

54 William Stokes, 'Medical education in the University of Dublin, a discourse delivered at the opening of the School of Physic in Ireland session 1864–65' (Dublin: Printed at the University Press by M.H. Gill, 1864), p. 32.

55 H. Macnaughton Jones, *Clinical teaching in hospitals* (Cork: George Purcell & Co., 1877), p. 21.

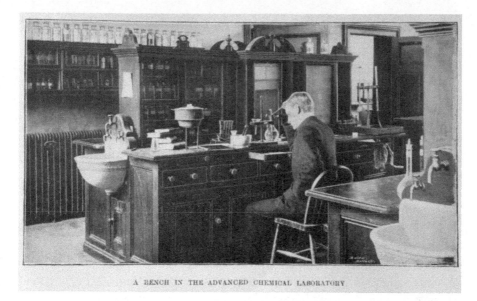

A BENCH IN THE ADVANCED CHEMICAL LABORATORY

3   'A bench in the advanced chemical laboratory'.
From *Guide to the Belfast Medical School for session 1903–4* (Belfast:
A. Mayne and Boyd, 1903). Courtesy of the RCPI Heritage Centre.

physiologists, such as Hughes Bennett and William Benjamin Carpenter, the microscopist Lionel Beale and many more men on the Continent, can 'afford us ample proof of the importance which the microscope possesses for us; nay further, it is absolutely necessary for every medical man to be familiar with the use of it, as well as with its past revelations'.[56]

Familiarity with the microscope and the observation of cell structures were important aspects of the curriculum from the late nineteenth century. At the Royal College of Surgeons during the 1880s, if not before, students were required to examine preparations of different objects under the microscope and to study these before being examined on them, as part of their second professional examination.[57] Similarly, students at Trinity College received practical laboratory instruction in chemistry and histology, with students studying histology being given their own place in the laboratory, a microscope and a full set of apparatus and reagents.[58] Laboratories were

56 W. Battersby, '"Medical education", an address delivered in the dining hall of Trinity College at the opening meeting of the second session of the Dublin University Medico-Chirurgical Society, November 27th, 1868 by the auditor W.E. Battersby, B.A. Med. Sch.' (Dublin: M. & S. Eaton, 1868), p. 22.
57 *Royal College of Surgeons in Ireland Calendar, January 1886*, p. 86.
58 *The Dublin University Calendar for the year 1885* (Dublin: Hodges, Figgis and Co., 1885), pp. 179–80.

costly to build and maintain. Laboratory fittings were expensive and often had an impact on the finances of a medical school.[59] The Catholic University in 1892 had its histology, physiology, chemistry and pharmacy laboratories provided with new fittings at a cost of £275. 11s., with £146. 13s. 5d. allotted for the public health laboratory fittings and instruments and £43. 3s. 9d. for the cost of the chemistry laboratory.[60] A bacteriological laboratory was set up in the Catholic University at the request of the chair of pathology in 1893.[61] Students at Queen's College Belfast complained in 1900 about the parsimony that characterised many of the departments of the medical school there, in particular in the departments of natural history, zoology and botany, which were viewed as 'dead and uninteresting' and which 'cannot be learned, unless book-work go hand-in-hand with practical work in the Laboratory'. The chemistry and physics departments were also criticised for the lack of new apparatus, and while it was acknowledged that improvements had been made in the teaching of anatomy and physiology, new instruments were urgently required.[62] In 1902, the fitting of the new laboratories for practical physiology made the news in the Trinity College student press, with students writing that they would now have the 'satisfaction of knowing that the Trinity School of Medicine is keeping well up to the times'.[63] Likewise, the new pharmacy laboratory at University College Cork made the student news in 1914, which also reported that the medical museum had been properly organised and catalogued. According to one student, 'these improvements are a good sign, and show that the "powers that be" are at last beginning to recognise that the Medical School is in need of attention in many respects'.[64] However, just a year later, medical students complained again about the state of the medical building where 'beautiful cultures of fungus may be observed in graceful spirals along the side walls and windows'.[65]

By the early twentieth century, professors at Irish medical schools were acknowledging that the laboratory had come to have an even more prominent place in the medical curriculum and this meant that students were more

59 W.F. Bynum, *Science and the practice of medicine in the nineteenth century* (Cambridge: Cambridge University Press, 1994), p. 181.
60 'June 14, 1892', Catholic University School of Medicine Governing Body Minute Book, 1892–1911 [UCD Archives, CU/14]. These expenses were paid from the bequest of the late Patrick Lynch MD.
61 '21st of October 1892 and January 27th, 1893', Catholic University School of Medicine Governing Body Minute Book, 1892–1911 [UCD Archives, CU/14].
62 'The College from a student's standpoint – 1. medical', *Q.C.B.* 1(6) (1900) p. 7.
63 'News from "the schools": medical school by "Scalpel"', *T.C.D.: A College Miscellany* 8(139) (8 November 1902), p. 126.
64 'Medical notes', *Quarryman* 1(2) (January 1914), p. 24.
65 'Medical notes', *Quarryman* 2(3) (February 1915), p. 65.

drawn to the medical school than formerly.[66] At the same time, it is evident that some members of the medical profession felt a tension between new advances in laboratory science and clinical observation. In an address to students at St Vincent's Hospital in 1880, Dr Quinlan referred to the ophthalmoscope, laryngoscope, spectrum analysis and microscope as aids to medical science; 'but while they carefully studied them, it would be a grievous error to rely unduly upon them, and to neglect the careful painstaking clinical observation of disease'. Quinlan compared the physician who relied on the former and neglected the latter to Aesop's astronomer 'who fell into the pit while he walked along, his eyes fixed upon the stars, but unobservant of the common objects in the path on which he walked'.[67] Similarly, writing in the *Irish Journal of Medical Science*, in 1911, W. Thompson suggested that 'not a few of the present generation of clinical teachers have little sympathy with laboratory work. They have not been brought up on it; and it does not appeal to them'.[68] As L.S. Jacyna has argued, clinical medicine proved itself 'remarkably resistant to the newer laboratory science', suggesting that 'the crucial aspect of surgeons' education, the experience that shaped their attitudes and established their predominant patterns of practice, remained their initiation in clinical methods on the wards'.[69] For most medical students, in both the nineteenth and twentieth centuries, the hospital remained the most important sphere of their educational experience.

The hospital

Writing in *St. Stephen's* magazine in 1904, one medical student described his first day of clinical experience in the following way: 'How shall I ever forget my first entrance into a General Hospital! And, apropos of that, what pleasure, what wealth, what happiness can equal the student's joy on the first day he possesses a stethoscope? A stethoscope! His own!! His very own!!!'[70]

It is evident that, even by the early twentieth century, clinical teaching was still viewed as the most significant part of a medical student's training. From the 1840s, with the emergence of the laboratory, clinical medicine was thought by some to be 'too limited in its notion of the foundation of

66 Thompson, 'More about medical education', p. 186.
67 'Abstracts of the introductory addresses delivered at the Dublin Hospitals and Medical Schools, session 1880–81', *Lancet*, 13 November 1880, p. 791.
68 Thompson, 'More about medical education', p. 188.
69 L.S. Jacyna, 'The laboratory and the clinic: the impact of pathology on surgical diagnosis in the Glasgow Western Infirmary, 1875–1910', *Bulletin of the History of Medicine* 62(3) (1988), p. 405.
70 'First impressions', *St. Stephen's: A Record of University Life* 2(9) (1905), p. 194.

medicine'.[71] However, it is clear that laboratory medicine faced scepticism and outright hostility.[72] In Britain and the United States, 'scepticism of the utility of laboratory teaching for most medical students was deep and abiding' among their teachers.[73] As Jacyna has shown for Edinburgh in the period from 1875 to 1910, it was surgeons' initiation in clinical methods on the wards that was the crucial aspect of medical education and which 'shaped their attitudes and established their predominant patterns of practice'.[74] By the 1900s, as Christopher Lawrence has illustrated, many doctors disputed the relevance of the new laboratory sciences to their clinical practice and 'were not anxious to modify their analysis of bedside skills in accordance with these new disciplines'.[75] Although science was 'routinely invoked ... as the foundation of medicine', it was thought to have only a 'limited role in clinical practice'.[76] Clinicians often advised students that once they began their clinical studies at the bedside, 'they would find that their scientific book-learning had been very little preparation for the clinical art'.[77]

Certainly, many students remarked on the sense that 'real' medical training did not start until a student started his or her clinical experience. One's first entrance to the wards of a hospital for clinical teaching was often marked as a momentous occasion. Robert Blackham commented that in Dublin in the 1880s, 'The title "Doctor" was bestowed somewhat lightly', 'and from the day he became a student in a Dublin Hospital, the embryo Irish medico was addressed by his teachers and his patients as "Doctor"'.[78] J. Johnston Abraham found himself in a quandary in his first year of medical studies in 1894 and began to 'wonder if medicine really was my life work, if I would not be happier as a writer'.[79] He went to discuss his dilemma with Professor Edward Dowden, the professor of oratory and English Literature at Trinity, who advised him that Almroth Wright, the famous British bacteriologist and immunologist, had had the same conflict as a student but that 'He found that he had chosen his real vocation once he began hospital work. You haven't started hospital yet! No! then you may find the same. But if you don't, talk to me again'.[80] Carrying on with his medical studies into his second year, Abraham found that once he started hospital he was happier and

71 Jacyna, 'The laboratory and the clinic', p. 384.
72 Jacyna, 'The laboratory and the clinic', p. 386.
73 Bonner, *Becoming a physician*, p. 275.
74 Jacyna, 'The laboratory and the clinic', p. 405.
75 Christopher Lawrence, 'Incommunicable knowledge: science, technology and the clinical art in Britain, 1850–1914', *Journal of Contemporary History* 20 (1985), p. 510.
76 Lawrence, 'Incommunicable knowledge', p. 504.
77 Lawrence, 'Incommunicable knowledge', p. 510.
78 Blackham, *Scalpel, sword and stretcher*, p. 2.
79 Abraham, *Surgeon's journey*, p. 55.
80 Abraham, *Surgeon's journey*, p. 56.

began to see how the preliminary lectures he had been attending, in subjects such as anatomy, chemistry, zoology and physiology, which he found 'all a bit wearisome at times except Anatomy, Botany and Zoology – were essential if one was to understand the nature of disease and the methods of combating the ills that man, and especially woman, had to suffer. I knew I had found my vocation'.[81] Similarly, John Biggart, a student at Queen's who started his clinical experience at the Royal Victoria Hospital in the early 1920s, remarked, 'for the first time we felt that we were really becoming engaged in our profession. I suppose for most of us it meant something to do with patients and their ailments, and we had a rather mystical conception of what the doctor could do'. He recalled one of his greatest difficulties being 'the overcoming of the shyness of bodily and physical intimacy ... yet somehow or other, almost unconsciously, we slowly acquired the art of medicine'.[82] John Lyburn, who studied at Trinity College, remarked on his amazement as he witnessed his first surgical operation.[83] There was a sense that once the student entered the hospital wards and began to engage with the practice of seeing patients that he or she was now seen as a member of the profession.[84]

Professors also recognised the important transformative role of clinical experience in the education of the practitioner. For example, in an address to students at the Meath Hospital in 1905, Sir John W. Moore explained that although a

ripe and practical knowledge of anatomy and a sound acquaintance with physiology, and histology, chemistry and physics are essential ... when all is said and done, the preparation of your life-work will have to be carried on in the out-patient department, the clinical wards, the operating theatre, and the post-mortem room of a well-equipped general Medico-Chirurgical hospital, such as that within the walls of which we are assembled.[85]

William Doolin (1887–1962), the Irish surgeon and editor of the *Irish Journal of Medical Science* from 1925, believed that hospital work was integral to the education of the Irish doctor. Doolin noted that if the student had successfully completed his pre-clinical studies then he would 'start his

81 Abraham, *Surgeon's journey*, p. 58.
82 John A. Weaver, 'John Henry Biggart, 1905–1979: a portrait in respect and affection: presidential address to the Ulster Medical Society, 1st November 1984', *Ulster Medical Journal* 54(1) (1985), p. 6.
83 Lyburn, *The fighting Irish doctor*, p. 58.
84 Blackham, *Scalpel, sword and stretcher*, p. 2.
85 Sir John W. Moore, *'Clinical case-taking', reprinted from the Dublin Journal of Medical Science, November 1905* (Dublin: John Falconer, 1905), p. 4.

hospital work with his faculties of observation and generalisation sufficiently developed, and with a keen interest as to the ultimate result of each clinical experiment in which he is permitted to participate'. Doolin viewed the hospital as 'the laboratory of the clinical teacher who is a scientist inasmuch as he is pledged to the critical scrutiny of facts' and drew links between the hospital and the laboratory, stressing that both involved the process of solution through observation, deduction and experiment.[86] Indeed, there was a sense that the laboratory and the clinic could be complementary. John Wynne Foot, speaking to students in 1913, spoke of the 'two pillars which support the Temple of Aesculapius', which were knowledge and experience, and encouraged students to 'seek to acquire both'.[87] However, while he acknowledged the importance of 'a ripe and practical knowledge of anatomy and a sound acquaintance with physiology and histology, chemistry and physics are essential'. 'When all is said and done', he stressed, 'the preparation for your life-work will have to be carried on in the out-patient department, the clinical wards, the operating theatre, and the post-mortem room of a well-equipped general Medico-Chirurgical Hospital, such as that within the walls of which we are assembled'.[88]

Universities arranged their timetables so that students in the clinical years could obtain their hospital experience in the morning and have lectures back at the medical school in the afternoon. For instance, at Trinity College, in 1908, arrangements were made so that no lectures were given between 9 a.m. and 11 a.m. and that during the third year no classes were held before 1 p.m.[89] At the Adelaide Hospital, weekday mornings were dedicated to clinical instruction or lectures on medicine, surgery and diseases of women, and from 10 a.m. students could attend the extern departments. Tuesday mornings were kept aside for operations.[90] Similarly, at Sir Patrick Dun's Hospital in the 1920s, students could undertake clinical instruction from 9 a.m. until 11.30 a.m. For students who were just starting their hospital studies, special classes were held in the winter months which embraced 'the elements of Medicine and Surgery, including note-taking'. All students also had the opportunity to observe operations and to attend the medical and surgical out-patient departments, and special demonstrations on fevers and pathology, as well as the departments of X-ray, ophthalmology,

---

86 William Doolin, 'Medical education, reprinted from "Studies"', September 1925, pp. 12–13 [UCD Special Collections].

87 Moore, 'Clinical case-taking', p. 13.

88 Moore, 'Clinical case-taking', p. 6.

89 Letter from the Registrar's Office, School of Physic, Trinity College, 4 December 1908 [RCPI Heritage Centre, DCHC/2/10].

90 The Adelaide Medical and Surgical Hospitals: arrangements for Clinical teaching during the winter session 1880–81 [TCD Manuscripts, IE TCD MS 11270/8/1/2].

dentistry, anaesthetics and venereal diseases. Teaching fees from students were significant. Hospital fees were £12. 12s. 0d. for the winter and summer sessions combined, or £8. 8s. 0d. for the winter session (six months) and £5. 5s. 0d. for the summer session (3 months).[91] Hospitals were often obliging with regard to the payment of fees. Although students in the late nineteenth century usually had to pay a pound on enrolment, they did not have to pay their fee for attending the institution until they required the certificate of attendance.[92]

Students frequently had to travel in order to get to their chosen hospital. J. Johnston Abraham recalled that 'Hospital rounds were at nine in the morning, so after a hurried breakfast cooked in my rooms – there were no breakfasts in Hall for undergraduates in my time – I used to sprint across the College Park on my way to meet the Great Man, the professor of surgery, in the Front Hall'.[93] R.W.M. Strain, a student at Queen's in the 1920s, wrote that from third year, medical students' mornings were devoted to clinical medicine and they would make their way 'by shortcuts through back streets and alley ways' to the Royal Victoria Hospital.[94] There were some disadvantages to having to travel for hospital experience away from the location of the medical school. Fourth- and fifth-year medical students at University College Cork complained in 1914 that they were inconvenienced by the timing of lectures at midday in the college which meant that they had to leave the hospital at 11.30 a.m., a problem 'all the more accentuated by the fact that clinical instruction does not begin, in at least two of the city hospitals, until 10.30 a.m. on the average'. This inconvenience was made all the more annoying by the fact that occasionally after a 'daily record-breaking walk through short cuts and lanes of evil repute' they arrived at the lecture theatre to find a notice telling them that their professor would not be meeting them on that day.[95]

Students in Dublin could attend a range of hospitals including the Richmond, Whitworth and Hardwicke Hospitals, the City of Dublin Hospital, Meath Hospital, Adelaide, Sir Patrick Dun's (connected with Trinity College Dublin), the Mater Misericordiae, Mercer's, Jervis Street, St Vincent's, Steevens' Hospital in addition to specialised hospitals such as the Rotunda Hospital, Coombe Lying-In Hospital, Cork Street Fever Hospital, Dublin Orthopaedic Hospital and the National Eye and Ear Infirmary. In Cork, students could attain clinical instruction at the North and South infirmaries,

91 Pamphlet from 1922 giving details of medical training available at SPD Hospital: session 1922–23 [RCPI Heritage centre, PDH/5/3/1].
92 Blackham, *Scalpel, sword and stretcher*, p. 26.
93 Abraham, *Surgeon's journey*, p. 58.
94 Strain, *Les neiges d'antan*, p. 17.
95 'Medical notes', *Quarryman* 1(4) (March 1914), pp. 83–4.

the Mercy General Hospital, the Maternity Hospital, the Children's Hospital, the Eye and Ear Infirmary and the Cork District Lunatic Asylum. In Belfast, students could choose from the Royal Victoria Hospital, the Belfast Union Hospital, Belfast Maternity Hospital, Ulster Hospital for Women and Children, Belfast Hospital for Sick Children, the Belfast Ophthalmic Hospital, Ulster Eye, Ear and Throat Hospital, Belfast District Lunatic Asylum and, from 1909, the Mater Infirmorum Hospital. Students at the Cork medical school could obtain their clinical experience at a few institutions, including the South Charitable Infirmary and County Hospital, where clinical instruction was provided daily in the wards by a physician and surgeons, operations took place daily and there were also special lectures provided.[96] Students could also attend classes at the North Charitable Infirmary and the Cork District Hospital, where students had 'unlimited opportunities of acquiring a practical knowledge of disease by the comparison of many similar cases under the guidance of the Medical and Surgical Staff'.[97] Cork students could also attend two smaller hospitals; the Mercy Hospital, where medical, surgical and ophthalmic cases were treated daily in the extern department, and where there were two wards reserved for the treatment of diseases of women, and the Eye, Ear and Throat Hospital, where clinical instruction was provided on a more irregular basis, with 'evening demonstrations from time to time in the use of the Ophthalmoscope, Laryngoscope etc., whereby students may acquire a practical knowledge of these instruments'.[98] Students could also attend the Victoria Hospital for Diseases of Women and Children, the Cork District Lunatic Asylum and the Cork Fever Hospital for more specialised clinical experience.[99] For maternity cases, students attended the County and City of Cork Lying-in Hospital and the Cork Maternity.[100]

Students in Galway were more limited with regard to their clinical experiences. They attended the Central Hospital for their clinical lectures and students usually went to a larger hospital in Dublin in their fifth year of study. The Galway medical school faced criticisms throughout the nineteenth and early twentieth centuries for the lack of clinical experiences available to students. Thomas Laffan, writing in 1888, remarked that the school of medicine in 'this College is as regards staff and clinical service, decidedly inferior to those of the other Colleges'.[101] Thomas Garry, who had

---

96   'The Cork School of Medicine', pp. 13–14.
97   'The Cork School of Medicine', pp. 16–17.
98   'The Cork School of Medicine', p. 19
99   'The Cork School of Medicine', p. 21.
100   'The Cork School of Medicine', p. 22.
101   Thomas Laffan, '"The medical profession in the three kingdoms in 1887", the essay to which was awarded the Carmichael Prize of £100 by the Council of the Royal College of Surgeons, Ireland, 1887' (Dublin: Fannin & Co., 1888), pp. 195–201.

been a student in Galway in the 1880s, was more defensive of the advantages of studying in Galway. He wrote that in Galway 'opportunities for practice in hospital were very limited but it had considerable advantages as regards purely theoretical work. The professors as a rule were only too willing to assist and encourage the student, conditions which did not always exist in the medical schools in Dublin'. In contrast, when he moved to Dublin to complete his medical studies he found that there 'the professors in all the Dublin schools delivered the prescribed lectures and then disappeared as soon as they could to attend to their hospital or private practice ... The upshot was that students were left to their own devices or else to place themselves under the guidance of a "grind" or coach, a most pernicious form of cramming'.[102]

The clinical teaching at the Central Hospital was under the direct control and supervision of the Medical Faculty and fees were paid to the College. In this way, students' clinical experiences were different from those in Dublin or Cork. In Galway, according to a report on the medical school published in 1925, students were more closely supervised with regard to their hospital experience and were required to show their 'quota of attendances while in Dublin it is a different matter as the student is not under the same compulsion or supervision'. The advantage of being based in Galway, according to the report, was that 'the relatively small classes help in no small degree to ensure individual instruction to the members of the class and thus give them confidence that can only be ensured by frequent contact with the patient', while in Dublin students were left to their own guidance. Students in Galway attended hospital lectures six mornings a week. They were also expected to attend at the local Tuberculosis Sanatorium in the 1920s. Because the Central Hospital in Galway was small, medical students were obliged to attend a 'larger medical centre for some months in their fifth year'.[103] Students were required to have 27 months' attendance at a recognised general hospital, including the clinical lectures given therein, and no more than 18 of the 27 months could be taken in Galway – 'for the remaining nine months a certificate of attendance at a recognised Metropolitan Hospital must be presented'.[104]

Undoubtedly, a large number of students from Galway, Cork and Belfast went to Dublin for additional clinical training, and were often encouraged to do so by their professors. In a paper given by Dr McMordie, the demonstrator in anatomy at Queen's College Belfast, to the Belfast Medical

102 Garry, *African doctor*, pp. 10–11.
103 *University College Galway: Report on the Galway Medical School* (Galway: O'Gorman Printing House, 1925) [NUI Galway Special Collections, p. 8].
104 *University College Galway: Report on the Galway Medical School*, p. 22.

Students' Association (later BMSA), in 1902, he mentioned that it was 'profitable to visit Dublin on account of the opportunities it afforded one of meeting teachers and students of different views, it was well to bear in mind that the clinical teaching was not better, if indeed it was as good, as that in Belfast'.[105] Indeed, occasionally students from the provincial medical schools moved to Dublin to complete their medical training. In his report on the progress of the Catholic University Medical School in 1907, when asked about the decrease of students in Cork compared with the increase in students at the Catholic University Medical School, Monsignor Molloy explained that 'a small number of students may have come in recent years from Cork to Dublin to complete their medical course, on account of the special advantages offered by the hospitals in Dublin, and, possibly, attracted by the increasing reputation of our School'.[106]

According to the *Medical Press and Circular*, in Ireland, 'the student goes to any school he pleases and any hospital he pleases, and enters his name for any number of lectures he pleases … it is, in fact, but seldom that an Irish student confines his studies to a single hospital and, in order that he may be perfectly free to seek his education where he thinks he can best obtain it'.[107] In England, hospitals usually had an attached medical school and students received all of their education at these. In Dublin, the hospitals and schools were entirely separate, with the exception of Sir Patrick Dun's Hospital, which was officially connected with Trinity College. According to the *Medical Press and Circular*, 'as might be expected, religion, social rank, and locality of residence have their influence in causing certain classes of students to resort to schools and hospitals suitable to their condition'.[108] However, Irish hospitals had religious affiliations. Oliver St John Gogarty, who studied at Trinity College, remarked somewhat glibly that in Dublin disease was a '*modus vivendi* and it therefore assumes a religious aspect. There are Protestant, Catholic and Presbyterian diseases in Dublin'.[109] Religious affiliation, therefore, often played an important role in choice of hospital, while university medical schools often acted as 'feeders' for certain hospitals. For example, students attending lectures at the Catholic University Medical School tended to attend the Mater Misericordiae and St Vincent's Hospital, which were both Catholic hospitals.[110] The perceived quality of medical staff was also important. Robert Blackham, who enrolled

105 'Belfast Medical Students' Association', *Q.C.B.* 3(3) (25 January 1902), p. 45.
106 *Progress of the Catholic University School of Medicine, 1907* (Dublin: Humphrey and Armour Printers, undated), p. 20 [UCD Special Collections].
107 'Students' number', *Medical Press and Circular*, 24 September 1879, p. 266.
108 'Students' number', *Medical Press and Circular*, 24 September 1879, p. 266.
109 Gogarty, *It isn't this time of year at all!*, p. 29.
110 'Ireland: I. Education', *Medical Press and Circular*, 22 September 1886, p. 239.

in the Ledwich School of Medicine in 1883, decided to go to the Adelaide Hospital for his clinical experience, 'not because I was an ardent admirer of its Protestant proclivities, but because I considered its medical staff better than that of most of its rivals.' He then completed his clinical training at the Richmond Hospital, because it was closer to the Rotunda Hospital which he also had to attend for midwifery experience.[111] John Lyburn, who began his studies at Trinity in 1922, chose to attend the Richmond Hospital, which he felt was 'the best equipped and gave the student the most practical application of medicine', while he was also inspired by the staff members who included Sir Thomas Myles and Sir Conway Dwyer.[112]

If a student was unhappy with the quality of teaching, it was understood that he or she could go elsewhere, and, as Chapter 1 illustrated, students were not shy about complaining about the standards of the education provided. An article in *St. Stephen's* in 1903 drew attention to the 'scandalous condition' of the resident pupils' rooms in the Coombe in comparison with the 'luxurious apartments' of the Matron and Assistant Master. The student further complained:

It is a well-known fact in the School that the Hospital has been boycotted by a great section of the students this year, and as resident pupils pay nearly twice what is paid in the Coombe Hospital, they expect to get at least proper attention. The Hospital is a Catholic one, and deserves every support from Catholic University students, but something must be done by the proper authorities to remove existing grievances'[113]

This article had some effect: in the next issue of *St. Stephen's* the magazine reported that the 'luxurious furniture' in the rooms for the Assistant Master and Matron were their own property, but also that the Committee of the Hospital had 'done a great deal to better the condition of the students' rooms, and further improvements are promised'.[114] One Dublin student in 1904 referred to some of the grievances of students attending St Vincent's Hospital, where students suffered from the lack of a students' waiting-room and were forced to 'lounge about [in] cold draughty halls and corridors, sneezing and using their handkerchiefs till the arrival of the belated professor', in contrast with the Mater, where students were 'generously provided with a comfortably heated waiting-room', a fact which 'indirectly acts as an

111 Blackham, *Scalpel, sword and stretcher*, pp. 26–7.
112 Lyburn, *The fighting Irish doctor*, p. 57.
113 'News from the Schools', *St. Stephen's: A Record of University Life* 1(10) (February 1903), p. 222.
114 'News from the Schools', *St. Stephen's: A Record of University Life* 1(11) (March 1903), p. 244.

inducement to its students to attend classes'.[115] Cork students complained in 1914 of a lack of basic knowledge about minor surgery, and asked if it might be possible to have a junior hospital class on this topic, mentioning, 'it is pitiful at present to see how little we know of these subjects, even when we get well on towards our final, all because when we are junior students we are left more or less to pick up whatever little we can, without any instruction'.[116]

Students also took an interest in appointments to Irish hospitals. For instance, in 1901, students complained about a house surgeon appointment at the Royal Victoria Hospital where a Dublin student was chosen rather than a Belfast student. In a resolution passed by the Belfast Medical Students' Association, they explained that Belfast candidates should have prior claim to such positions because they had trained in Belfast and had worked as resident pupils in the hospital; their qualifications were equal to that of an outside candidate, and, finally, because the students felt that 'to appoint an outsider would cast a slur on the teaching of this School, and discourage the students attending it'.[117] Similarly, in 1903, there was an election for the position of assistant master at Holles Street Hospital, the Catholic maternity hospital. *St. Stephen's* reported that there had been four candidates in the field, one of whom was a past 'Rotunda' student 'who has never attended either lecture or case in Holles Street'. Fearing that this candidate would attain the position over one of the three 'Holles Street men', a testimonial was drawn up with 200 signatures. Explaining this action, the writer in *St. Stephen's* stated that:

> the home candidates have all had brilliant courses and, at least one of them, considerable experience in obstetric practice, no reason whatever existing for the infusion of strange blood into the place ... however, when we take into consideration the bigoted action of the 'Rotunda Board' in persistently refusing to recognise the claims of eminent Catholic physicians, we regard the issue as safe, and trust that the threatened vigorous action of the students will not be made necessary.[118]

To the joy of the writer of the 'Medical notes', Dr J.J. Walsh, late house surgeon at the Mater, and a former student of Holles Street, was chosen for the position.[119]

115 Correspondence: Letter to the Editor of *St. Stephen's*, *St. Stephen's: A Record of University Life* 2(8) (March 1904), pp. 70–1.
116 'Medical notes', *Quarryman* 1(4) (March 1914), p. 84.
117 Appointment of a Resident Surgeon to the Royal Victoria Hospital, *Q.C.B.* 2(7) (20 May 1901), p. 15.
118 'Medical notes', *St. Stephen's: A Record of University Life* 2(1) (December 1903), p. 18.
119 'Notes from the medical school', *St. Stephen's: A Record of University Life* 2(2) (February 1904), p. 33.

Hospitals were also the scene of friction between students. Junior medical students in the hospitals were criticised by two final-year students at Queen's College Belfast in 1916 for 'crowding round the beds, and the lecturer, to the complete exclusion and obliteration of those who are going up for their Final in March and June'. In the letter, which was directed 'as much to the lady medicals as to the budding Victor Horsleys, with the nice clean collars, and the wonderful stethoscopes', the author asked:

> Could you not shout 'Here, sir', as well from the back of the class and then fade quietly away and play 'Nap' or otherwise amuse yourselves while those who have temporarily sacrificed all such pleasures for the sake of their exam gather in the pearls of wisdom. Remember, we are not in these classes for fun – funny though they may sometimes be – and we should be only too glad to be finished with them.[120]

Likewise, students at Cork in the same year suggested that 'the students who are preparing for that inconvenient little detail – the final – at the end of the year should receive every consideration from the more junior students'.[121]

It is clear that clinical experience was viewed as a turning point in the medical student's education by students and professors alike. Observation still remained important, and this suggests that the tensions between the clinic and the laboratory were still prevalent in late nineteenth-century Ireland. Indeed, Irish clinicians had much in common with their English counterparts who from the 1880s emphasised the art and mysteries of clinical medicine, in contrast with German clinicians in the same period who focused on the possibility of clinical medicine becoming an exact science.[122] As Christopher Lawrence has suggested,

> To represent medicine as a method or discipline reducible to a body of knowledge which had precise rules for its implementation, was to imply criticism of the peculiar claims of these medical men to moral and cultural leadership of professional and national life. More tangibly, it was to place the superior claims of character and breeding on an equal footing with those of scientific merit when making appointments.[123]

Rawdon Macnamara, speaking to students in 1884, highlighted the importance of the sense of 'feeling': 'by this sense you derive knowledge

120 'Open letter to the "First-year Hospital" Students', *Q.C.B.* 18(1) (December 1916), p. 18.
121 'Medical notes', *Quarryman* 3(3) (February 1916), p. 53.
122 Lawrence, 'Incommunicable knowledge', p. 511.
123 Lawrence, 'Incommunicable knowledge', p. 507.

that cannot be imparted to you', emphasising that students should 'lose no opportunity of cultivating this sense, thereby alone can you obtain that which is most properly styled the "*tactus eruditus*"'.[124] R.F. Tobin, speaking to students at St Vincent's Hospital in 1887, warned of the dangers of an over-reliance on scientific diagnoses, stating that 'eyes ever bent on the ground may lose sight of what is above; minds occupied with scientific investigations may come to believe in science to the exclusion of all other teaching; men permitted to check the progress of disease and to stay the hand of death, may in their pride forget Him "by whom they live, move and have their being"'.[125] Arthur Wynne Foot highlighted the importance of students cultivating the faculty of observation and that this was the main means that they could truly develop their education and knowledge.[126] He expressed the advantages of students studying and recording cases, emphasising that this independent observation would help them to become autonomous and help them to 'cease to hang like a marsupial upon what falls from a teacher's lips'. Through independent observation, students would 'diminish the likelihood of selling your minds to the most cunning of all fiends – the demon of theory'.[127] Similarly, James Craig, speaking to students in the Meath Hospital in 1893, encouraged them to 'Get close to the bedside, and begin at once to use your hands and eyes and ears. Note carefully what is pointed out to you, observing the way your teacher proceeds to obtain the needed information from the patient, and then the methods he adopts in making an examination of the case'.[128]

Indeed, the hospital was viewed as the centre for the cultivation of good habits and gentlemanly manners and doctors' clinical art was 'grounded ultimately in his own experience which, of course, depended on his calibre as an individual'.[129] Professors' addresses to Irish students are indicative of these beliefs. Henry MacNaughton, speaking to students in 1877, advised them to carry a stethoscope, clinical thermometer, pocket measure, scissors, forceps, probe, small scalpel, lancet, silk and silver wire, litmus paper, clinical diagram and notebook and a pocket urinary test apparatus. Familiarity with

124 Rawdon Macnamara, 'An address, introductory to the session 1884–1885, delivered in the theatre of the Meath Hospital and County of Dublin Infirmary' (Dublin: J. Atkinson & Co., 1884), p. 12.
125 R.F. Tobin, 'An address delivered at St Vincent's Hospital, Dublin, introductory to the medical session 1887–8' (Dublin: John Falconer, 1887), p. 15.
126 Arthur Wynne Foot, 'An address delivered in the theatre of the Meath Hospital at the opening of the session 1887–88' (Dublin: John Falconer, 1887), p. 8.
127 Foot, 'An address delivered in the theatre of the Meath Hospital at the opening of the session 1887–88', p. 15.
128 James Craig, 'Introductory address delivered at the opening of the session of 1893–4 in the theatre of the Meath Hospital' (Dublin: John Falconer, 1893), p. 11.
129 Lawrence, 'Incommunicable knowledge', p. 512.

the microscope was also encouraged.[130] Attentiveness from the first day was advocated, with MacNaughton suggesting that it was 'By the bedside of your cases in hospital; examining patients for yourselves in the extern departments; taking careful notes; writing your own prescriptions; cultivating the great faculty of a good physician or surgeon – the power of close observation' that students could fit themselves for their 'future self-denying but noble profession'.[131] Evidently, the influence of Robert Graves, who pioneered bedside teaching in Ireland, was still felt even by the late nineteenth century. John T. Banks, professor of medicine at Trinity College Dublin, and then president of the Royal Academy of Medicine in Ireland, speaking to students at the Richmond Hospital in 1883, encouraged them to devote as much time as possible to attendance on the sick at the hospital, suggesting that by doing so they would 'gradually learn the physiognomy of disease and will acquire the power of distinguishing its features'.[132]

Students were encouraged to attend hospital regularly, and the importance of note-taking was advocated by their teachers.[133] A letter from an 'Irish Surgeon', which appeared in the *British Medical Journal* in January 1890, bemoaned the fact that there was no regular, methodical system of note-taking in Dublin hospitals, in contrast with the London hospitals where he claimed that notes were written up and kept by clerks and dressers. Although he acknowledged that the Irish system of medical education provided more hands-on clinical experience, in contrast with the London system. He argued that in London hospitals 'every student must of necessity take accurate notes of his cases, and he is, at any rate, taught to be systematic in his work'.[134] Members of the Irish medical profession were quick to defend these allegations, with one recent graduate defending the standards in Dublin, arguing that 'the instruction received at the bedside in Dublin is quite equal to that in any other part of the world' and, in his experience as a clinical clerk, having witnessed daily notes being taken of cases.[135] John Moore, in 1905, commented that the attendance of some students at hospital could be 'spasmodic and intermittent', which he attributed to the sessional examinations which students had to study for at the expense of hospital

---

130 H. Macnaughton Jones, 'Clinical teaching in hospitals' (Cork: George Purcell & Co., 1877), p. 21.
131 Macnaughton Jones, 'Clinical teaching in hospitals', p. 16.
132 John T. Banks, 'Introductory address delivered on the opening of the medical session, 1st November 1883 at the Richmond, Whitworth and Hardwicke Government Hospitals' (Dublin: Gunn & Cameron, 1883), p. 28.
133 Moore, *'Clinical case-taking'*, p. 9. James Craig, speaking to students in 1893, encouraged them to 'observe habits of strict regularity in attendance, and be among the first arrivals in the morning'. Craig, 'Introductory address', p. 11.
134 'Clinical teaching in Dublin', *British Medical Journal*, 11 January 1900, pp. 104–5.
135 'Clinical teaching in Dublin', *British Medical Journal*, 8 February 1890, p. 327.

attendance.[136] Gentlemanly conduct was seen as essential. Edward Hamilton, speaking to students in 1885, warned them to 'avoid the temptation to levity', stressing that students would be 'surrounded by the sick and the dying, who watch with bated breath each event of our visit, and scan with feverish curiosity the countenance of their attendant, trying to read their fate in every shade which passes over his features. Scenes like these are ill-suited to the ribald jest, the merry jibe, or the ill-timed practical joke'.[137]

In conclusion, it is clear that the hospital was viewed by most students and professors as being the place where real medical study began and where the important traits of the profession would be transmitted. In spite of the rise of the laboratory in the late nineteenth century, the emphasis on clinical or bedside teaching continued to be felt well into the twentieth century.

The medical student society

Medical student societies were an important agent of professionalisation, and through their meetings and social events helped to groom students into respectable and competent practitioners. The first Irish medical student society was the Medical Society of the University of Dublin (Trinity College) founded in 1814.[138] The society met every Saturday evening, and had two aims: to collect original information on all branches of medical science with a view to publishing these and 'to improve the junior members of the society, by their writing dissertations on medical subjects and publicly defending them'.[139] Over fifty years later, in 1867, the Medico-Chirurgical Society was established at Trinity College Dublin followed later by the Belfast Medical Students' Association (1886), the Queen's College Cork Medical Students' Association (1896) (later, QCCMSA), the Catholic University Medical Students' Debating Society (1901), the University College Galway Medical Society (1918), the Biological Society of the Royal College of Surgeons (date not known) and the Irish Medical Students' Association (1944), a national body of medical students. There is scant evidence of the Dublin Medical Students' Club (1882), a short-lived body founded 'for the benefit of Irish medical students and to afford them a place in which they may meet for general intercourse etc.'.[140]

136 Moore, 'Clinical case-taking', p. 8.
137 Edward Hamilton, 'Royal College of Surgeons inaugural address, session 1885–86' (Dublin: Gunn & Cameron, 1885), p. 15.
138 'Laws of the medical society of the University of Dublin' (Dublin: R. Smith, 1815).
139 'Medical Society of the University of Dublin', London Medical and Physical Journal 34 (1815), p. 81.
140 Letter: Dublin Medical Students Club to the President of Queen's College, Cork (undated but approximately 1882–3) [UCC University Archives. UC/COUNCIL/16/43].

Membership of these societies provided many tangible benefits for students. In 1880, Dr E.G. Little, the President of the Biological Association, outlined these as being largely educational, including 'to supplement the matter of our studies and to keep students out of too narrow a groove', and to 'make men think for themselves'.[141] Similarly, in 1898, the President of the Royal College of Surgeons, Dr Drury, remarked that he believed that medical student societies 'fulfilled one of the very highest purposes of education'. Alluding to the fact that associations allowed young medical men to forge connections and helped to foster camaraderie among the students, he commented that medical societies allowed for 'the cultivation of individuality and the friction which he was thrown into with his fellow men in that society was of the very highest value'.[142] In 1901, a member of the Catholic University Medical Students' Debating Society pointed out the necessity of medical students learning to speak fluently on their feet, and how such practice would aid them in their future careers. Thanks were given to the supportive members of the medical faculty who had donated subscriptions and provided a room for meetings.[143]

Medical student society committees were usually made up of a president, vice-president, secretaries, treasurer and council, containing a mix of members of the medical profession and students with a clear hierarchy. For example, the President of the Biological Association from 1879 to 1880, was Alexander Macalister, professor of anatomy, and the Vice-Presidents included eminent members of the Dublin medical profession such as Samuel Haughton. The council was composed of student members.[144] Meetings of these societies were usually attended by a mixture of students and junior and senior members of the profession. Daniel Kilbride has shown how professors and gentlemen physicians in Philadelphia in the same period mingled casually with students, with such socialising helping to prepare students to become both doctors and gentlemen.[145] Medical student societies were also responsible for organising social events. In 1902, a social club for Catholic University medical students called 'The Cecilians', after the

141 'November 19 1880', TCD Biological Association (Minute Book 1), November 1879– May 1885, pp. 45–6 [TCD Manuscripts Department].
142 'Biological Society', newscutting, *Daily Express*, 30 November 1894, TCD Biological Association (Minute Book 2), February 1894–December 1899 [TCD Manuscripts Department].
143 'CU Medical Students' Debating Society', *St. Stephen's: A Record of University Life* 1(1) (1 June 1901), p. 16.
144 'Officers and Committee for 1879–1880', TCD Biological Association (Minute Book 1), November 1879–May 1885, p. 1 [TCD Manuscripts Department].
145 Daniel Kilbride, 'Southern medical students in Philadelphia, 1800–1861: Science and Sociability in the "Republic of Medicine"', *Journal of Southern History* 65(4) (1999), pp. 727–8.

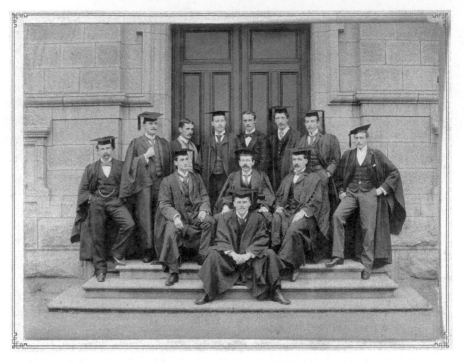

4   Photograph of the Dublin Biological Association, 1893.
Courtesy of the Wellcome Library, London.

location of the medical school on Cecilia Street, Dublin, was founded with
the support of the professor of anatomy Dr Birmingham. The aim of this
club was to 'supply the want, so keenly felt by Catholic students in Ireland,
for the social side of University life' and to further foster the *esprit de
corps* of the students attending the medical school. The society proposed
to organise three dinners in the winter session as well as musical evenings
and theatrical parties, while in the summer session it was expected that
cycling parties and picnics would be organised.[146] At an early meeting of
the society, Birmingham delivered a lecture illustrated by lantern slides of
a tour across Europe through the Rhine valley. Following this, the aims
and the principles of the club were outlined, which were summed up in
the motto, 'Enjoyment without Excess', a motto which perhaps indicates
professors' desires for students to behave respectably.[147] Despite these good
intentions, in 1907, it was brought to the notice of the medical faculty by

146 'Medical notes', *St. Stephen's: A Record of University Life* 1(9) (December 1902), p. 195.
147 'News from the School', *St. Stephen's: A Record of University Life* 1(10) (February
1903), p. 221.

Professor Coffey, the professor of physiology, that complaints had been made by parents of students with regard to 'certain irregularities following dinners' of the club. It was decided that in future all meetings of the Cecilians would be held in an institution where no alcoholic liquors were available for sale.[148]

Students were actively encouraged to present papers at meetings of these societies and the President of the Biological Association made a point in 1928 of encouraging all members to take an active part in the discussions, hoping that 'no members, especially those in their earlier years, would feel reticent about getting up and speaking at meetings of the association'.[149] The BMSA stressed that it was not a 'mere academic society for the discussion of transcendental philosophy or for the acquisition of fluency in the utterance of platitudes but a highly practical organisation having for its object the advancement of the interests of the Belfast Medical Students in all that directly or indirectly affects their professional training'.[150] Members of the Biological Society were awarded medals for best papers and best cases or exhibits.[151] Papers presented at meetings of these societies were usually on a scientific topic; however, debates, such as the common topic of women in the medical profession, were also held. Sport, medicine and the medical student society came together in 1905, when Dr S.T. Irwin read a paper at a meeting of the BMSA entitled, 'Some Accidents in the Football Field', with the minutes of the BMSA remarking on the keen interest 'which this paper excited'.[152] Members of medical student societies also occasionally contributed to professional matters. At a meeting of the Biological Association in 1900, a paper was read by the President on the 'Pathological Study of Insanity'. As a result of this contribution and the discussion which followed, a resolution was passed which urged the formation of a Central Laboratory for Asylums, a matter which was then taken up by the Medico-Psychological Association.[153] Furthermore, issues relating to proposed changes to medical education were regularly discussed.

Medical student societies also enabled students to air their grievances about the standard of their education and educational facilities. In 1895

148 'November 29, 1907', Catholic University School of Medicine Governing Body, Minute Book, 1892–1911 [UCD Archives, CU/14].
149 'November 20, 1928', TCD Biological Association (Minute Book 6), November 1921–October 1929 [TCD Manuscripts Department].
150 Secretaries' Report for session 1905–06, BMSA Minute Book, November 1898–November 1907 [QUB Special Collections].
151 'Sports, clubs and societies', *Mistura* 1(1) (winter term 1953), p. 17.
152 'Second general meeting – Dec. 14 1905', BMSA Minute Book, November 1898–November 1907 [QUB Special Collections].
153 'University Biological Association', *T.C.D.: A College Miscellany* 6 (103) (10 November 1900), p. 131.

and 1896, the QCCMSA wrote to the College Council with regard to the provision of physiological instruments for the purpose of study and to complain about the 'backward condition' of the Anatomical School.[154] In 1912, a deputation of the BMSA was sent to interview the Guardians of the Belfast Union Infirmary with regard to the question of pupilships in that institution, while their president, Dr Kerr, was asked to approach the professor of anatomy regarding additional seating accommodation in the dissecting room.[155] As will be discussed in more depth in Chapter 6, women were admitted to most of these medical student societies; however, the societies often served as a realm for women to defend their place in the profession.

In conclusion, medical student societies served three main purposes: educational, social and as a forum for protest. The societies also further helped to develop a cohesive identity for medical students by organising social events. Furthermore, through the attendance of members of the Irish medical profession at meetings, medical students were supervised in this mode of professionalisation.

Conclusion

From 1924, a pre-registration examination was introduced in Irish medical schools which meant that students had to pass an assessment before they could proceed to their first medical year. This meant that the medical programme was extended to six years.[156] Writing in 1925, William Doolin, extern surgeon to St Vincent's Hospital, Dublin explained:

> Our curriculum is now planned on the basis of six years' study, of which two and a half are devoted to the preclinical studies and three and a half to the clinical and allied subjects. There is a fundamental soundness in the arrangement of this curriculum as a whole, despite a certain lack of elasticity and a general over-attention to examinational requirements. Paradoxical as it may sound to the lay reader, the student can be 'taught' neither the art nor science of medicine; in our medical schools we cannot expect to produce fully trained doctors; at the most, we can but hope to equip our students with a limited,

154 'Copy of resolutions from QCCMSA meeting, February 13, 1895', and 'Copy of resolutions from QCCMSA meeting, February 26, 1896' [UCC University Archives, UC/COUNCIL/1/1/].
155 'November 19, 1912', BMSA Committee Minute Book, 1899–1925 [Royal Victoria Hospital Archives].
156 Murray, *Galway: a medico-social history*, p. 193.

fragmentary amount of knowledge, to train them in the method and spirit of scientific enquiry, and launch them forth into the world with such intellectual momentum as will make them active learners, observers, readers, thinkers, for years to come. The achievement of this aim depends on the teacher and the student rather than on the curriculum.[157]

Doolin's remarks illuminate the fact that even by the 1920s some doctors were suggesting that students could not be taught the art or science of medicine, but simply that university education would provide the rudimentary knowledge to underpin this. Arguably, it was through experience – in particular, clinical experience – that they would become true members of the medical profession.

Although educational experiences at Irish medical schools did not significantly change from the 1880s to the 1920s, it is clear that certain aspects of medical education held particular meanings for Irish doctors. Lectures in the pre-clinical years were often criticised and their relevance to some medical students remained unclear. Students demonstrated their lack of interest in and respect for these subjects through the disruption of classes and complaints. Other teaching spheres, such as the medical museum, began to decline in significance from the late nineteenth century. However, some spheres of teaching, such as the dissecting room, continued to be viewed as an important rite of passage for students. Students were active participants in their education, and were unafraid to complain about their educational experiences, while they also actively participated in acquiring new knowledge through their involvement in medical student societies. All of these shared experiences helped to cement a sense of collective identity.

It is evident that clinical experience was viewed as the most important part of a student's training throughout the period in question. It is clear, however, that clinical experiences varied depending on the medical school, and while Dublin provided an array of opportunities for medical students, students attending the provincial schools, in particular Galway, were more limited. Moreover, the choice of school was often dependent on one's religious affiliation, and medical schools became feeder schools for different hospitals. Additionally, the hospital also became the scene of friction not only between students but also over appointments. It is evident that newly initiated members of the medical profession felt they had a right to a say in these appointments and possessed a strong sense of loyalty to their

---

157 William Doolin, 'Medical education, reprinted from "Studies"', September 1925, p. 8 [UCD Special Collections].

own medical schools. Regardless of the rise of the laboratory in the late nineteenth century, the legacy of Graves' bedside teaching continued to be felt in Ireland well into the twentieth century, and it was clinical experience that was viewed as being the most important formative experience, by students and teachers alike.

5

'Boys to Men':
Rites of Passage, Sport, Masculinity and
Medical Student Culture, *c*.1880–1930

Writing in 1892, Henry Albert Hinkson, in a book entitled *Student life in Trinity College, Dublin*, described university years in the following way:

> It is a time when one stands on the very edge of life, eager for a plunge into life's joyous waters, when one has assumed the toga of one's manhood, and is yet a boy in heart. Despite the responsibilities of examinations and lectures, there is a delightful freedom and reckless gaiety in college life, and a *camaraderie* never felt in later years.[1]

Hinkson's description of university life draws attention to the role of universities in aiding the transformation of boys to men and the juxtaposition of the serious and more frivolous aspects of college life. Recent scholarship has explored these themes, illuminating how manliness became a crucial force in student life in the nineteenth and twentieth centuries.[2]

Although identity construction became an important part of the culture of medical schools, less work has been done on the performance of identity of medical students. While recent valuable studies have highlighted how the image of the medical student was improved in the nineteenth century

---

1 H.A. Hinkson, *Student life in Trinity College, Dublin* (Dublin: J. Charles & Son, 1892), p. 5.
2 In particular, Paul Deslandes' work on Oxford and Cambridge has highlighted the role of these universities in aiding the transition from boyhood to manhood while Carol Dyhouse has shown the prevalence of 'male culture' in the London medical schools in the interwar period. See Paul R. Deslandes, *Oxbridge men: British masculinity and the undergraduate experience, 1850–1920* (Bloomington: Indiana University Press, 2005) and Carol Dyhouse, *Students: a gendered history* (London: Routledge, 2005), p. 153.

and the importance of shared educational activities in helping to create cohesive bonds between future medical practitioners, less attention has been paid to how masculine ideals were passed on to medical students and how educational and extra-curricular spheres became centres of gendered performance and sites for the maintenance of hegemonic masculinity. Ultimately, as I will argue here, this identity construction, through various rites of passage, and social and educational activities, aimed to preserve Irish medicine as a masculine sphere. Women students, though largely treated in an inclusive manner for educational experiences, were generally excluded from these activities from their admission to Irish medical schools from the late nineteenth century up until at least the mid-twentieth century.[3] As Dyhouse has shown for British medical schools, 'women might be just about tolerable if they confined themselves to the role of spectators, when (whether in the operating theatre or in the sports field) their role was essentially one of admiring male *performance*'.[4]

According to Roy Porter, the 'boisterous, jovial sporting atmosphere of the all-male medical school with its student hi-jinks and horseplay' consolidated an '*esprit de corps* that helped doctors to present some kind of united front'.[5] Similarly, as John Tosh has shown, the public demonstration of masculinity occurs in three key areas: home, work and all-male associations, with the appeal of all-male conviviality being felt the most among young unmarried men 'who are temporarily denied the full privileges of masculinity'.[6] Medical students certainly fit into this category, occupying largely homosocial spaces. All-male settings 'sustained gender privilege, while at the same time imposing a discipline on individuals in the interests of patriarchal stability'.[7] As sociologist Sharon R. Bird has surmised, drawing on the work of Chodorow, Gilligan and Johnson, homosociality helps to perpetuate hegemonic masculinity in three main ways: emotional detachment, competitiveness and sexual objectification of women.[8] All three

3   Laura Kelly, '"Fascinating scalpel-wielders and fair dissectors": women's experience of medical education, *c*.1880s–1920s', *Medical History* 54(4) (2010): 495–516.

4   Dyhouse, *Students: a gendered history*, p. 152.

5   Roy Porter, *The greatest benefit to mankind* (London: HarperCollins, 1997), p. 356. Similarly, James Garner has drawn attention to how London medical schools were places where the 'the hard-drinking, hard-living, rugby-playing, public-school educated medic achieve[d] ubiquity, with all his attendant machismo and preposterous ritual' reigned. James Garner, 'The great experiment: the admission of women students to St Mary's Hospital Medical School, 1916–1925', *Medical History* 41 (1998), p. 74.

6   John Tosh, 'What should historians do with masculinity? Reflections on nineteenth-century Britain', *History Workshop* 38 (1994), p. 184.

7   Tosh, 'What should historians do with masculinity?', p. 187.

8   Sharon R. Bird, 'Welcome to the men's club: homosociality and the maintenance of hegemonic masculinity', *Gender & Society* 10(2) (1996), pp. 121–2.

of these aspects can be applied when exploring medical student activities in Ireland in the late nineteenth and early twentieth centuries from a gendered perspective.

I will illustrate how rites of passage in medical education became imbued with masculine tropes. In this way, the transformation of student to practitioner was often symbolised as the transformation of boy to man. Masculine displays and the cultivation of the image of the medical student as a rowdy, boisterous and predominantly male individual therefore became an important force in segregating men and women students. Manliness was a crucial force running through the initiation and often ritualistic rites of passage that made up the five to six years of medical study at Irish universities. Heather Ellis has shown how the University of Oxford in the first half of the nineteenth century perceived its role to be 'that of turning boys to men', with manliness being seen as an ideal and 'defined by the possession of maturity, both moral and intellectual, and constructed primarily in opposition to notions of boyishness, rather than overtly gendered ideas of femininity or effeminacy'.[9] This is what I will take manliness to represent for the purposes of this chapter.

Medical education for many marked a transition from boyhood to manhood. Different aspects of medical studies were described as 'rites of passage' or hardships, competitive feats that students had to get through in order to complete their metamorphosis from medical student to fully fledged member of the profession. These rites of passage were couched in increasingly masculine terms and students' spaces became centres for the performance of masculinity. The spaces I will focus on here include the lecture theatre, dissecting room and the sports field. The dissecting room was viewed as an important rite of passage for students in garnering emotional detachment, while the lecture theatre, though regimented, was a common site of student pranks and boisterous behaviour. Finally, the sports field was important in helping to create a well-rounded medical student, cultivating ideals such as strength of nerve and fostering competition, while for later generations the Officers' Training Corps (OTC) and Pearse Regiment also helped to solidify the importance of manly traits.

9 Heather Ellis, '"Boys, semi-men and bearded scholars": maturity and manliness in early nineteenth-century Oxford', in S. Brady and J.H. Arnold (eds), *What is masculinity? historical dynamics from antiquity to the contemporary world* (Basingstoke: Palgrave Macmillan, 2011), p. 267.

The transformation of the 'gyb' and rites of passage

First-year students, often referred to as 'gybs', were characterised in the student press as being jovial in nature, 'youths with strange and weird notions of student life', 'outspoken and boisterous', 'young hooligans' before they settled down into hard work as the years progressed.[10] They were also commonly referred to as 'boys', with one piece in 1911 describing their 'school-boy shyness'.[11] Other pieces remarked on the 'appearance of stupidity and awkwardness' which marked the first stage of the development of 'the medicus'.[12] Articles in the student press by more senior medical students often disapprovingly remarked on the boisterous behaviour of the younger students. A piece in 1903 encouraged the first-year student to cultivate 'a less bumptious demeanour that at present characterises him. Of course, he is young and will settle down in time but a speedy recognition of his exact importance in the College will conduce both to his own future comfort and that of his seniors'.[13] In this sense, first-year or pre-clinical students were characterised as 'boys' before undertaking a transformation as a result of their clinical experiences.

Members of the medical profession frequently wrote about this transformative process. Rawdon Macnamara, a professor at the Royal College of Surgeons, and surgeon to the Meath Hospital, in an introductory address to students at the Meath Hospital in 1884, remarked how students came to the wards 'rough, selfish, thoughtless, unsympathetic'. However, 'after a very short time, let occasion arise, who so gentle, who so thoughtful, who so sympathetic, who so self-denying, who so tender-hearted? What a wonderful transformation!'[14] After this transformation had taken place, the medical practitioner had an important, heroic role to play in society, binding and healing 'not merely the limbs of their patients, but the more formidable fractures which separate class from class'.[15] Similarly, a student writing in 1912 shared this perspective, outlining how the early years of medical study were filled with pranks before a transformation which produced a more subdued and serious graduate: 'But we are all changed since then. Medicine

10 'As others see us' and 'Advice to freshmen', *T.C.D.: A College Miscellany* 44(763) (28 October 1937): 4 and 8. 'Pre-reg notes', *University Annual: University College Galway* 5(4) (1927–8), p. 55.
11 'First impressions', *St. Stephen's: A Record of University Life* 2(9) (1905), p. 13.
12 'The medicus', *Q.C.C.* 3(1) (January 1907), p. 5.
13 'The Schools: the medical school', *Q.C.B.* 5(1) (26 November 1903), p. 12.
14 Rawdon Macnamara, 'An address, introductory to the session 1884–1885, delivered in the theatre of the Meath Hospital and County of Dublin Infirmary' (Dublin: J. Atkinson & Co., 1884), p. 10.
15 Rawdon Macnamara, 'Abstract of the introductory addresses delivered at the Dublin Hospitals and Medical Schools, session 1881–82' *Lancet*, 26 November 1881, p. 912.

to her students is not always a goddess fair; sometimes she seems a vampire sucking the life of her victims, draining from them every particle of every form of vitality except what is needed for her work'.[16] For this student, the jovial aspects of the earlier years of study were soon replaced by hard work, resulting in a more serious graduate at the end of the degree. Similarly, Nevin, a character in G.M. Irvine's novel *The Lion's Whelp*, explained this transformation in the following way: 'From contemplating disease and deformity in our hospitals, we go into the streets to see only deformity and disease – the more ghastly the more interesting to us – and so, for four or five years, what is sweet and wholesome in our fellows is crushed out of our lives. I wonder if we ever recover this loss. Not entirely perhaps'.[17] Nevin's statement draws attention to the hardening effects of medical study and the idea that students experienced a certain loss of innocence through their educational experiences. Students also used terms such as 'chrysalis', 'pupa' or 'embryo' to describe the medical student prior to conversion into a qualified practitioner.[18] For many medical students, this transformation involved not just conversion from boy to man but also involved becoming more civilised as a result of integration into city life, with student magazines regularly referring to students 'coming up to Dublin' from the country. Universities were, and are, settings not only for rites of passage, but also for secular ceremonies, cultural performances and rituals of reification, of revitalisation, resistance, incorporation and investiture, amongst others.[19] Additionally, as Kathleen Manning has argued, rituals are crucially important for allowing for the development of a group identity among university students, causing the 'I' to become 'we'.[20]

Hardship was an important element in cultivating a manly identity among students. Sir Thomas Myles (1857–1937), an Irish surgeon, speaking at a meeting of the Belfast Medical Students' Association in 1912, remarked that 'the medical student must always remain apart from the genial mass of mankind. Death and suffering were always with him. What were tragedies to others were commonplace to him'.[21] Experiences at medical school were cloaked in language of hardship and suffering – the idea that students had to overcome difficulty and adversity before they could mature into medical

16 'The last lecture', *Q.C.B.* 13(8) (June 1912), p. 13.
17 G.M. Irvine, *The lion's whelp* (London: Simpkin, Marshall, Hamilton, Kent & Co. Ltd., 1910), p. 34
18 'As others see us', p. 4.
19 Kathleen Manning, *Rituals, ceremonies and cultural meaning in higher education* (Westport, Conn.: Bergin & Garvey, 2000), pp. 3–8.
20 Manning, *Rituals, ceremonies and cultural meaning in higher education*, p. 120.
21 'Belfast Medical Students' Association', *British Medical Journal*, 3 February 1912, p. 270.

practitioners. As discussed earlier in the book, medical students often lived together in digs during university. These were often depicted in student magazines, and subsequently in doctors' memoirs, as another hardship which students had to endure.

As described in Chapter 4, the most important rite of passage was undoubtedly the first entrance into the dissecting room. One student writing in 1911 described the student's introduction to the dissecting room in the following way:

> Acting under competent advice he robes himself in faultlessly ironed apron and sleeves of a dangerous and steely brightness, and finally, with a Birmingham [Ambrose Birmingham's illustrated *Notebook of Anatomy* (1902)] clasped tightly 'neath his axilla, makes his entrée to a place, which, for two years, will be, or should be, his almost constant habitation'.[22]

Following the student's first day in the dissecting room, notably aided by a 'lady medical' who helped him with his tasks, 'he trots off dutifully to the digs – a new man. He is no longer the one who feared to enter the dissecting room, he is now a medical, his step is more assured, and his Birmingham more prominent than is really compatible with his year'.[23]

The physical appearance of medical students also underwent transformation and each stage of the student's maturation was characterised by an item of clothing. Initially, the students wore a clean, 'faultlessly ironed' apron in the dissecting room, sold to them by 'the fatherly porter'.[24] This became covered in dirt and blood after their initiation in the dissecting room. Upon entering third year of their studies, entering the hospital and the next stage of their development, 'scalpel, forceps and greasy dissecting coats have been discarded; likewise, the catcalls and boisterousness of other days. Our social standing and a new hat weighs heavily upon us – lovely men to be sure'.[25] Similarly, a poem published in 1917 remarked that a month or two after the first entrance into the dissecting room there had been a change 'since his initiation', and that the student's 'new white dress has now been sloped in many a mess; he thinks it recreation!'[26] Male medical students were often marked out by their dirty aprons. In 1917, the Royal College of Surgeons requested that students ensure that their dissecting coats were always

---

22 'First impressions', *National Student* 2(6) (December 1911), p. 12.
23 'First impressions', p. 13.
24 'First impressions', p. 12.
25 'Medical notes', *Galway University College Magazine* 2(9) (1922–3), p. 21.
26 'First impressions', p. 12.

clean and white. One student commented that he, like the majority of his counterparts, with the exception of the ladies, had made his coat last all term without washing it.[27]

Smoking was an important part of the dissecting room experience and served to reinforce notions of masculinity while also helping to ease the nerves that went along with the practice of dissection.[28] Indeed, as Nye has argued, for members of the medical profession, smoking was part of 'the unholy trinity of smoking, drinking and profanity' which 'were salient expressions of male exclusivity if not aggression'.[29] Recognising the popularity of smoking among their students, many of the Irish medical schools provided smoking-rooms for students from the 1880s.[30] Smoking while dissecting was a common practice among the male students and was permitted by university professors. Medical students at Trinity College Dublin in 1900, for example, were presented in the following way:

the groups of youthful anatomists discussing football, politics &c, while they cut and chop – the eager student, heedless of all around, with his pipe hanging listlessly between his teeth as he vigorously plies scalpel and forceps, and last, but surely not least, the far-famed 'stove class'.[31]

J. Johnston Abraham recalled students in the dissecting room at Trinity College in the 1890s working 'away steadily, smoking as we did so', and even until the 1950s this practice still appears to have been commonplace.[32] Thomas Hennessy, who studied at University College Dublin in the 1950s, referred in his autobiography to the anatomy professor permitting students to smoke in the dissecting room 'because some people found the smell of

27 'College Notes', *R.C.S.I. Students' quarterly* 1(3) (November 1917): 44 [RCPI Heritage Centre, TPCK/6/7/12].
28 One student remarked in 1911 that 'the consumption of tobacco is certainly enormous, and the bright gas jets dependent from on high give to the whole an appearance of comfort that a sudden entry without cannot but help to appreciate'. 'First impressions', p. 12.
29 Robert A. Nye, 'Medicine and science as masculine "Fields of Honor"', *Osiris* 12 (1997), p. 76.
30 Walter Rivington, '"The medical profession of the United Kingdom", being the essay to which was awarded the First Carmichael Prize by the Council of the Royal College of Surgeons in Ireland, 1887' (Dublin: Fannin & Co., 1888), p. 700. In 1909, for example, University College Galway provided students with a refurbished combined smoking and reading room. *U.C.G.: A College Annual* 1(1) (February 1909), p. 24.
31 'News from "The Schools"', *T.C.D.: A College Miscellany* 6(103) (10 November 1900), pp. 129–30.
32 J. Johnston Abraham, *Surgeon's journey: the autobiography of J. Johnston Abraham* (London: Heinemann, 1957), p. 46.

formaldehyde a little difficult to take'.[33] Hilton's research on smoking in popular culture in Britain has shown through his study of Mass Observation questionnaires that 'the cigarette became important in public displays of masculinity' and that the 'proffering of cigarettes to friends and colleagues helped define the group', helping to cultivate a group identity through which masculinities could be defined.[34] Illustrating this point, a law student who visited the dissecting room in Trinity in 1927 felt isolated from the medical students' group dynamic because 'Everyone was smoking and I had no cigarettes; I didn't like to ask for one because I know a medical student is always smoking his "last one" and I didn't care to embarrass anyone'.[35] Similarly, at a 'smoker' concert organised by the BMSA in 1937, it was agreed unanimously by the student committee that non-medicals would be admitted to the concert but that the distribution of cigarettes would be confined to medical students.[36] Smoking thus had particular meanings for medical students. Not only was it seen as a peculiarly masculine activity, and in this way, further served to segregate men and women students, but it also helped to cover the smell of formaldehyde and acted as a tool in calming the nerves associated with one's first experience in the dissecting room.

As well as entry to the dissecting room, student magazines and doctors' memoirs often singled out examinations as being an important rite of passage. By the late nineteenth century, examinations were longer and more likely to be written and practical in format than oral. Students were not only tested in the preliminary scientific subjects but also faced examinations on their scientific and clinical subjects.[37] In Ireland, from 1886, students wishing to take the primary medical degree of the National University of Ireland were required to take four main examinations during their time at university.[38] Similarly, at Trinity, efforts were made in the late nineteenth century to bring some order to the structure of the medical syllabus with an officially recommended sequence of lectures and examinations.[39] Deslandes has shown

---

33 Thomas Hennessy, *My life as a surgeon: an autobiography* (Dublin: A. & A. Farmar, 2011), p. 69.

34 Matthew Hilton, *Smoking in British popular culture, 1800–2000* (Manchester: Manchester University Press, 2000), p. 130.

35 'My impressions of the Dissecting Lab by a Man of Law', *T.C.D.: A College Miscellany* 304 (587) (24 November 1927), p. 50.

36 'Committee meeting 21 Jan. 1937', BMSA Minute Book, 1932–48 [Royal Victoria Hospital Archives].

37 W.F. Bynum, *Science and the practice of medicine in the nineteenth century* (Cambridge: Cambridge University Press, 1994), p. 181.

38 James Murray, *Galway: a medico-social history* (Galway: Kenny's Bookshop and Art Gallery, 1994), p. 193.

39 R.B. McDowell and D.A. Webb, *Trinity College Dublin, 1592–1952: an academic history* (Cambridge: Cambridge University Press, 1982), p. 330.

how competitive examinations were viewed as tests of character and 'could be manipulated symbolically to allow undergraduates to vent competitive spirits; formulate, express and preserve gender identities; and articulate some of the primary concerns of late adolescents on the cusp of manhood'.[40] Examinations were constructed as 'horrific ideals, tests of character, and sacred masculine rituals'.[41] As Michael Brown's work has shown, militarism and heroism came to play a crucial role in British physicians' writings in the nineteenth century.[42] Similarly, medical examinations were often described in martial terms by students. Q.C.G. in 1902 reported of 'hostilities between Examiners and Medicals at Earl's Fort' (a play on 'Earlsfort Terrace' in Dublin, where examinations were held), explaining that the 'Medical forces are pretty strong ... the preparation of their full war equipment is being rapidly pushed forward, and they are expected to be ready to take the field towards the middle of April'.[43] These types of strategies helped to define examinations as a masculine activity, which was increasingly important once women undergraduates began sitting for examinations in the late nineteenth century.[44]

Certainly, in the Irish context, the achievements of women in examinations were often referred to in the student press in a competitive way. An article in *St. Stephen's* in 1902 commending the successes of some of its women students in gaining medals in the national examinations, asked, 'What a pity it is that "the Boys" don't begin work a short time before the School Examinations!'[45] In this way, women were seen as competitors. Masculinity thus became more important to students at this point as a way of reaffirming their place in the profession in the wake of increasing numbers of women students. Occasionally, such book-worming on the part of the women medical students was called out by their male counterparts. Q.C.C. in 1906 remarked that few women students attended the student dance that year and asked whether this was on account of them working too hard.[46] However, for medical students, examinations were also viewed as important in the transformation of the gyb. One former student at Queen's College Belfast

40 Paul R. Deslandes, 'Competitive examinations and the culture of masculinity in Oxbridge undergraduate life, 1850–1920', *History of Education Quarterly* 42(4) (2002), p. 556.
41 Deslandes, 'Competitive examinations', pp. 577–8.
42 Michael Brown, '"Like a devoted army": medicine, heroic masculinity, and the military paradigm in Victorian Britain', *Journal of British Studies* 49(3) (July 2010): 592–622.
43 'War threatened in the extremely near east', *Q.C.G.* 2(2) (February 1904), p. 52.
44 Deslandes, 'Competitive examinations', pp. 577–8.
45 'News from "The School"', *St. Stephen's: A Record of University Life* 1(8) (November 1902): p. 172. Other descriptions remark on their studious nature, with one in *Q.C.B.* remarking that the 'lady medical' was 'more diligent, assiduous' than the male student ('Winsome woman', p. 7).
46 'Aphroditiana', *Q.C.C.* 2(3) (23 March 1906), p. 58.

remarked that after first-year summer examinations students 'were now ready to take our places as the senior students in the dissecting room. We knew that we were no longer freshmen, and that we could afford to look with a kindly eye on those youngsters who had just arrived raw from school'.[47] Examinations also served to civilise rowdy first-year students. Q.C.B. in 1900 remarked that after the visit to Dublin to undertake their examinations the 'boisterous' freshmen now had a 'dejected and subdued appearance'.[48]

Failure to pass examinations had important consequences and meant that students would not progress to the target state of qualified practitioner but instead could be resigned to what was described as the 'chronic student'. Chronic students were ones who took several years to qualify with a medical degree, if they even did so, and appear to have been a feature of Irish medical school life up until at least the 1940s.[49] These students failed to progress past their first or second year of medical study, were often prone to drinking, and may be viewed as a step down in the hierarchy of medical student masculinities, denied the full privileges of masculinity. Arthur Wynne Foot, in a lecture to students in 1873, described the 'chronic' as 'incurable … an unwholesome and a dangerous member of a profession ashamed to own him'.[50] Chronics were similarly referred to in derogatory terms in both the student press and in doctors' memoirs. A 1923 poem criticised the chronic, 'the hoary veteran', for his lack of knowledge ('can't find an acid radicle, or tell it from its base') and inability to pass the 'annual stunt' of examinations.[51] In this way, chronic students were seen as less manly. Doctors' memoirs also criticised chronics for taking advantage of naive students. J. Johnston Abraham described the chronic as 'a nuisance and a great corrupter of innocence', while Thomas Garry explained that they 'lay in wait for new students who were generally unsophisticated and had plenty of money. Like all addicts whether of drink or drugs, they took immense delight in dragging others down to their own level'.[52] There are clearly class issues at play here:

---

47 R.W.M. Strain, *Les neiges d'antan. a two-part story: recollections of a medical student at the Queen's University of Belfast, 1924–30 and of a houseman, the Royal Victoria Hospital, Belfast, 1930–31* (Truro: R. Strain, 1982), p. 9.

48 'The Schools: the medical school', *Q.C.B.* 2(1) (20 November 1900), p. 9.

49 From the 1940s, Irish universities took measures to eliminate the problem of chronic medical students. For instance, at University College Cork, from 1946, students were given two years to pass each of the first three examinations in medicine ('Limiting the number of medicals' by President Alfred O'Rahilly, *Cork University Record* 7 (summer term 1946), p. 24).

50 Arthur Wynne Foot, 'An introductory address delivered at the Ledwich School of Medicine, November 1st, 1873' (Dublin: John Falconer, 1873), p. 17.

51 'The same old second-medical', *Fravlio-Queens* (June 1923), p. 6.

52 Abraham, *Surgeon's journey*, p. 46 and Thomas Garry, *African doctor* (London: John Gifford, 1939), p. 15.

chronic students evidently had the means to repeat their examinations, while students of more limited means had more incentive not to engage in drinking and to focus instead on more respectable extra-curricular activities, such as sport. However, bad behaviour was not unique to the chronic students and prank-playing and student rags remained an important rite of passage well into the twentieth century, and one which also served again to segregate men and women students.

Pranks and rags

Prank-playing was an important initiation rite for medical students and one that is alluded to in both the contemporary student magazines and in the memoirs of Irish doctors. Challenges to authority at universities in the twentieth century, although usually quite benign and ritualised, were, according to Dyhouse, 'both frequent and frequently tolerated as part of the construction of masculinity, part of the "natural order of things"'.[53] Medical students were usually singled out in the student press for being the perpetrators of such pranks. This extract from *Q.C.B.* in 1914 describes 'the ideal medical student' in the following way:

> But to him, the very highest form of humour consisted in gathering a large body of fellow students, and going out with them to cause as much trouble and annoyance as possible in places where there was no danger of receiving any damage themselves. He was, in short, an ideal medical student.[54]

Such representations of boisterous male medical students persisted late into the twentieth century. Prank-playing became an accepted part of medical student life for students in their early years of study. Although arguably student pranks were not distinctive to medical students, they nevertheless occupy a particular place in accounts of medical student life in student newspapers and doctors' memoirs, and because medical students studied for the longest period they had something of a 'delayed adolescence' compared with other students. Students from other faculties frequently commented on this. One piece in *Q.C.B.* in 1900 remarked that 'sober Artsmen sidle past, filled with reverent awe at the bold independence of the medical chrysalis and feeling in comparison with such glory their lives are but nothing'.[55] The

53 Dyhouse, *Students: a gendered history*, p. 177.
54 'A medical biography', *Q.C.B.* 16(4) (February 1914), p. 10.
55 'As others see us', p. 4.

lecture theatre was often a setting for displays of bad behaviour and some of this appears to have been tolerated to a large degree by the professors. In 1903, *Q.C.G.* reported that two medical students had pinned a duster to the tail of one of the professors, which 'elicited roars of laughter, especially from the perpetrators'.[56] By the 1930s, there were similar reports, with James Lloyd Turner Graham, a first-year student at the Royal College of Surgeons, noting in his diary in 1933 that 'The lectures are generally of a rowdy character. The fellows kick up a din if the lecturer says anything funny and also when he does not'.[57] At Queen's College Belfast, in the first half of the twentieth century, medical students traditionally threw missiles and caused general havoc at the introductory lecture of the professor of botany on the first day of term.[58] More serious pranks directed at professors could have negative consequences. In 1919, Thomas Sheehan, a second-year medical, along with Gerard O'Farrell, an engineering student, was charged in court for stealing the camera of Bertram Windle, President of University College Cork and an eminent member of the Irish medical profession. Sheehan was discharged conditionally 'on his entering into a recognisance in the sum of £5 and one Surety in £5 to be at good behaviour'.[59] The pair were also suspended from the college for the remainder of the year.[60]

Although prank-playing was, of course, part of general student life, regardless of discipline, it held particular meaning in the world of medical students. In the cases of Oxford and Cambridge, contained within 'humorous acts were more serious messages about the abilities of undergraduates to disrupt and unsettle figures of authority and briefly subvert Oxbridge institutional and masculine hierarchies'.[61] Importantly, students were rarely disciplined for such acts and professors showed a remarkable degree of tolerance towards them. Such pranks were generally benign in nature, yet enabled students to disrupt the hierarchy, albeit momentarily. In this way they may be viewed as acts of rebellion, or just one of the stages in the transformation of medical students from boys to men. Women, notably, did not take part in these rites of prank-playing, but were occasionally the targets of these activities. In 1912, *Q.C.B.* remarked on first-year students answering

56 'Medicine', *Q.C.G.* 1(2) (February 1903), p. 42.
57 James Lloyd Turner Graham diary, 7 December 1933 [RCPI Heritage Centre, BMS/48].
58 Denis Biggart, *John Henry Biggart: pathologist, professor and Dean of Medical Faculty, Queen's University, Belfast* (Belfast: Ulster Historical Association, 2012), p. 23.
59 Certificate of Order, Petty Sessions District of Cork, dated 11 December 1919, Academic Council various correspondence March–April 1923 [NUI Galway Archives and Special Collections, 1/23].
60 Letter from the President of University College Cork addressed to the Registrar, University College Galway, dated 29 January 1920, Academic Council various correspondence, March–April 1923 [NUI Galway Archives and Special Collections, 1/23].
61 Deslandes, 'Competitive examinations', p. 92.

to each other's names out of turn for the roll-call and second-year students squeaking 'Here, Doctor' when a female student's name was called.[62]

Pranks directed at fellow students were not uncommon and, again, they highlight the rowdy nature of medical student life. Oliver St John Gogarty and his friends once sold an extremely intoxicated medical student to the Royal College of Surgeons as a corpse. The unconscious student was placed by the porter among the other cadavers in the dissecting room. The other students waited outside for some hours, until the unfortunate student, now fully sober, came running into the street, shouting, 'It's the last time I'll die to pay for your drink'.[63] Such accounts, particularly prevalent in doctors' autobiographies, could be read as conforming to stereotypes; however, similar examples of masculine bravado are not uncommon in the archival sources. In 1895, William McCarthy wrote to the President of Queen's College Cork to complain about fellow student D. Cagney. McCarthy reported that he sold Cagney three books for 9s. 5d., and that Cagney promised he would pay him the next day. Cagney did not pay him the money and had allegedly been bragging to his friends about the deed. He boasted that McCarthy was very foolish in trusting his word and that he never had any intention of paying him the money. McCarthy added that he did not mind the loss of the money but regretted 'being gulled so outrageously, and the swindler glorying in his infamy'. He reported that 'the tone of a section of the college is so low that actions of the sort I have named above are not considered at all dishonourable but rather the other way'.[64] McCarthy's testimony suggests that Cagney's actions were applauded by his fellow medical students.

Pranks took on a more organised format in yearly student rag days, in which medical students were taking an active part by the 1920s and which provide an interesting insight into the student–professor dynamic.[65] Rags owe their roots to the Medieval Feast of Fools, in which novices and choirboys parodied and mocked their superiors.[66] Cultural performances such as rags enabled students to celebrate their community while challenging the usual modes of behaviour.[67] Students dressed in strange costumes on rag days, often depicting political or celebrity figures of the day and a noisy procession through the city was arranged. In Belfast, rags were held for charity causes but also for famous visitors or new appointees to chairs in the medical

62 'The Last Lecture', Q.C.B. 13(8) (June 1912), p. 13.
63 Ulick O'Connor, Oliver St John Gogarty (London: Mandarin, 1990), p. 22.
64 Letter: William McCarthy to J. Slattery, President QCC, 2 December 1895 [UCC University Archives, UC/PRESIDENT/18/72].
65 For more on rags, see Dyhouse, Students: a gendered history, pp. 186–203.
66 John R. Gillis, Youth and history: tradition and change in European age relations, 1770–present (New York: Academic Press, 1974), pp. 25–6.
67 Manning, Rituals, ceremonies and cultural meaning in higher education, p. 84.

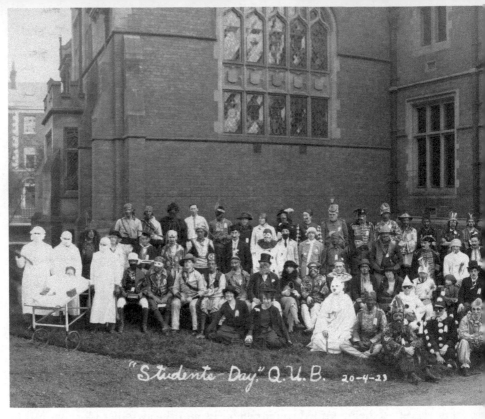

"Students-Day" Q.U.B. 20-4-23

5 Students' Day, Queen's University Belfast, 1923.
Courtesy of Trinity College Dublin Manuscripts Department.

faculty.[68] A photograph of Belfast students on 'Students' Day' 1923 depicts a large group in an assortment of costumes, including Charlie Chaplin, 'black and white minstrels' and clowns. To the left of the photograph is a group of three students dressed as surgeons, with a patient on a tray. One of the 'surgeons' is wielding a large blade-like instrument.[69]

Student rags frequently disrupted city life but were excused to an extent by the fact that the proceeds from the day were donated to charity.[70] Moreover, professors often participated in the initiation rituals as part of these proceedings. For example, in 1923, three new medical professors, C.G. Lowry, W.W.D. Thomson and Andrew Fullerton willingly took part in a special initiation ritual for the rag day in Belfast. Lowry was made to ride a donkey bareback down to the centre of the city while Thomson and Fullerton 'were captured between lectures, dressed in their pyjamas, gowns and mortarboards … they rode in a brougham drawn by long ropes manned

68 Biggart, *John Henry Biggart*, p. 32.
69 Photograph of Students' Day at Q.U.B., 20 April 1923 [TCD Manuscripts, MUN/MED/25/22].
70 T.F. O'Higgins, *A double life* (Dublin: Town House, 1996), pp. 52–3.

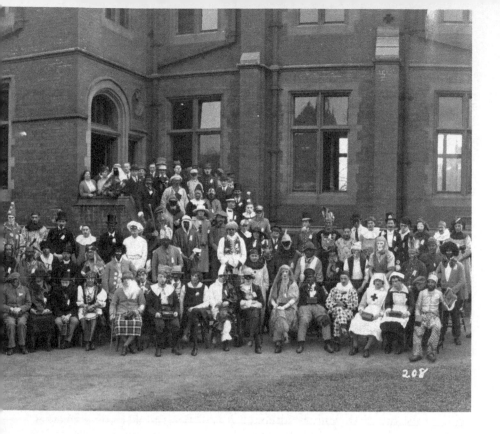

by students'.[71] The two professors were forced to drink champagne and were anointed with oil over a laurel crown.[72] This act is revealing. The students were evidently in control of initiation of the professors and in this way turned the trend of student transformation into doctors on its head. The professors willingly gave up their power temporarily, and were anointed into the student body. In 1927, a rag was organised by the BMSA to commemorate the knighthood of the bacteriologist Sir Thomas Houston. More than 100 students took part, with a large group forming a 40-foot-long microbe with green skin and huge jaws which was surrounded by a guard of smaller microbes. Houston rode on a lorry behind the microbe dressed in mail and 'entered wholeheartedly into the affair', afterwards having a duel with the microbe which was 'finally despatched with a great syringe'.[73] There is a certain amount of symbolism in this act, reflecting the students' membership of a professional and scientific group interlinked with a celebration of the triumphs of modern science.

71 Biggart, *John Henry Biggart*, p. 32.
72 Ian Fraser, 'The first three professors of surgery', *Ulster Medical Journal* 45(1) (1976), p. 39.
73 'Belfast students' humour: great microbe slain by medical knight', *Irish Times*, 27 February 1927, p. 3.

Doctors and students at hospitals also occasionally organised rags jointly, reinforcing the group dynamic. In 1921, the Jervis Street Hospital, Dublin held a rag to raise money for the hospital with students and doctors alike dressed in costumes.[74] Medical students armed themselves with the motifs of their profession, often wielding the masculine instruments of blades and scalpels. Mary Semple, an arts student at UCD in the 1930s, recalled that on rag days six to ten carts with tableaux would parade through the city and that the medical students usually did a 'mock-up of an operating theatre with a recumbent figure and surgeons brandishing fearsome instruments'.[75] Student rags could often take on an element of hooliganism, and during the 1930s it appears that bad behaviour escalated. In 1933, during the Trinity College rag, policemen were shelled with eggs after which the 'ragging of the shops commenced'.[76] In 1936, it was reported that at the previous rag 'eggs in various stages of decay, tomatoes and the other missiles usually devoted to such occasions whistled through the air in an obnoxious super-abundance to the dismay of spectators and in not a few cases to the detriment of their apparel'.[77] Such activities led to the cancellation of the Trinity rag day in 1939.[78]

Alcohol consumption was often associated with medical student culture well into the twentieth century, although it is difficult to determine whether drinking was a common practice. According to his biographer, Oliver St John Gogarty and his friends, including James Joyce, tended to drink in Nighttown, an area of Dublin famous for its brothels.[79] This group of medical students are immortalised in the chapter 'Oxen of the Sun' in Joyce's *Ulysses*, where Stephen Dedalus is seen drinking with Buck Mulligan and other medical students at the maternity hospital where Mina Purefoy is in labour. Following the delivery of the baby, the group proceeds to drink in a pub. The drunken debate between the characters in this section focuses on themes in obstetrics and forensic medicine, with a number of scenarios lifted out of contemporary medical debates.[80] Despite being an incident of fiction, the practice of medical students drinking while undertaking clinical experience may not have been an uncommon practice. In her memoirs,

---

74 'Ragging for charity', video at www.britishpathe.com/video/ragging-for-charity, accessed 8 April 2013.

75 Mary Semple, 'Going hatching', in Anne Macdona (ed.), *From Newman to new woman: UCD women remember* (Dublin: New Island, 2001), p. 13.

76 James Lloyd Turner Graham diary, 12 June 1933 [RCPI Heritage Centre, BMS/48].

77 Correspondence, *T.C.D.: A College Miscellany* 42(740) (21 May 1936), p. 162.

78 Editorial, *T.C.D.: A College Miscellany* 46(813) (6 June 1940), p. 181.

79 O'Connor, *Oliver St John Gogarty*, p. 54.

80 Vike Plock, *Joyce, medicine and modernity* (Gainesville: University Press of Florida, 2010), pp. 71–2.

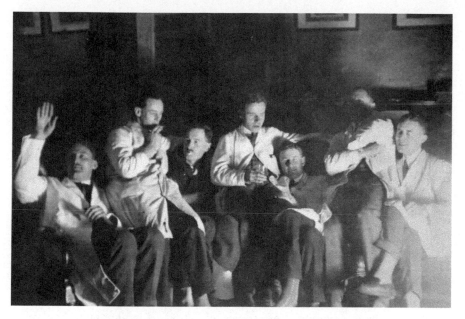

6   Group of Trinity College medical students, *c.*1920s.
From the Francis Joseph O'Meara Collection.
Courtesy of the RCPI Heritage Centre.

Sidney Croskery, a Belfast-born doctor who trained at the University of
Edinburgh, wrote of her clinical experiences at the Coombe Hospital in
Dublin in the early twentieth century. She was partnered up with a male
Egyptian student and wrote: 'I was very glad I had to work with him and not
with one of the other male students. Not all, but some of these, who came
from English and Scottish universities, seemed to have come to Ireland to
have a good time and kick over the traces, drinking and making a noise
in our Common Room night and day'.[81] She wrote of a tragedy that had
occurred at the undergraduate quarters of the Coombe shortly before she
arrived there. A medical student who had been out drinking with a crowd
at the pub near the gate of the hospital had fallen backwards off his seat.
His friends had brought him home and put him to bed. The student was
found 'dead in his bed in the morning, with a fractured skull'. According
to Croskery, 'I was told he was a quiet, decent fellow but just not used to
drinking spirits. Possibly if his pals had not been fuddled themselves and
he had been taken to hospital, a trephining operation might have saved his
life'. When Croskery's younger sister Lil went to the Rotunda Hospital for
clinical experience, she found that the male students there behaved similarly,

81 Sidney Elizabeth Croskery, *Whilst I remember* (Dundonald: Blackstaff, 1983), p. 23.

reporting that some of the undergraduates were irresponsible and 'drank even when on call'.[82]

The pastime of drinking could have important consequences for both students' finances and their education. One writer for *Galway University College Magazine* explained how he and his fellow medical students' philosophy could be summed up in the words: 'Drink to-day, for to-morrow you die'. Squandering of finances could lead to a visit to the pawn shop. According to this student, he had been revolted by the thought of visiting pawn shops, which seemed to him 'a most disreputable thing', but soon all his earthly goods became represented by small slips of paper.[83] Likewise, Ouseley and his fellow medical students in Oliver St John Gogarty's semi-autobio-graphical novel *Tumbling in the Hay* engage in the practice of pawning. After pawning his cufflinks, a family heirloom, Ouseley feels intensely guilty, stating: 'I felt a sense of degradation. My friends repelled me. If my mother knew! The very thought of a pawn office! They saw nothing bad in it. They took it as a joke, a grim one at the worst, inseparable from the life of a "medical"'.[84] Bridget O'Brien, a student at UCD in the 1930s, recalled some medical students pawning their copies of *Gray's Anatomy* on a Friday 'in the hope of redeeming it on a Monday when their money from home came through'.[85] However, by the 1940s and 1950s, as will be discussed in more detail in Chapter 7, it appears that medical students were trying to revoke the negative image painted by their predecessors. By this time, students were also becoming more involved in charity work and rag events seem to have placed more emphasis on raising money for good causes, thereby perhaps improving the reputation of medical students.

Why were pranks, drinking and occasions of rowdiness given so much attention in the student press and subsequently in doctors' memoirs? It is possible that, moving into the twentieth century, when medicine was becoming increasingly clinical and doctors were being criticised for their lack of bedside manner, that they wanted to portray themselves as fun-loving and well-rounded individuals, not as cold and lacking in compassion. Indeed, professors' addresses from the early twentieth century hinted at the need for students to cultivate a good bedside manner, and not, in the words of Humphrey Rolleston, 'to regard the patient as a machine out of order and an interesting problem in pathology'. Students needed to get inside their patients' minds, 'so as to think their thoughts, feel their feelings and thus

82 Croskery, *Whilst I remember*, p. 23.
83 'The Autobiography of a medical student', *Galway University College Magazine* 3(10) (1924–5), pp. 39–40.
84 Gogarty, *Tumbling in the hay*, p. 15.
85 Bridget O'Brien (Carroll), 'In Dublin's fair city', in Anne Macdona (ed.), *From Newman to new woman: UCD women remember* (Dublin: New Island, 2001), p. 16.

understand their mentality and anxieties so thoroughly … there must be calmness without coldness, decision without dour dogmatism, friendliness – but firmness'.[86] In an introductory lecture to students at the Royal College of Surgeons in 1903, Sir Lambert Ormsby encouraged students to 'Take care in starting that you are equipped with all the necessary armour and weapons for the counter upon which you have entered … Let your one aim and end be always to achieve the enviable reputation of a good doctor and a courteous gentleman'.[87] A 1915 *Irish Times* piece on the essential qualifications for anyone considering a career in the medical profession summarised these as a love of study, a scientific bent, a kindly disposition and good bedside manner, the business instinct and good health.[88] Writing in his 1939 memoirs, Thomas Garry, who had trained in Galway and Dublin, believed:

> it is the wildest and most adventurous students who often turn out the best, most humane and generous doctors. I have little taste for the man who boasts that he never entered a pub in his life or took part in the riotous assemblies inseparable from student life at all times in all countries. He is not the sort of man who makes a good doctor with wide human sympathies and becomes the friend and confident of his fellow men.[89]

As some doctors' memoirs have suggested, boisterous activities also allowed medical students to get any 'rowdyism' out of their system before they went on to become professional men. Moreover, returning to my earlier point about medical studies being viewed as a struggle or time of hardship, such pranks or displays of rowdy behaviour also served to counteract feelings of despondency at the more difficult aspects of medical education. For this reason, it appears that prank-playing and mischief were for the most part excused. In his memoirs, J. Johnston Abraham commented that bad behaviour was 'the result of coming up against pain and suffering and the gruesome side of life at a time when the only way they can react against it is to rush to the other extreme and hilariously ignore it'.[90]

Likewise, in his novel *The Lion's Whelp*, which follows the life of a Belfast-trained doctor, G.M. Irvine excused the medical student for being

86 'Doctor and his patient: great physician's advice to students', *Irish Times*, 3 October 1927, p. 8.
87 Sir Lambert Ormsby, 'The ideal physician: his early training and future prospects', *Irish Journal of Medical Science* 116 (December 1903), pp. 449–50.
88 'Careers for boys and girls: I. The medical profession', *Weekly Irish Times*, 13 February 1915, p. 5.
89 Garry, *African doctor*, p. 17.
90 Abraham, *Surgeon's journey*, p. 44.

'full of animal spirits' because of the fact that he had been 'just freed from the restraint of the family and of school'.[91] Moreover, he justified such bouts of rowdyism by claiming that such periodic occurrences were a compensation for days and weeks of 'monotonous book-worming'.[92] One student at Queen's College Galway stated that the work of the medical student 'is so monotonous and his Exams so tiring, that his levity seems an outlet of Nature for maintaining his mental equilibrium'.[93] Similarly, a professor in Gogarty's novel *Tumbling in the Hay* excused the students' 'merriment' on his rounds at the Whitworth Hospital, Dublin that morning and ignored the 'many, very many manifestations of ill-manners and bad breeding' because, in his view, these were simply 'indications of ignorance and lack of experience, and I know that these are but transitory manifestations in any man who at heart is sound'.[94] Again, this implies that rowdyism was excused because it was viewed as being part of the transformative process. Displays of bad behaviour may also have been tolerated by professors, perhaps because they themselves had acted similarly in their student days and this was seen as something which one had to engage with in order to complete the transformation from student to fully fledged practitioner. However, these pranks also served another function: they helped to define who was a member of the group and who was not. Crucially, women did not partake in prank-playing and had a limited role to play in student rags. These activities served further to separate them from the men students.

Sport

The main extra-curricular activity which effectually segregated male and female medical students was sport. Sport became an integral aspect of the gentleman's training in the Victorian and Edwardian periods.[95] According to Richard Holt, 'Team-sports provided emotional as well as physical rewards. Being in a team was to be "one of the lads"; it gave warmth, simple shared values and objectives, and an endless source of banter'.[96] Sport was not just

91 Irvine, *The lion's whelp*, p. 21.
92 Irvine, *The lion's whelp*, p. 20.
93 'Medicine', *Q.C.G.* 5(2) (February 1907), p. 50.
94 Gogarty, *Tumbling in the hay*, pp. 225–8.
95 See J.A. Mangan, *Athleticism in the Victorian and Edwardian public school* (London: Frank Cass, 2000). For rugby and masculinity, see John Nauright and Timothy J.L. Chandler (eds), *Making men: rugby and masculine identity* (London: Routledge, 1999).
96 Richard Holt, *Sport and the British: A Modern History* (Oxford: Oxford University Press, 1990), p. 155.

important for reasons of fitness or competitiveness, it was also important for the traits of duty, solidarity and service that it encouraged in its players, and this is why team-sports were preferred to individual ones by both educationists and army leaders.[97]

Historians such as Dyhouse and Garner have noted the importance of sport, in particular rugby, in the culture of British medical schools.[98] Indeed, medical students and young doctors were keen sportsmen and the first rugby club in the world was founded at Guy's Hospital, London in 1843.[99] Heaman has suggested that, at St Mary's Hospital Medical School in London, sports clubs and games 'were intended to foster these "social and tender feelings" and make students and the doctors they would become meet as comrades rather than committee members'.[100] Indeed, more broadly, university societies and sports clubs helped to foster kinship among students.[101] Taken at face value, sports teams may be viewed as a means of helping to bond students together. As Messner has convincingly argued in his study of masculinity and sport, sports teams present the image of a 'family' with the shared goal of winning which helps to unite its members. However, this public face masks the reality of intense and constant competition which is part and parcel of athletic participation.[102] Therefore, like examinations, sport also served to encourage competition and may be viewed as another aspect of homosociality within medical schools. Historians of medicine have neglected this and other important aspects of sport for medical students. Sport not only helped to promote physical fitness, but encouraged what Tosh has described as 'character-building qualities of courage, self-control, stoical endurance, and the subordination of ego to the team', qualities which resonated with the character formation common in conventional middle-class households where 'pain and emotion were repressed, and individuality curtailed, in the cause of producing a type'.[103] Moreover, sport also served to further segregate male and female students.

Rugby appears to have been the most popular sport among medical students in the period of this chapter. Cricket, which had been popular in the 1870s and 1880s began to decline later in the nineteenth century owing

97 Holt, *Sport and the British*, p. 205.
98 Dyhouse, *Students: a gendered history*, p. 152. Garner, 'The great experiment', p. 84.
99 Holt, *Sport and the British*, p. 85.
100 E.A. Heaman, *St. Mary's: The history of a London teaching hospital* (Liverpool: Liverpool University Press, 2003), p. 85.
101 Tomás Irish, 'Fractured families: educated elites in Britain and France and the challenge of the Great War', *Historical Journal* 57(2) (June 2014), p. 512.
102 Michael A. Messner, 'Like family: power, intimacy and sexuality in male athletes' friendships', in Peter M. Nardi (ed.), *Men's friendships* (Newbury Park, Calif.: SAGE, 1992), p. 219.
103 Tosh, 'What should historians do with masculinity?', pp. 188–9.

to a lack of the establishment of a governing body to oversee the game in Ireland, or other attempts at regulation such as the organisation of national competitions or a calendar of play.[104] Competition from other sports and the impact of the Land Wars have also been blamed for the decline of cricket.[105] Rugby, on the other hand, began to become consolidated as '*the* game of the middle classes across Ireland', and in elite schools such as Clongowes and Castleknock College, soccer, which was viewed as unsuitable for middle-class boys, largely owing to reports of violent conduct at soccer matches, was abandoned by the students in favour of rugby.[106] There is ample evidence of the important part that rugby played in the lives of Irish medical students. John A. Murphy has argued that there was a 'virtual interchangeability at the turn of the twentieth century between rugby, college and the medical faculty', noting that nineteen out of the twenty students playing rugby for Queen's College Cork in 1876 went on to have medical careers.[107] *Q.C.C.* in 1907 referred to 'the "lunaticus footballus"', with his 'ears still filled with the applause of watching hundreds, eyes ever seeing the flying ball, and burning with a mad desire to do for that —— idiot who plays so beastly foul!'[108]

Professors at Irish medical schools were active in promoting sport at university level. Although Waddington has argued that the impetus for the founding of sports clubs usually came from medical students themselves, professors played an important role in supporting sport at university level in Ireland.[109] At Queen's College Cork in 1906, five out of the seven guarantors of the rugby football club were professors in the medical faculty, while Professor Pearson, the professor of surgery, was commended for changing the hour of his Wednesday lecture from 4 p.m. to twelve noon to allow the students Wednesday afternoons free for football.[110] Irish medical schools actively advertised their sports facilities as a means of encouraging prospective students. For example, the prospectus for the Belfast medical school in 1903 boasted that its playing fields were 'one of the finest grounds in Belfast for this purpose, fully formed and enclosed, and situated in close proximity to the College'.[111] This indicates the type of men that medical

104 Rouse, *Sport and Ireland: a history*, p. 214.
105 Tom Hunt, *Sport and society in Victorian Ireland: the case of Westmeath* (Cork: Cork University Press, 2007), pp. 113–14.
106 Rouse, *Sport and Ireland: a history*, p. 215.
107 John A. Murphy, *Where Finbarr played: a concise illustrated history of sport in University College Cork, 1911–2011* (Cork: Cork University Press, 2011), p. 89.
108 'The medicus', p. 6.
109 Waddington, *Medical education at St Bartholomew's Hospital*, p. 251.
110 Report read at opening general meeting for the season 1906–07, Rugby Football Club Minutes QCC 1905–1912 [UCC University Archives, UC/MB/CS/RF/1].
111 *Guide to the Belfast Medical School for session 1903–4* (Belfast: A. Mayne and Boyd, 1903), p. 24.

schools were trying to attract to their courses: sporty, middle-class men who were robust, healthy and disciplined.

Sport was advocated by professors as being important for the promotion of good health and to counteract bad behaviour. As early as 1868, E.D. Mapother, professor of anatomy and physiology at the Royal College of Surgeons, remarked on the importance of training 'the physical as well as the mental faculties, which are closely interdependent' in order to combat the threat of contagious diseases to which medical students were often exposed. He argued that every medical school should provide facilities for the playing of sport and suggested that students' spare time should be spent in the ball-court, gymnasium or cricket field, rather than 'smoking at the dissecting room fires, or in the taverns to which want of occupation will tempt them'.[112] In the Victorian period, as Holt has argued, concepts of the healthy mind and body 'merged into a garbled Darwinism that was itself often intermingled with notions of Christian and imperial duty'.[113]

Students also seem to have been aware of the importance of exercise to their mental health. In 1879, in a letter to the Medical Board, students at the Adelaide Hospital spoke of how they felt 'very keenly the want of outdoor exercise' due to spending the majority of their time within the bounds of the hospital.[114] There is therefore a sense that sport could help to combat stress while also encouraging discipline and hard work. Similarly, Philip Crampton Smyly (1838–1904), former president of the Royal College of Surgeons, illustrated to students how the discipline, self-control and skills learnt through playing rugby could be applied to their studies and future careers:

> Similar laws and training, similar earnestness and self-control, ensure similar results. The bodily training must be perfect; too much at once or too little is equally futile. It is the same with the mind. You would not have your cup this year had you trained your bodies as some of you try to train your minds for your examinations. Give something of the same training to your hands and minds as you do to your feet and bodies. You will then be successful, and win, not only the hospital challenge cup, but you will be successful men – men of the hand –surgeons.[115]

112 E.D. Mapother, *The medical profession and its educational and licensing bodies* (Dublin: Fannin & Co., 1868), p. 117.
113 Holt, *Sport and the British*, p. 85.
114 Letter to the Medical Board dated 1st of July 1879, Adelaide Hospital Medical Board Minute Book, 17 September 1875–8 May 1880 [Trinity College Manuscripts, IE TCD MS 11270/2/3/3/2].
115 Philip Crampton Smyly, '"Is it true?" An address delivered in the theatre of the Meath

In this instance, male students were encouraged to play rugby because the same skills could be applied to the practice of surgery, which was seen as a fundamentally male domain of practice. There is also a sense that playing sport could help to encourage discipline and camaraderie among the students, qualities which would be useful in their future careers. Rugby would have been more appealing to medical students and their professors than a sport such as cricket because it was a more collective team sport; cricket was seen as a sport where there was more scope for individualism.[116] Rugby, fundamentally, 'seems to have promoted a strong male group conformity and a certain social conservatism wherever it was played'.[117]

James Craig encouraged students at the Meath Hospital in 1893 to take part in rugby and 'win renown' by helping to attain the 'much-coveted' Hospitals' Cup again.[118] The Hospitals' Cup was a rugby tournament founded in 1884 with the establishment of the Dublin Hospital Football Union which was composed of representative doctors from each of the Dublin hospitals.[119] The competition was an important fixture in the medical student's calendar, with matches never failing 'to excite a considerable amount of interest in student circles'.[120] In London, similar competitions existed between the rugby teams of the hospitals there.[121] These events also acted as valuable fundraising events for hospital charities and 'worthy causes'.[122] Students were dedicated to these competitions and success in sport was believed to reflect positively on the reputation of the medical school, shedding 'lustre on the College and on the faculty'.[123] Intense rivalries developed between different teams, particularly, it seems, between the 'Mater Boys' and 'Vincent's'.[124] Such rivalries would certainly have helped to cement students' sense of collegiality. Success in the Hospitals' Cup competition was also positively reinforced by medical staff. In 1921, the Honorary Secretary of the Medical

Hospital and Co. Dublin Infirmary on Monday, October 3, 1890, introductory to the session of 1890–91' (Dublin: John Falconer, 1890), p. 4.
116 Holt, *Sport and the British*, p. 155.
117 Holt, *Sport and the British*, p. 228.
118 James Craig, 'Introductory address delivered at the opening of the session of 1893–4 in the theatre of the Meath Hospital' (Dublin: John Falconer, 1893), p. 7.
119 Dublin Hospital Football Union Minute Book, 1884–1901 [RCPI Heritage Centre, BMS/2/3].
120 'News from the school', *St. Stephen's: A Record of University Life* 1(11) (March 1903), p. 244.
121 Keir Waddington, *Medical Education at St Bartholomew's Hospital, 1123–1995* (Woodbridge: Boydell Press, 2003), p. 253.
122 Roberta Park, '"Mended or ended?": football injuries and the British and American medical press, 1870–1910', *International Journal of the History of Sport* 18(2) (2001): 118.
123 'Medical notes', *Galway University College Magazine* 3(1) (1924–5), pp. 85–6.
124 'Notes from the medical school', *St. Stephen's: A Record of University Life* 2(2) (February 1904), p. 33. The Mater and St Vincent's were two Dublin hospitals.

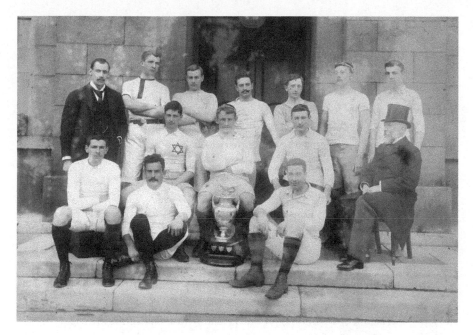

7   Sir Patrick Dun's Hospital rugby football team with the Hospitals' Cup in 1895.
Courtesy of the RCPI Heritage Centre.

Board of the Meath Hospital was directed to organise a picnic in connection
with the Football Club as an acknowledgement of their success in winning
the Hospitals' Cup.[125]

Occasionally there were tensions between sport and academic life. In
1898, the BMSA, in cooperation with the college sports clubs, approached
the College Council to request a Wednesday half-holiday for the purpose
of allowing students to play sport.[126] In 1908, the medical faculty at Trinity
College was petitioned to change the 'Half' examinations to April or
May and for afternoon lectures to be rearranged to the morning so that
medical students could partake in cricket practice.[127] Moreover, dedication
to sporting pursuits could sometimes have negative consequences for
students. P.A. Greene, a medical student and top athlete at University
College Galway, failed his second medical examination in autumn 1930. The
Students' Representative Council wrote to the Academic Council of UCG

125 'Meeting of the Medical Board June 23rd 1921', Minute Book, Medical Board of Meath
     Hospital, 1899–1937 [National Archives of Ireland].
126 Secretaries' Report of year 1898–9, BMSA Minute Book, November 1898–November
     1907 [QUB Special Collections].
127 'College Clubs: Cricket: the increasing demands of the professional schools', T.C.D.: A
     College Miscellany 14(241) (13 May 1908), p. 73.

requesting that Greene be allowed to pursue his third year lectures because he was 'among the foremost athletes in U.C.G. ... and highly esteemed for his social activities' among the students.[128] Somewhat surprisingly, but perhaps recognising Greene's importance to the athletics of the College, the Registrar of the university wrote to the National University of Ireland to request permission for Greene to pursue his course of study. Nonetheless, the Standing Committee responded with a letter stating that students who had not passed the second-year examination in medicine could not be permitted to continue into third year.[129] However, professors were not always so sympathetic. In 1908, J.P. Pye, the professor of anatomy and physiology at University College Galway, wrote a letter to the College Council in which he claimed that the working of his classes that session had been so unsatisfactory that he felt it his duty to write such a report. He complained about a lack of attendance at lectures and 'a change in tone' which he attributed directly to 'the encouragement given by the College to Athletics. I do not think the students who come here are in a position to indulge in the luxury of athletics ... but this is not all. I cannot help noticing certain concomitants of athletics which are an unmitigated evil, as well as a considerable nuisance to other people. It is the duty of the College to take note of such things'.[130] For the month of February, he noted six occasions when he had been present to give lectures on experimental physiology and the entire class had been absent.[131]

Nevertheless, in spite of these tensions, rugby remained popular amongst the students. Analogies between sport and war were prominent at British universities in the early twentieth century.[132] Rugby was often described by Irish students in militaristic terms, perhaps in an attempt further to promote an image of the doctor as heroic. In 1904, in one student magazine, it was depicted as 'jerseyed combat', while another piece, 18 years later, described how students in Galway carried a 'wounded comrade' with a 'bloody gash received on the rugger field' to the anatomy room where he was laid 'on a grimy

128 Letter from Students' Representative Council to the Academic Council of University College Galway, dated 1 October 1930 [University Archives, NUI Galway. Academic Council Minutes, 1/47].
129 Letter from the National University of Ireland Dublin to the Registrar, University College Galway, 16 October 1930 [University Archives, NUI Galway. Academic Council Minutes, 1/47].
130 Special report of the professor of anatomy and physiology, 10 March 1908 [NUI Galway Special Collections, BU/B/274].
131 Special report of the professor of anatomy and physiology.
132 Sonja Levsen, 'Constructing elite identities: university students, military masculinity and the consequences of the Great War in Britain and Germany', *Past & Present* 198 (2008), p. 154.

table beside the mutilated remains of what was once a man'.[133] The secretary's report for University College Cork's rugby club in 1909–10 described the game in militaristic terms: 'I can assure you that the red and black jerseyed brigade will be a force in Munster football, add lustre to College football fame and gladden the heart of many a veteran who on many a land fought and gathered the laurels of victory for the grand "old skull and cross bones"'.[134]

Rugby became central to an ideology of manliness in sport, as it promoted unselfishness, fearlessness and self-control.[135] These were qualities which were also expected of doctors in the period. There was also an important class element to the playing of rugby. Rugby was for the most part 'a homogenous, middle-class sport', with the exception being Limerick City, where rugby was more widely popularised owing to superior organisation there than in other cities in Ireland and a different ethos amongst its organisers 'towards the spread of the game'.[136] Murphy has suggested that at Queen's College Cork rugby 'had everything to do with hereditary professional position, exclusive education, leafy suburbs and desirable residences'.[137] Students were encouraged to play rugby because it fitted in with ideals and notions of respectability which were particularly important to the Irish medical profession. In 1914, a fictional letter from 'A Proud Parent to his son, a medical gyb' appeared in the *Quarryman*, stating:

> We all derived the hugest amusement from your account of the football matches. College men are famous the world over as footballers, and now that you are a full-blown member of their celebrated Rugby Club, you will naturally take a special pride in their achievements. The subscription (one guinea) *was* a bit thumping, but this only proves the select nature of the club, so don't worry about it. When a select club admits you to membership, you must not groan if such a club should make you pay through the nose for the privilege.[138]

Although fictional and satirical in nature, the piece emphasises the exclusive nature of the rugby teams of Irish medical schools and the fact that those

---

133 'Notes from the Medical School', *St. Stephen's: A Record of University Life* 2(2) (February 1904): 33 and 'Medical notes', *Galway University College Magazine* 2(9) (1922–3), p. 22.

134 Secretary's report, 1909–10, QCC Rugby Club Minutes [UCC University Archives, UC/MB/CS/RF/1].

135 J.A. Mangan, *The games ethic and imperialism: aspects of the differences of an ideal* (Harmondsworth: Viking, 1986), p. 23.

136 Rouse, *Sport and Ireland: a history*, p. 187.

137 Murphy, *Where Finbarr played*, p. 89.

138 'Letter from a Proud Parent to his son, a Medical Gyb', *Quarryman* 1(4) (March 1914), p. 87.

playing it were coming from a certain class. Indeed, rugby also had important cultural and class connotations: it was primarily viewed as an English sport, and one with associations with the professional classes. Although this period witnessed the popularisation of Gaelic sports, which McDevitt has argued were created as a means of refuting British influence, there is little evidence to suggest that medical students took a great interest in these.[139] The Gaelic Athletic Association (GAA), founded in 1884, enacted barriers to promote Gaelic sports in opposition to 'foreign games' such as cricket and rugby, such as between 1901 and 1905 when it decreed that anyone who played, promoted or attended 'foreign games' could not participate in the GAA.[140] In spite of this, rugby continued to be the sport of medical students and this continued even after the creation of the Irish Free State in 1922. The popularity of rugby may have been for a few reasons: first, rugby was more successful at embodying the characteristics expected of the Irish medical profession in the period and was a more bloody game than the Gaelic sports where the 'intellectual aspects of the game were paramount';[141] secondly, its class associations; and, finally, the fact that Irish practitioners were reliant on the British market for posts may have meant that they were less inclined to reject British games.[142] Nevertheless, not all medical students readily conformed to the stereotype of the sporting male student. The writer of a fictional account in 1913 mentioned 'a prolonged spell of hospital' following his first practice game.[143] Noël Browne, who studied at Trinity College Dublin in the 1930s, reluctantly played rugby 'mainly for the companionship'. He also hesitantly joined the boxing team but resigned from the 'silly and dangerous sport' after being filled with remorse after knocking another boxer unconscious.[144]

Involvement in sport occasionally had positive social and career consequences for budding doctors.[145] Smith, a medical student in *The Lion's Whelp*, gained popularity at Queen's for 'being a jolly fellow and a good football player'.[146] Bethel Solomons, captain of the Trinity College rugby

---

139 Patrick F. McDevitt, 'Muscular Catholicism: nationalism, masculinity and Gaelic team sports, 1884–1916', *Gender & History* 9(2) (1997), pp. 262–84.
140 Rouse, *Sport and Ireland: a history*, p. 210.
141 McDevitt, 'Muscular Catholicism', p. 278.
142 McDevitt has suggested that Gaelic sports and the opposition of British games marked the first step towards freedom from British control ('Muscular Catholicism', p. 278).
143 'The impressions of one "Abdullah"', p. 43.
144 Noël Browne, *Against the tide* (Dublin: Gill & Macmillan, 1986), p. 61.
145 M. Jeanne Peterson has suggested that for the London medical schools in the mid-nineteenth century 'more than one medical student's activities and prowess in the athletic realm brought him recognition as a sportsman and introductions that benefited his professional career' (*The medical profession in mid-Victorian London* (Berkeley: University of California Press, 1978), p. 62).
146 Irvine, *The lion's whelp*, p. 20.

team in the 1900s, went on to gain ten international caps for the Irish national team. He noted that being a good rugby player could affect one's choice of hospital and future career, remarking that 'scouting parties of housemen and senior students would visit the dissecting rooms to try and enlist good Rugby players' to join particular hospitals.[147] Following qualification, Solomons' sporting life influenced his career path. Because he was captain of the university football club, it was expected that he would remain in Dublin. He was also offered a commission in the Royal Army Medical Corps, 'like most other international rugby players at that time'.[148] Again, this suggests that the Irish medical profession was trying to encourage well-rounded, healthy men.

Women medical students were very much excluded from this male sporting world. 'Lady medicals' had the option of joining hockey and tennis clubs if they wished to take part in sporting activities, but there is little sense from the contemporary sources that they were involved to a great degree in these in the period in question. In fact, one critical editorial in *T.C.D.* in 1924 suggested that the 'corporate spirit is not inculcated in girls as it is in boys' and that '*esprit de corps* is lacking from their vocabulary'.[149] In response, a woman student argued that women had fewer facilities available to them for extra-curricular activities than men while also pointing out that the women's residence was several miles away from the College unlike the men's on-campus accommodation. Furthermore, she remarked that women students were 'firmly excluded from the real life of College' but that when 'any chance is given to them they only too willingly rise to meet the occasion'.[150] Ironically, it was often the female medical students who fundraised for improved sports facilities for the men students. In 1907, a group of Belfast medical students, in conjunction with their professors, organised a fete to raise money for a new athletic field; however, the president of the Students' Representative Council complained that the women students were the only ones showing a 'proper amount of zeal by organising a stall'.[151]

The Officers' Training Corps

Finally, it is also important to mention the Officers' Training Corps (OTC), which was established at Queen's College Belfast in 1908 and at the Royal College of Surgeons and Trinity College Dublin in 1910.[152] The point of

---

147 Bethel Solomons, *One doctor in his time* (London: Christopher Johnson, 1956), p. 41.
148 Bethel Solomons, 'Medical memories', *Irish Times*, 7 July 1952, p. 6.
149 Editorial, *T.C.D.: A College Miscellany* 29(507) (24 May 1923), p. 158.
150 Correspondence, *T.C.D.: A College Miscellany* 29(508) (31 May 1923), p. 176.
151 'Fete news: medical students' stall', *Q.C.B.* 8(4) (February 1907), p. 14.
152 'Officers' Training Corps: The Dublin Contingent', *Irish Times*, 10 May 1910, p. 9.

these was to provide students with military training with the idea that they would eventually apply for commissions in the Special Reserve of Officers or in the Territorial Force.[153] Men then wishing to serve in the army could be exempted from part of the probationary training or some examinations. The overall aim of the OTC was to ensure that there was a surplus of potential junior officers.[154] University professors were actively involved in these organisations. For instance, at the Royal College of Surgeons, Richard Dancer Purefoy, president of the College, and Frederick Conway Dwyer, professor of surgery and vice-president, acted as ex-officio members of the military education committee. Sir Thomas Myles, Sir Lambert Ormsby and other eminent members of the Irish medical profession acted as ordinary members of the military education committee.[155] Writing in 1921, H.E.R. James, Lieutenant-Colonel of the RAMC, advocated the benefits of the Officers' Training Corps to medical students and suggested that there should be specialised training for medical students to fit them with the skills necessary for field service as an army medical officer. This training, he suggested, 'should be as recreational as possible and calculated for the mental enlargement as well as the physical culture of the student'.[156] Furthermore, the benefits of involvement in an OTC for the student were thought to be numerous. James argued that students acquired an insight into subjects of 'supreme value' to a position in a State Medical Service, while the training received also helped to fill gaps in the ordinary curriculum. Moreover, students' organisational and discipline skills were developed, their 'habits of punctuality and the realisation of duty and responsibility' were also fostered, while they also received 'an annual airing in camp without expense, and with the greatest benefit to his health. He is a member of a corporate body within the University and his social relations with his comrades are of the pleasantest and most healthy kind'.[157]

The OTC instilled the traits of efficiency and discipline in students. At the Royal College of Surgeons, cadets were expected to attend at least 15 instructional parades each year, and to attend 30 of these if at recruit level. They were also expected to attend Camp for 15 days and to be present at

153 *Regulations for the Officers Training Corps, 1912* (London: Harrison and Sons, 1912), p. 7.

154 *Royal College of Surgeons, Ireland, Officers' Training Corps, Handbook, July 1913* (Dublin: Alex. Thom & Co., Abbey Street), p. 7.

155 *Royal College of Surgeons, Ireland, Officers' Training Corps, Handbook July 1913*, p. 1.

156 H.E.R. James, 'The best form of instruction for medical students to fit them to take their part in case of national emergency', *Proceedings of the Royal Society of Medicine* 14 (1921 (War Sect.), pp. 29–30.

157 James, 'The best form of instruction', p. 33.

the annual inspection and to obtain a uniform.[158] After one year's training, students could apply for Certificate A, and after two years for Certificate B.[159] In order to attain a certificate, students would undergo a written and an oral examination which addressed various aspects of army life, such as cavalry, artillery, infantry and medical concerns.[160] Uptake by students at the Royal College of Surgeons appears to have been enthusiastic. In 1918, there were three officers and 120 members in other ranks.[161] In 1917, a student at the Royal College of Surgeons claimed that the Officers' Training Corps characterised the *esprit de corps* of the medical school. That year, rates of recruitment had never been higher, and attendance at drills, parades and field days was also 'exceptionally good'.[162] Revealingly, this also gives an insight into the separatism that existed between the men and women students, with the men being involved in more 'masculine' activities such as the OTC and women in more suitably 'feminine' activities such as the Hockey Club. The formation of an Officers' Training Corps at University College Dublin was a contentious issue, and in 1929 a protest meeting was organised by students against the setting up of an OTC in the university.[163] The students who organised the meeting argued that the purpose of the university should be solely educational 'and that the obtrusion of a militaristic policy was invidious and not in keeping with the purposes for which the College was maintained as a national institution'. Moreover, the students argued that the formation of an OTC would produce disunity among the students.[164] The OTC continued to operate at the Royal College of Surgeons and Trinity College into the 1930s. In 1935, it was replaced by the Regiment of Pearse, which was part of the Volunteer Force.[165] There were Regiments of Pearse at University College Dublin, Trinity College, the Royal College of Surgeons, University College Cork and University College Galway.[166] These regiments further instilled the value of masculine traits in medical students while also reinforcing separatism between men and women.

158 *Royal College of Surgeons, Ireland, Officers' Training Corps, Handbook July 1913*, p. 4.
159 James, 'The best form of instruction', pp. 29–30.
160 *Regulations for the Officers Training Corps, 1912*, pp. 41–51.
161 'RCSI OTC Notes', *R.C.S.I. Students' Quarterly* 2(2) (June 1918), p. 16.
162 'Esprit de corps', *R.C.S.I. Students' Quarterly* 1(2) (May 1917), p. 28. Kirkpatrick collection: Clubs and Associations [RCPI Heritage Centre, TPCK/6/7/12].
163 'The Free State O.T.C.: Dublin students' opposition', *Irish Times*, 16 November 1929, p. 9.
164 'Students and O.T.C.: A resolution of protest', *Irish Times*, 22 November 1929, p. 8.
165 Terence O'Reilly, 'The FCA, 1946–2005', *History Ireland*, 19(4) (2011).
166 *Royal College of Surgeons in Ireland: Schools of Surgery, including Carmichael and Ledwich Schools handbook* (Dublin: University Press by Ponsoby and Gibbs, 1938 and 1939), p. 19.

Conclusion

The chapter has illustrated how various aspects of medical student culture were couched in a highly masculine rhetoric in the student press and subsequently in recollections in doctors' memoirs. Although women were treated in an egalitarian manner with regard to their educational experiences at Irish institutions, the increased emphasis on masculine activities and representations in student magazines which reinforced the male–female divide, and on rites of passage and transformation of boys to men, suggests underlying fears about the introduction of women to the medical profession. As Brown has suggested, in the nineteenth century, medical invocations of military masculinity might be seen as 'an attempt to construct medicine as an exclusively masculine domain to divest it of its domestic associations and to harvest forms of symbolic capital that were significantly less accessible to women'.[167] In the same way, it could be argued that with increasing numbers of women medical students entering Irish institutions from the 1880s onwards, sport and activities of a boisterous nature came to play a more prominent role as medical practitioners, amidst fears of an already overcrowded medical marketplace, attempted to cultivate a masculine image of the doctor. Furthermore, with increasing concerns about bedside manner, male medical students were increasingly encouraged to partake in sport in order to be better rounded, while doctors' memoirs and autobiographies highlight the playing of sport and pranks in order to support this image.

As Chapter 6 will illustrate, representations of men and women medical students in the student press were highly polarised, with male medical students generally represented as rowdy, boisterous and sport-loving, and women depicted as de-sexed, cold and studious, but always ready to play a supportive role to their male counterparts. Educational activities such as anatomy dissections and examinations were also described in masculine terms, while activities such as pranks, drinking, rags and sport further served to segregate women medical students from the men. All of these aspects display the hallmarks of homosociality – competition, emotional detachment and sexual objectification – and ultimately characterised Irish medicine as a largely male preserve. Segregation also played out subsequently in the careers of women doctors. Of a sample of women doctors who matriculated at Irish universities between 1885 and 1922, only 16 per cent were working in hospital appointments five years after graduation, with 70 per cent working in general practice.[168] As will be explored in more depth in the following

---

167   Brown, '"Like a devoted army"', p. 495.
168   Laura Kelly, *Irish women in medicine, c.1880s–1920s: origins, education and careers* (Manchester: Manchester University Press, 2012), p. 112.

chapter, although the first generation of Irish women doctors had broken new ground in entering medical schools, they found themselves subject to the confines of hegemonic masculinity in their student lives.

6

'This Feminine Invasion of Medicine': Women in Irish Medical Schools, c.1880–1945

Writing in his diary on 25 March 1935, James Lloyd Turner Graham, a student at the Royal College of Surgeons in Dublin, mused on the question of women in the medical profession:

Arose at 7:55. Went into college in Mr Robert's car. The anatomy room discussion, in one crowd, this morning was whether girls are successful doctors. I wonder do they. One never hears of them doing anything brilliant, but then there is only very few of them compared with fellows. Some say they are too tempremental [*sic*]. Some of them in the college do not seem to be very brilliant, yet they always pass their exams. I think they do not put much attention to anything too fickle, yet when it is necessary they can concentrate on the one thing and are strong-willed enough to exclude everything else. A fellow is not so strong willed and is more easily drawn away.[1]

Graham's remarks on women in the medical profession were nothing new. Since the question of women's admission to the medical profession had emerged in the late nineteenth century, women's suitability for medical study had been hotly debated by members of the medical profession and the general public. Arguments against women studying medicine were rooted in Victorian beliefs about women's physical, mental and emotional natures which found their origins in physiological theories from the late nineteenth century.[2] At the same time, those arguing in favour of women studying medicine suggested

---

1 Diary of James Lloyd Turner Graham, 1935 [RCPI Heritage Centre, BMS/48].
2 Laura Kelly, *Irish women in medicine, c.1880s–1920s: origins, education and careers* (Manchester: Manchester University Press, 2012), p. 22.

that women's emotional temperaments made them eminently suitable for a career in the field, particularly in the areas of women's and children's health, and that there were also opportunities for women doctors in the missionary field and in India.[3] Irish women's rise in the professions was slow. In the 1900s, teaching was the main option for female university graduates, and it was not until the First World War that a discernible change in attitude occurred with regard to women doctors in Britain and Ireland.

This chapter aims to explore the history of women in Irish medical schools from the 1880s up until the 1940s. I will provide some background regarding the history of women's entry to Irish medical schools, suggesting that Irish institutions, albeit in some cases for financial reasons, were largely supportive of women's admission to medical schools as well as hospitals for clinical experience. I will then outline women's educational and social experiences while studying medicine, suggesting that although women were for the most part treated in an egalitarian manner, they affirmed an identity which was very much separate from that of the male students. Moreover, the way in which women medical students were represented in Irish university magazines suggests that they were viewed by the male students in a specific way, and that even by the 1940s older concerns about the de-sexing effects of medical study on women were still prevalent. Finally, I will briefly discuss the experiences of medical missionary sisters who began to be a noticeable presence in the Irish medical student body from the 1940s. Ultimately, this chapter will highlight the experiences of the first generations of women medical students in Ireland. It will suggest that although they were readily integrated into the Irish student body and that Irish medical schools and hospitals appear to have welcomed them, women medical students occupied a separate sphere from the male students with regard to their social experiences.

Women's entry to Irish medical institutions

Historians of higher education in Ireland have drawn attention to the challenges and obstacles that women faced in gaining access to university education in the nineteenth century.[4] The Irish movement for the higher education of women was strongly inspired by the English movement which

---

3 Kelly, *Irish women in medicine*, pp. 24–7.
4 See, for instance, Judith Harford, *The opening of university education to women in Ireland* (Dublin: Irish Academic Press, 2008); Susan M. Parkes, *A danger to the men: a history of women in Trinity College Dublin, 1904–2004* (Dublin: Lilliput Press, 2004); Eileen Breathnach, 'Women and higher education in Ireland (1879–1914)', *Crane Bag* 4(1) (1980), pp. 47–54.

had been led by pioneers such as Emily Davies.[5] Although women were not admitted to Irish universities, from 1869, they could take Examinations for Women in both Trinity College and the Queen's Colleges. These were aimed at secondary school level, but nevertheless demonstrated to university authorities that women were capable of academic excellence. In addition, the activism of pioneering women such as Isabella Tod and Margaret Byers, who established the Ladies Collegiate School (1859) and the Belfast Ladies Institute (1867) respectively, also helped to pave the way for women's inclusion in higher education in Ireland.[6] With the foundation of the Royal University of Ireland in 1879, women could now take the examinations of that body, following private study, but they could not attend university classes at the Queen's Colleges until the 1880s, while Trinity College did not admit women until 1904.[7]

The difficulties that British and American women faced in gaining medical qualifications and access to medical education has been well documented.[8] In Britain, Dr Elizabeth Blackwell, who had studied at Geneva College, New York became the first woman doctor to have her name placed on the Medical Register in 1858 because of a special clause that allowed those in possession of a foreign degree to register.[9] The second was Elizabeth Garrett Anderson. Garrett Anderson had faced a huge amount of opposition in her quest to study medicine, not only from medical schools, which refused to admit her, but also from British licensing bodies which would not permit her to take their examinations.[10] She studied privately and eventually became a licentiate of the Society of Apothecaries, which allowed her to sit their examinations, and had her name placed on the Medical Register in 1865. The Society of Apothecaries refused to admit persons who had undertaken private study after this, and with no way of gaining a medical qualification, British women had no means of having their names placed on the Medical Register.[11] What followed was almost a decade of credentialist and legalistic

5 Susan M. Parkes and Judith Harford, 'Women and higher education in Ireland', in Deirdre Raftery and Susan M. Parkes (eds), *Female education in Ireland, 1700–1900: Minerva or Madonna* (Dublin: Irish Academic Press, 2007), p. 105.
6 Parkes and Harford, 'Women and higher education in Ireland', p. 107.
7 Parkes and Harford, 'Women and higher education in Ireland', pp. 109–10.
8 See, for instance, Catriona Blake, *Charge of the parasols: women's entry into the medical profession* (London: Women's Press, 1990); Anne Witz, *Professions and patriarchy* (London: Routledge, 1992); Regina M. Morantz-Sanchez, *Sympathy and science: women physicians in American medicine* (Chapel Hill: University of North Carolina Press, 1985); Ellen Singer More, *Restoring the balance: women physicians and the practice of medicine, 1850–1995* (Cambridge, Mass.: Harvard University Press, 1999).
9 Witz, *Professions and patriarchy*, p. 80.
10 Witz, *Professions and patriarchy*, pp. 80–3.
11 Witz, *Professions and patriarchy*, p. 83.

tactics by aspiring British women doctors who wished to gain entry to the medical profession.[12]

Although it has been argued that aspiring women doctors in Ireland 'met the same determined opposition and prejudice from the medical establishment' as elsewhere, it is evident that the first generations of women doctors found the Irish medical hierarchy to be peculiarly open-minded with regard to the question of women's admission and with regard to their educational experiences.[13] The King and Queen's College of Physicians in Ireland (KQCPI), later the Royal College of Physicians of Ireland, was the first institution in the United Kingdom to take advantage of the Enabling Act and admit women who had undertaken their medical studies abroad to their licentiate examinations in 1877. The role of the KQCPI in the registration of early British women doctors has been seriously underplayed by historians. The first women to take advantage of the KQCPI's leniency were British doctors who had studied abroad. Eliza Louisa Walker Dunbar was the first to qualify with a licence from the KQCPI in January 1877.[14] She was followed by many others, including the English doctor Sophia Jex-Blake, a leading campaigner for women's admission to the medical profession. Jex-Blake had been encouraged to study medicine after working at the New England Hospital for Women and Children in Boston in 1862 and being inspired by Lucy Sewell, a pioneer American physician. Jex-Blake applied to study medicine at Harvard University in 1867 but was rejected. She returned to Britain and was accepted by the medical school of the University of Edinburgh in 1869. However, as has been well documented by historians, Jex-Blake and her cohort, later named 'The Edinburgh Seven', encountered many obstacles and difficulties while studying at Edinburgh and were told in 1873 that they would not be allowed to qualify with medical degrees from the university.[15] Jex-Blake and some of her colleagues went to the University of Bern. She graduated with an MD

---

12 Witz, *Professions and patriarchy*, pp. 86–99.
13 F.O.C. Meenan, *Cecilia Street: the Catholic University School of Medicine 1855–1931* (Dublin: Gill & Macmillan, 1987), p. 81. Similarly, more recently, Irene Finn has argued that the Irish medical profession, with the exception of the King and Queen's College of Physicians in Ireland (KQCPI), held a hostile view towards women in medicine (see Irene Finn, 'Women in the medical profession in Ireland, 1876–1919', in Bernadette Whelan (ed.), *Women and Paid Work in Ireland, 1500–1930* (Dublin: Four Courts Press, 2000), pp. 102–19).
14 Kelly, *Irish women in medicine*, p. 39.
15 Kelly, *Irish women in medicine*, p. 20. For more on the story of the 'Edinburgh Seven', see Anne Crowther and Marguerite Dupree, *Medical lives in the age of surgical revolution* (Cambridge: Cambridge University Press, 2007), pp. 152–75. For Sophia Jex-Blake, see S. Roberts, *Sophia Jex-Blake: a woman pioneer in nineteenth-century medical reform* (London: Routledge, 1993).

degree in 1877. However, owing to the regulations of the Medical Act, a 'foreign' degree would not enable a doctor to practise medicine in Britain. Meanwhile, two politicians, Russell Gurney and William Francis Cowper-Temple, who supported women's admission to the medical profession, actively campaigned for legislation to allow this. In 1876, Gurney's Enabling Act was passed by the British parliament, 'enabling' all of the nineteen recognised medical examining bodies to accept women but stating that they were not obliged to do so. The KQCPI became the first institution to take advantage of this new legislation, thus offering women doctors a means of qualifying as registered medical practitioners.[16] Sophia Jex-Blake described this decision as 'the turning point in the whole struggle'.[17] The decision of the KQCPI was arguably the result of a combination of factors: an atmosphere of liberality with regard to women's higher education which existed in Dublin; the fact that women were already being admitted to Irish hospitals to gain their clinical experiences; and, finally and probably most significantly, the question of the financial gain which the KQCPI could make from the fees charged to women graduates.

Dublin institutions had a history of open-mindedness with regard to women in higher education. Women had been admitted to the Museum of Irish Industry which organised public lectures and courses on scientific subjects from the 1850s.[18] Women were also admitted to the Royal College of Science in Dublin from its opening year in 1867.[19] One writer to the Irish newspaper *The Freeman's Journal* in 1870 commented that Dublin had 'achieved honour in other countries by its liberality to ladies in connection with the Royal College of Science' and hoped that the Dublin medical schools would soon follow the example set by Paris and (briefly) Edinburgh.[20] The Royal College of Science offered a Diploma Associate and the RUI also recognised some of the courses offered by the college.[21] Moreover, Catholic and Protestant secondary schools for girls which emerged in the late nineteenth century were also crucial in helping to spearhead the Irish

16 Kelly, *Irish women in medicine*, p. 20.
17 Sophia Jex-Blake, *Medical women: a thesis and a history* (Edinburgh: Oliphant, Anderson & Ferrier, 1886), p. 204. For more on this, see Laura Kelly, '"The turning point in the whole struggle": the admission of women to the King and Queen's College of Physicians in Ireland', *Women's History Review* 22(1) (2013): 97–125.
18 Clara Cullen, 'The museum of Irish industry, Robert Kane and education for all in the Dublin of the 1850s and 1860s', *History of Education* 38(1) (2009), p. 106.
19 Clara Cullen, 'The museum of Irish industry (1845–1867): research environment, popular museum and community of learning in mid-Victorian Ireland' (unpublished PhD thesis, University College Dublin, 2008).
20 'Letter to the Editor', *Freeman's Journal*, 28 January 1870, p. 4. This was before the University of Edinburgh changed its mind with regard to women medical students.
21 Parkes and Harford, 'Women and higher education in Ireland', p. 117.

women's higher education movement.[22] As Parkes and Harford have shown, the development of higher education for women in Ireland was closely connected with the expansion of intermediate education for girls in the country.[23] Catholic and Protestant schools instilled a sense of vocation in young women but also encouraged their students to pursue educational goals and university education.

More generally, it could be said that women also played an important and visible role in Irish hospitals. Catholic sisterhoods had a crucial role in the secondary education of young women in Ireland but were also responsible for the management of Irish hospitals. In contrast with Britain, the majority of hospitals in Ireland were founded by Catholic sisterhoods.[24] Within these hospitals, the religious sisters were responsible for the nursing care, hygiene and hospital management.[25] As Sioban Nelson's comparative study of religious sisters in nineteenth-century hospitals has shown, nuns 'pioneered the path for women through the moral contagion of sickness', illustrating that women could be trusted in roles of authority, while also demonstrating how women 'could work among male bodies and the sick poor without loss of status'.[26] In Ireland, religious sisters occupied a semi-separate sphere in the context of hospital management and nursing in Ireland while male doctors were responsible for the medical care. Recognising the vital role of nuns in the management and nursing care within Irish hospitals, it is possible that the Irish medical and religious hierarchy recognised a role for women as doctors and the need for women doctors to tend to women patients. There were important class distinctions between medicine and nursing, however. Nursing was not always viewed as being a suitable career for middle-class women in the nineteenth century. Aside from the nursing work done by nuns in the late nineteenth century, the rest was undertaken mostly by poor women without training who were remunerated for their work with maintenance within the hospital.[27] This began to change from the 1890s with the emergence of nurse training schemes in Dublin hospitals and the

---

22 Judith Harford, 'The movement for the higher education of women in Ireland: gender equality or denominational rivalry?', *History of Education* 35 (2005), pp. 499–500.
23 Parkes and Harford, 'Women and higher education in Ireland', p. 105.
24 For example, the Irish Sisters of Charity founded St Vincent's Hospital in 1833 for the care of the sick poor in Dublin. The Sisters of Mercy founded the Mercy Hospital in Cork in 1857 and the Mater Misericordiae Hospital in Dublin in 1861 (see Gerard M. Fealy, *A history of apprenticeship nurse training in Ireland* (New York: Routledge, 2006), p. 9).
25 Fealy, *A history of apprenticeship nurse training in Ireland*, p. 9.
26 Sioban Nelson, *Say little, do much: nursing, nuns and hospitals in the nineteenth century* (Philadelphia: University of Pennsylvania Press, 2003), p. 164.
27 Maria Luddy, *Women and philanthropy in nineteenth-century Ireland* (Cambridge: Cambridge University Press, 1995), p. 51.

emergence of the 'lady nurse'.[28] However, medicine still remained a more financially lucrative career choice for middle-class women and would also have provided some with a means of social mobility.

Another significant reason for the liberality of the KQCPI, however, was arguably the financial gain that the institution could make from fees from women students. As Samuel Haughton, member of the Council of the KQCPI remarked in 1879, when asked about the question of women's admission to other licensing bodies:

> There are two doors open for women in England, and one in Ireland, and there is no chance whatever of their being closed; the College of Physicians in Ireland will receive them all, and the Apothecaries' Hall in England will receive them, and so will the University of London; and I have no doubt whatever that as soon as it becomes generally known that there is money to be made on them, some of the Scotch bodies will open their doors too.[29]

The KQCPI relied significantly on fees from licences and the potential income to be derived from female doctors may have been important in their decision. Also important in the story of women's admission to the KQCPI is the fact that the College Council in the 1870s was composed of senior members of the Irish medical profession who happened to be in favour of the admission of women to the profession, among them Samuel Haughton, Aquilla Smith and Samuel Gordon.[30]

The KQCPI was integral in the licensing of early British women doctors in the late nineteenth century. Of the first twenty-six women to have their names placed on the Medical Register, twenty-four had received their licences from the KQCPI.[31] Following the admission of women to the King and Queen's College of Physicians, Irish medical schools soon followed suit and admitted women to study medicine in their classes. In October 1879, the College Council of Queen's College Galway decided to allow women to enter the university, although no woman studied medicine there until 1902. Queen's College Cork permitted the admission of women from 1883, although its first female medical student enrolled in 1890. Women could attend the Royal College of Surgeons from 1884. The first female medical student at Queen's College Belfast began her studies in 1888. Women

---

28 Fealy, *A history of apprenticeship nurse training in Ireland*, pp. 68–9.
29 Special report from the Select Committee on the Medical Act (1858) Amendment (no.3) Bill [Lords], together with the proceedings of the committee, minutes of evidence and appendix, 1878–9 (320), Q. 3507, p. 245.
30 Kelly, 'The turning point', pp. 16–17.
31 Kelly, *Irish women in medicine*, p. 11.

could attend the Catholic University Medical School at Cecilia Street from 1898.[32] Trinity College lagged behind, admitting women to its classes from 1904. Lily Baker became the first medical graduate from Trinity College in 1906.[33] By contrast, the majority of British universities did not admit women until the 1890s and 1900s, with the exception of the University of London, which permitted women to take medical degrees from 1878. There were no graduates from that university until 1882, however, when Mary Ann Scharlieb and Edith Shove graduated following study at the London School of Medicine for Women which had been established by Sophia Jex-Blake in 1874. Other British universities were slower to open up their medical classes to women. The University of Bristol admitted women in 1891, the University of Glasgow in 1892, and the University of Durham in 1893, while Oxford and Cambridge allowed waited until 1916 and 1917 respectively.[34]

Representations of 'lady medicals'

The number of women students matriculating at Irish medical schools was initially low. In the ten-year period between 1885 and 1895, only 41 women matriculated at Irish medical schools.[35] However, numbers attending university were low nationally in this period. In 1901, just 3,259 people out of a population of 4.5 million were at university; of these, 91 were women.[36] The number of women medical students gradually increased during the early years of the twentieth century, peaking, as they did in Britain, during the First World War, before declining again after the war. At Queen's College Belfast, for example, 1 in 20 medical students in 1912 was female, while by 1918 this was 1 in 4.[37] Women medical students, being in the minority, stood out in the medical student body and were often characterised in a certain way. The student press allows an insight into constructions of femininity and masculinity. As Sarah Jane Aiston has shown in her study of the student press at the University of Liverpool between 1944 to 1979, women students were represented as the 'other' and tended to be stereotyped in a negative manner up until 1959. Female students were represented in the student press as being

32 Kelly, *Irish women in medicine*, p. 44.
33 Kelly, *Irish women in medicine*, p. 174.
34 Kelly, 'The turning point', p. 100.
35 Kelly, *Irish women in medicine*, p. 68.
36 Susan M. Parkes, 'Higher education, 1793–1908', in W.E. Vaughan (ed.), *A New History of Ireland*, vol.6, *Ireland under the Union II, 1870–1921* (Oxford: Clarendon Press, 1996), p. 540.
37 Kelly, *Irish women in medicine*, p. 69.

unattractive and at university in order to find a husband.[38] In Ireland, women medical students were often thought to have a 'civilising' effect on the male student body. Janthe Leggett, who studied at Dr Steevens' Hospital in the 1870s, remarked in a letter to Sophia Jex-Blake, that Professor Macnamara, the president of the Royal College of Physicians, believed that the presence of women students 'would refine the classes'.[39] In the contemporary student press, women medical students were often figures of fun. Crucially, there were important distinctions between representations of male and female medical students. As Raewyn Connell has argued, 'masculinity' does not exist except in contrast with 'femininity', with men and women being treated as the 'bearers of polarized character types'.[40] Furthermore, depictions of medical students were fundamentally different from those of students from other disciplines. In the world of Irish universities, medical students were a noticeable presence, standing out from the rest of the student population, and a variety of accounts describing the 'typical' male medical student exist in student magazines of the early twentieth century. Usually in these accounts, the male medical student is depicted as boisterous, sporty and extremely sociable. For example, *Q.C.B.* in 1907 highlighted the importance of medical students to the social life and collegial culture of the university:

> However we account for it, the fact remains that the medical student is the living force in Queen's College. Whether it is Students' Night or a concert in the Ulster Hall he shows his loyalty to Queen's in that impressive way which attracts the attention of the merchant princes of the city no less than the tram conductor. His soul and body are in the College – the souls of some men are in the clouds. He is proud of the Medical School of Belfast, and the distinguished Professors at its head. He glories in the athletic triumphs of the College and his ardent wish is to see Queen's second to none in all manly sports.[41]

While the medical student here is depicted as a sociable character, proud of his university and willing to partake in a range of social activities from students' nights to concerts to sports, other sources singled medical students out for their enjoyment of mischief and prank-playing.

38 Sarah Jane Aiston, '"A woman's place …": male representations of university women in the student press of the University of Liverpool, 1944–1979', *Women's History Review* 15(1) (2006), pp. 3–34.

39 Sophia Jex-Blake, *Medical women: two essays* (Edinburgh: William Oliphant & Co., 1872), p. 143.

40 R.W. Connell, *Masculinities*, 2nd edn (Berkeley: University of California Press, 2005), p. 68.

41 'The medical student (by an outsider)', *Q.C.B.* 8(6) (April 1907), p. 5.

Women medical students, on the other hand, were generally represented as being better behaved, more studious and harder working than their male counterparts. Medical professors also upheld such representations. Speaking to students of the London School of Medicine for Women in 1938, Lord Thomas Horder (1871–1955) commented that 'women were more thorough, more industrious, more studious and, as a sex, were more curious than men. This curiosity, he pointed out, had already borne fruit in the hands of those women who had made their names in research'.[42]

As Alison Bashford's work has shown, women doctors in the nineteenth century presented themselves as scientific experts in order to differentiate themselves from unprofessional groups such as midwives and nurses. However, this meant that women doctors also gained a reputation for being cold and came to be seen as de-sexed.[43] The perceived dehumanising and de-sexing effects of medical study on women were regularly referred to in the student press. One article in *Q.C.B.* in 1905 remarked that the discharge of the duties of a doctor or surgeon would result in a loss of womanliness for the female doctor.[44] 'Lady medicals' were commonly characterised as 'aloof' and cold, with one article in the *National Student* in 1913 referring to one female student as 'learned in the extreme and preserving the dignified hauteur, not to say aloofness, which appertains to her position as an Arts Graduate'.[45] Such descriptions of women medical students helped to mark them out as the other. A poem published in 1917 from the perspective of a male student described how his medical student girlfriend had become cold due to her studies, and any attempts by him to romance her were met with scientific-sounding responses.[46] In 1918, a piece in the *National Student* mocked the cold demeanour of the 'lady medical'. In a fictional incident that occurred between a student named 'Cherubia', whose subject in the dissecting room began speaking to her, Cherubia retorted to the cadaver 'Sir!!!! Perhaps you are not aware that in U.C.D. an unwritten law allows a man to speak to a *lady* only when they have been introduced at least seven times'.[47]

'Lady medicals' were also sexually objectified as objects of romantic interest. A poem published in *T.C.D.* in 1922 from the perspective of a male student whose girlfriend had started in the medical school, mentioned how

42 'Inadequate training facilities', *Irish Examiner*, 7 October 1938, p. 7.
43 Alison Bashford, *Purity and pollution: gender, embodiment, and Victorian medicine* (London: Macmillan, 1999).
44 'Winsome woman at Q.C.B.', *Q.C.B.* 6(3) (20 January 1905), p. 7.
45 'The impressions of one "Abdullah", first year student of medicine', *National Student* 3(2) (May 1913), p. 43.
46 For instance, on being asked if he could press her 'hand of snow', the female student replied 'Your brachial artery is half a beat too slow'. 'To a surgeon's girl', *RCSI Students' Quarterly* 1(1) (February 1917), p. 12.
47 'A celebrity in Cecilia Street', *National Student* 8(20) (March 1918), p. 15.

she now 'chatters of death with an air quite cool' and spent her time talking about spleens, ducts and foramina.

'Sic Transit ...'

My Lady is now in the Medical School,
Woe is me! Woe is me!
And she chatters of death with an air quite cool,
Woe is me! Woe is me!
She trips every morning, slender and sweet,
To explore a grey corpse in a winding sheet,
And she carries old bones in her reticule –
For My Lady is now in the Medical School.
Ah, woe is me!
My Lady is dressed in a long white coat,
Woe is me! Woe is me!
She looks upon me as a regular goat,
Woe is me! Woe is me!
She talks about spleens, not omitting to ram in a
Word here and there about ducts and foramina,
An Arts' man she thinks has his head filled with wool,
For My Lady is now in the Medical School.
Ah woe is me!
She passes me by with a haughty stare,
Woe is me! Woe is me!
With an I-know-something-that-you-don't-air
Woe is me! Woe is me!
She gave me a parcel one day on the train
I thought it held sweets – who'd have guessed at a brain,
And she horribly laughed when I flinched like a fool,
For My Lady is now in the Medical School,
Ah, woe is me!
My Lady greets me no more in the square,
Woe is me! Woe is me!
My Lady, still so stabbingly fair,
Woe is me! Woe is me!
I once asked her humbly why did she think that o'me
And she quoted a passage from someone's Anatomy.
Yet I weep for her still, though our love has grown cool,
When I think of her down in the Medical School.
Ah, woe is me![48]

48 'Sic transit ...', *T.C.D.: A College Miscellany* 29(496) (23 November 1922), p. 30.

Although a comical poem, it nevertheless gives an insight into contemporary fears about the hardening effects of medical education on women and the idea that women might become too masculine through the study of medicine. Such poems, which used humour to convey the idea that medical education would potentially result in a loss of womanliness, also reinforced the male/female divide.

Conscientiousness was also thought to come at a cost to these women's physical appearances. Oliver St John Gogarty, in his autobiography, referred to two female students in his class in the 1900s as 'breastless, defeminised, with dry hair'.[49] In a ballad entitled 'Ragtime Ballade for 1st year medicals', which appeared in *T.C.D.* magazine in 1917, women medical students 'trotted' to class, 'with big suit-cases, and unwashed faces, lest they should miss the first roll-call'.[50] Less common were pieces which portrayed women medical students as being obsessed with their appearance and the pursuit of a husband. A 'diary fragment' of one female student, published in the *R.C.S.I.: A Students' Quarterly* in 1917, portrayed the fictional 'lady medical' as being more interested in her physical appearance than her studies and also easily swayed by the comments of men. For instance, when a man tells her he 'didn't appreciate the taste' of her face powder, she made a note to 'get good juicy lemon at Knowles to-morrow and add a few drops per box'.[51] In 1931, in the *Northman*, a short-lived student newspaper of Queen's College Belfast, a deeply sexist poem entitled 'Lines written on the new lady doctor of Ballykinskeeny, Co. Antrim', written from the perspective of a local man from the village, lamented the replacement of the old village doctor, Doctor Bell, with a new lady doctor called Muir. Muir was criticised for her short skirts, affinity for cocktails and physical appearance ('bandy legs'), with the author stating: 'The country roun' it laughs and gegs at "doctors" now'. The poem also claimed that the reason she became a doctor was because she 'failed tae hook a man'.[52] Women students were often judged on their appearances – in particular, first-year students. In 1901, *St. Stephen's* reported the arrival of 'three or four of the fair sex', commenting: 'if one can judge from appearances, the new-comers may be relied upon to keep up the good record which their predecessors have made'.[53] Similarly, in 1915, the

49   Oliver St John Gogarty, *It isn't this time of year at all! An unpremeditated autobiography* (London: Sphere Books, 1983), p. 31.
50   'Ragtime Ballade for 1st year medicals, entitled Dixie', *T.C.D.: A College Miscellany* 23(395) (7 February 1917), p. 68.
51   'Diary fragment', 'College Notes', *R.C.S.I. Students' Quarterly* 1(3) (November 1917), p. 53.
52   'Lines written on the new lady doctor of Ballykinskeeny, Co Antrim', *The Northman* 3(1) (January 1931), p. 29.
53   'Notes from "The School"', *St. Stephen's: A Record of University Life* 1(3) (December

Quarryman reported, 'as for the new lady medicals, why – bless their pretty faces! – we have a record crowd of them this session ... We also watch with interest the growing rivalry for their favours between the 1st and 3rd year men'.[54]

Despite the fact that women medical students were often represented as studious, bookish, and at times, cold and defeminised, they were nonetheless viewed as having a supportive and nurturing role to play – 'always ready to oblige a young man when in difficulties'.[55] In this way, female medical students could be said to have been complying with patriarchy through emphasised femininity.[56] In spite of their often derogatory comments towards female medical students, authors regularly conceded that they had a positive role to play in university life. 'Lady medicals' at *Q.C.B.* in 1905 were commended for the patronage of the magazine, their support of the Union, and 'in affording "Mere man" a splendid opportunity at showing the world what a tolerant individual he is'.[57] Women assisted men, for example, through going to football matches or through organising fundraising efforts for male activities. *T.C.D.* reported in 1925 that although the women took no part in the 'rag' that year, 'their presence and their evident appreciation and enjoyment of the actions and speeches of the different characters made everything much more pleasant than it would otherwise have been'.[58]

It was perceived that there were opportunities for women to carve out a niche of practice for themselves, in spite of an increasingly overcrowded medical marketplace from the late nineteenth century onwards. *The Ballina Herald* reported in 1930 that the number of female students was considerably lower that year than it had been a decade previously, this being a result of 'the prevailing financial distress in the professional classes ... a medical training being lengthy and far from inexpensive'. Nevertheless, it acknowledged that 'Medicine as a career for girls, however, appears to be promising, all qualified women having plenty of work to do'.[59] Furthermore, there was still a demand for women doctors in the missionary field. Reverend Dr Kennedy, the Protestant Bishop of Chota Nagpur, India, speaking at the annual meeting of the Women's Work, S.P.G., in Dublin in 1934, commented that the lack of provision of hospital and medical facilities for Indian women was 'scandalous' and that he 'could not understand why

1901), p. 56.
54 'Medical notes', *Quarryman* 3(1) (December 1915), p. 15.
55 'Types of medical students', *Q.C.B.* (April 1915), p. 19.
56 R.W. Connell and James W. Messerschmidt, 'Hegemonic masculinity: rethinking the concept', *Gender & Society* 19(6) (December 2005), p. 848.
57 'Winsome woman', p. 7.
58 Editorial, *T.C.D.: A College Miscellany* 31(545) (11 June 1925), p. 181.
59 'Women medical students', *Ballina Herald*, 9 August 1930, p. 1.

the medical women in Ireland and England could be content to take the jobs that most of them had – looking after schoolchildren's eyes and teeth – while their sisters in India suffered for want of the facilities they could give them'.[60]

Educational experiences

Florence Stewart, who began her studies at Queen's University Belfast in 1927, wrote in her memoirs: 'When I studied in 1927 there were 10 girls and possibly 50–60 men. We sat in the front row of the lecture theatre, the only occasion I can remember is when we were asked to leave the room when some sex problems were to be discussed'.[61]

Stewart's recollections highlight a few interesting points – that female students were in the minority, but that the programme of lectures was inclusive with the exception of a class on 'sex problems', which appears to have been deemed too indelicate for female students' ears. Her quote also draws attention to the fact that even though male and female students were educated together, female students occupied a separate space in the lecture theatre. This practice appears to have been common at other Irish medical schools. A photograph of a class of medical students at University College Cork in 1918, for instance, shows a class of 67 students with five women seated in the first seats of the front row with two men at the end (Figure 8). The rest of the male class are seated in the rows behind.[62]

Historians of women in the medical profession have drawn attention to the sense of separatism that women doctors faced in their educational experiences and later in their professional lives.[63] Unlike many British and American medical schools, Irish women were educated alongside male students. For instance, in Britain, women were initially educated at single-sex medical schools such as the London School of Medicine for Women (founded in 1874) and the Edinburgh School of Medicine for Women (founded in 1886). These two institutions were largely responsible for the medical education of British women up until the opening of other British medical schools from the 1890s. However, even when medical schools opened their doors to women students it remained the case that women were

60 'India wants women doctors', *Irish Independent*, 18 October 1934, p. 11.
61 Florence Stewart memoirs [PRONI D3612/3/1].
62 Photograph of medical students at University College Cork, *c.*1918 [Medical Mission Sisters Archives, London].
63 See, for example, Virginia G. Drachman, 'The limits of progress: the professional lives of women doctors, 1881–1926', *Bulletin of the History of Medicine* 60(1) (1986), pp. 58–72.

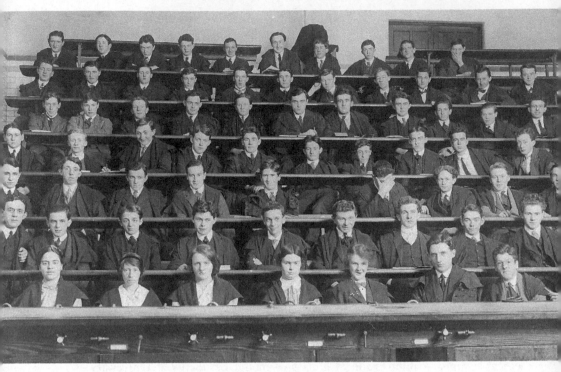

8   Group of students, including Anna Dengel
(bottom row, first from the left), at University College Cork c.1918.
From the Anna Dengel collection.
Courtesy of the Medical Missions Sisters Archive.

educated separately. For example, at the University of Birmingham, women students were educated separately from the men when they were admitted in 1900.[64] Irish medical schools do not appear to have taken any issue with educating men and women students together, with the exception of anatomy dissections. Monsignor Molloy, in a report on the Catholic University Medical School in 1907, reported that he had 'taken pains to ascertain whether any practical inconvenience has arisen from having women in our Medical School and I am informed that there has been none whatsoever', although he mentioned that the school had limited space due to the high number of medical students.[65] The *Irish Times* reported in 1922 that at Trinity College, University College and the Royal College of Surgeons,

64 Jonathan Reinarz, *Health care in Birmingham: the Birmingham teaching hospitals, 1779–1939* (Woodbridge: Boydell Press, 2009), p. 161.
65 *Progress of the Catholic University School of Medicine, 1907* (Dublin: Humphrey and Armour Printers, undated), p. 25.

'men and women are trained together without the slightest awkwardness'. The *Irish Times* argued that an objection to the mixed teaching of medical students 'is as belated as would be nowadays an objection to women cyclists or women hockey-players'.[66] Referring to her experiences of mixed classes at the Royal College of Surgeons in Dublin, student Clara Williams remarked very positively that, 'Here the classes have been found productive of nothing but good, and they are helping in a large measure to destroy the prejudice against women studying medicine. The present generation of medical men having been educated with women, regard them exactly as their other fellow-students, and respect them according to their merits and capabilities, which is all any of us desire'.[67]

The British Medical Journal in 1931 lamented that in London

the only schools open to medical women students are the London School of Medicine for Women and, to a modified extent, University College Hospital and King's College Hospital, which last-named has again opened its doors to women students during the past year. It is felt that such a state of affairs can only be temporary and hopes can be entertained that in the near future the principle of co-education will prevail in the capital.[68]

However, Irish hospitals also allowed women students on their wards apparently without any difficulties. For example, at Dr Steevens' Hospital in Dublin, Janthe Leggett, a student at the University of Edinburgh, was admitted to the hospital for its clinical classes from November 1869 to summer 1873. In a letter to Sophia Jex-Blake, Leggett explained that she had been granted the unanimous consent of the Board of Dr Steevens' Hospital to pursue her clinical studies there. Moreover, she had been treated in a civil manner by the male students at the hospital.[69] In 1887, two women students applied to get access to the Adelaide Hospital, and the Medical Board agreed to this and expressed that they wished it to be understood that 'Lady Students will be treated in all respects as the other members of the class, and that the clinical teaching shall in no respect be modified or changed on account of the presence of ladies'.[70] Similarly, at the Royal Victoria Hospital in Belfast, the question of the admission of female students was

66 'Women medicals', *Irish Times*, 3 March 1922, p. 4.
67 Clara Williams, 'A short account of the school of medicine for men and women, RCSI, by Clara L Williams', *Magazine of the LSMW and RFH* 3 (January 1896), p. 109.
68 'Women in medicine', *British Medical Journal*, 5 September 1931, p. 453.
69 Jex-Blake, *medical women*, p. 143.
70 Medical board meeting, 30 September 1887, Medical Board Minute Book: 5 May 1880–7 June 1900, p. 237 [TCD Manuscripts, IE TCD MS 11270/2/3/3/3].

brought up at a meeting in September 1889, and the members of the board decided that there should be no restrictions or objections made on their admission.[71] Likewise, at the Meath Hospital, a student named Miss Greene was allowed to enter the hospital for clinical experience after the passing of a resolution by the medical board that 'female medical students be admitted to the practice of the hospital on precisely the same terms as male medical students'.[72] Additionally, women were able to hold the positions of clinical clerks and surgical dressers in the same way as men.

It is possible again that the lucrative issue of fees tempted Irish hospitals to open their wards to women students. Many of the Irish voluntary hospitals were in a poor financial state in the late nineteenth and early twentieth centuries, as is attested in their institutional histories. These hospitals, which included St Vincent's, as well as the Mater Misericordiae, the Adelaide Hospital, the Rotunda Lying-In Hospital, Dr Steevens' Hospital, the Coombe Lying-In Hospital and the Royal Victoria Eye and Ear Hospital, all located in Dublin, had been founded by philanthropic bodies. The institutions were run by a committee of local subscribers, with additional funds coming from grants from grand juries or municipal corporations. Accordingly, therefore, the admission of women students to the wards of Irish hospitals made sound financial sense, as it increased income from teaching fees.[73] Irish hospitals could also gain from fees paid by British women doctors who were unable to gain clinical experience in British hospitals. Octavia Wilberforce went to the Rotunda Hospital in July and August 1918 in order to gain practical midwifery experience. While there, she remarked on the pervading atmosphere of equality between the sexes:

> The best part of this place is the way men and women work together, and the younger men, Simpson, Gilmour and English make one feel just as capable as the men students ... Here in Dublin, men and women students have worked together at Trinity College for years. At Arthur Ball's hospital [Sir Patrick Dun's] I was so pleased to see the perfect naturalness and equality of men and women. They forget half the time that there's any difference between the men and women students, and that's what you need in Medicine. Equality and absence of sex.[74]

71 Royal Victoria Hospital, Medical Staff Minutes, 1875–1905, 10 September 1889, p. 205 [Royal Victoria Hospital Archives].
72 Meeting of Medical Board, 29 November 1888, Meath Hospital Medical Board Minutes (Rough), 30 October 1879–27 November 1902, p. 324 [National Archives of Ireland].
73 Kelly, *Irish women in medicine*, p. 92.
74 Pat Jalland (ed.), *Octavia Wilberforce: the autobiography of a pioneer woman doctor* (London: Cassell, 1994), p. 101.

The one instance where women were separated from the male students during their years of medical education was for anatomy dissections. As Alison Bashford's work has shown, the issue of anatomy dissections was a complex one. It is clear that there was 'considerable cultural investment in a gendered and sexualised understanding of dissection in which the masculine scientist/dissector penetrated, came to "know" the feminised corpse in a dynamic shot through with all types of desire'.[75] When women medical students entered the dissecting room, they disrupted and reversed 'the gendered subjectivities and the sexualised dynamics which operated there'.[76] In the United States, it was believed that the practice of dissecting would have a hardening effect on women students.[77] Opponents of the medical education of women, such as Harvard's Professor Ware, believed that dissection would guarantee the 'defilement of women's moral constitution'. On the other hand, advocates of women's medical education argued that the practice had the potential to 'fortify the character and moral sensibilities of the physician in training'.[78] However, Irish institutions appear to have taken issue specifically with the idea of men and women dissecting together and the sexualised nature of anatomy dissections.

The practice of dissection was also thought to have a de-sexing effect on women students. For example, an article which appeared in the *Medical Press and Circular* in 1870, written by a Dublin-based male medical student, argued that the dissecting room fire was no place for women students, given the types of conversations which occurred there. Moreover, he argued that 'it is scarcely consistent with the laws of morality or society that a lady should be busy dissecting the perinæum of a male subject with a gentleman sitting at her elbow reading the steps of the dissection'.[79] Others believed that the subject of anatomy was indelicate for women to concern themselves with. Writing in his memoirs, William M. Hunter, a student at Queen's College Belfast in the 1890s, remarked that 'The first lady student was received in silence in the Dissecting Room, we thought it was no place for women'. However, because the student was 'good natured', Hunter and his fellow students 'gradually accepted her as a chum and passed no remarks'.[80] One of the main issues appears to have been that of men and women dissecting together. For instance, the *British Medical Journal*

75 Bashford, *Purity and pollution*, p. 114.
76 Bashford, *Purity and pollution*, p. 114.
77 John Harley Warner and Lawrence J. Rizzolo, 'Anatomical instruction and training for professionalism from the 19th to the 21st centuries', *Clinical Anatomy* 19(5) (2006), p. 404.
78 Warner and Rizzolo, 'Anatomical instruction', p. 405.
79 'Lady doctors' (letter to the Editor), *Medical Press and Circular*, 9 March 1870, p. 199.
80 William M. Hunter, 'Private life of a country medical practitioner', p. 7.

commented in 1870 that it was 'an indelicate thing for young ladies to mix with other students in the dissecting-room and lecture theatre',[81] while at the University of Edinburgh, the issue of men and women dissecting together resulted in a famous riot at the institution in 1870.[82] The male students at the University of Edinburgh medical school protested that women dissecting alongside men signified a 'systematic infringement of the laws of decency'.[83]

In order to try and resolve concerns about women and men dissecting together, Irish universities, like their counterparts worldwide, had separate dissecting rooms constructed for male and female students. In 1897, for instance, the Catholic University Medical School built a separate dissecting room with a waiting room for female medical students and the College Council reported that 'the results have proved most satisfactory and encouraging, and the Faculty are satisfied that the step taken in this decision is one which will add considerably in the future, to the success and usefulness of the School'.[84] Separation of medical students for anatomy dissections took place in all of the Irish medical schools. For instance, the Royal College of Surgeons had a ladies' dissecting room built in 1892 while Trinity College built one at the cost of £1,000 which remained in use until 1937.[85]

Why were anatomy dissections so problematic? We may gain an insight into Victorian attitudes of feminine 'delicacy' by examining the case of English anatomy museums.[86] At some anatomy museums in England, such as Kahn's Museum in the 1850s, women were permitted to attend the display on certain days, a practice that the *Lancet* objected to at the time because it was believed to undermine one of the most common arguments against women studying medicine: that they would find anatomy distressing.[87] However, the key issue seems to have been that university authorities were not favourable to the idea of men and women dissecting together. Revealingly, Queen Victoria, who disapproved of women in the professions, had a particular dislike of the 'awful idea of allowing

81 'Lady surgeons', *British Medical Journal*, 2 April 1870, p. 338.
82 Bashford, *Purity and Pollution*, p. 112.
83 Bashford, *Purity and Pollution*, p. 112.
84 'Annual report of the faculty: May 20th 1898', Catholic University School of Medicine, Governing body minute book, vol.1, *1892–1911* [UCD Archives, CU/14].
85 Kelly, *Irish women in medicine*, p. 95.
86 See A.W. Bates, '"Indecent and demoralising representations": public anatomy museums in mid-Victorian England', *Medical History* 52(1) (2008), pp. 1–22 and A.W. Bates, 'Dr Kahn's museum: obscene anatomy in Victorian London', *Journal of the Royal Society of Medicine*, 99(12) (2006), pp. 618–24.
87 Bates, 'Indecent and demoralising representations', p. 11.

young girls and young men to enter the dissecting room together, where the young girls would have to study things that could not be named before them'.[88] As observed above, in 1870, the *British Medical Journal* considered it 'indelicate' for male students to share the dissecting room with 'young ladies'.

The sight of corpses and the dissection of them may also have been seen as a corrupting influence on 'lady medicals' if they were working alongside the male students. The dissecting room may have been viewed as a place where sexual thoughts were liable to develop. By separating the women from the men, university authorities might have felt that they were protecting the 'delicate' female students from the threat of male advances, or perhaps even from male humour and seedy discussion that may have been particularly prevalent in such a context.[89] There were also concerns about the impropriety of women dissecting a male corpse, and likewise of men dissecting female corpses; historians have drawn attention to the highly sexualised nature of anatomy dissections in general.[90] As Bashford's work has shown, through the process of dissection, female students 'came to know' the male body. They penetrated it with scalpels, and in this way the power was handed over to the female dissector.[91] Even into the 1950s, it appears that at Irish universities male students were assigned male cadavers and female students female cadavers.[92] The action taken by Irish medical schools surrounding the practice of dissection clearly indicates that this was one aspect of medical education which remained problematic.

The separation of men and women for dissections appears to have come to an end by the late 1930s. Women's entry to the male dissecting room in Galway from the 1930s was said to have resulted in a 'romantic atmosphere' where 'in the presence of the dismembered frames of an earlier generation we find budding romances and broken hearts', the effect of which was that in time men 'must inevitably become more effeminate and the ladies more demoralised'.[93] At Trinity College, when separation of men and women for dissection came to an end in 1937, it was claimed that women were

---

88 A.M. Cooke, 'Queen Victoria's medical household', *Medical History* 26(3) (1982), p. 308.

89 For bawdy dissecting room ballads, see Daragh Smith, *Dissecting room ballads from the Dublin Schools of Medicine fifty years ago* (Dublin: Black Cat Press, 1984).

90 Waddington, 'Mayhem and medical students', p. 53 and Bashford, *Purity and Pollution*, p. 114.

91 Bashford, *Purity and pollution*, p. 114.

92 E.B. McKee, *Doc: revelations of a reluctant Yank studying medicine among the Irish* (Narragansett, RI: Ebook Bakery Books, 2013), p. 139.

93 'Medical', *The university annual: University College Galway* 8(9) (1933–4), p. 83.

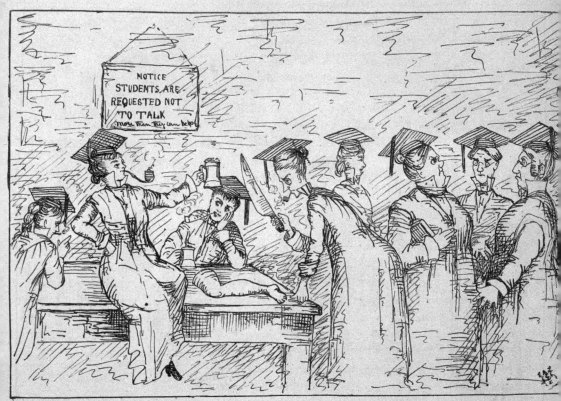

THE FAIR STUDENTS

Shade of Æsculapius !!!look here ! !!!!

9   Drawing of women in the dissecting room, entitled 'The Fair Students'.
From *Higher education of women: mental, by a junior moderator*
(publication date unknown). Courtesy of the National Library of Ireland.

only allowed to 'poke around with the female anatomy'.[94] Although Irish
medical students were educated together for all other subjects and there
were no issues with clinical training in the same way that there were in
Britain, it is evident that the practice of dissections was a complex one.
But in separating men and women for dissections, Irish universities were
only following international concerns of the times.

94 'An Irishwoman's diary', *Irish Times*, 21 July 1992, p. 9.

Social lives

Joyce Delaney, who studied at University College Dublin in the 1940s, wrote that the 'social life of the university was a great disappointment' to her.[95] She recalled the proportion of men to women students being ten to one, but in spite of this she felt that being a female medical student meant that she was less appealing to the male students than 'what used to be known as a "glamour girl"'. Writing about the university dances, she remarked:

> Our main meetings with the men took place at the university 'hops' or dances. There we female medical students had to submit to the indignity of watching the men make a dive for the decorative little shop girls and secretaries. To a girl we all wished for points off our Intelligence Quotients and even more off our ankles! Although we assuaged our battered pride by deciding the pretty outsiders were 'cheap', we all knew inwardly that they were more attractive.[96]

In her words, the female medical students became attractive to the men once the pubs had shut and 'the drinkers, rendered unselective by liquor, rushed in and whirled us on to the dance floor'.[97] Similarly, E.B. McKee, a student at the Royal College of Surgeons in the 1950s, wrote in his memoirs of his student days that 'accompanying women to these dances did not imply a romantic interest. They were classmates who wanted to attend and needed an escort. A good time was had but once the evening was over, it was over. The following day you reverted to classmate status'. In spite of this, he did acknowledge that occasionally romances did develop within his class, but, for the most part, relationships 'developed outside the college setting'.[98] Female students often complained about the lack of social life at university. One correspondent to *T.C.D.: A College Miscellany* in 1939, for instance, argued that there was not a 'great deal of mental activity to be found in the College' outside of activities such as games, the cinema and gossip.[99] The T.C.D. Women's social survey found in 1944 that the sports of tennis and hockey were popular among women students, as well as the watching of sporting events, while the cinema, theatre and dances were also common social activities.[100]

95 Joyce Delaney, *No starch in my coat: an Irish doctor's progress* (London: Cox & Wyman Ltd., 1971), p. 16.

96 Delaney, *No starch in my coat*, p. 16.

97 Delaney, *No starch in my coat*, p. 16.

98 McKee, *Doc*, p. 188.

99 Correspondence, *T.C.D.: A College Miscellany* 45(801) (16 November 1939), p. 43.

100 'Women's social survey, 1944', *T.C.D.: A College Miscellany* 51(893) (December 1944), pp. 92–3.

It was argued by some that women students missed out on the social side of medical school life because they did not play rugby, which, as the previous chapter has shown, was crucial in helping to develop a well-rounded identity among male medical students. Indeed, British physician John Powell-Evans suggested that 'one reason why women students are not welcomed at hospital is because they cannot play Rugby football'. Remarking on this, the *Irish Times* commented that 'the connection between prowess in this science and in the science of medicine is, to the lay mind, anything but clear. Perhaps Rugby football develops a constitution, and indeed a temperament, that may be of value later in the operating theatre. Perhaps it is professional etiquette that those who themselves will maintain the supply of doctors should assist also to maintain the demand'. Taking a critical view of these comments, the *Irish Times*, suggested that Powell-Evans' theory made him 'no better than a heretic' and that the only course of action was to urge upon all women medical students 'the necessity of taking up the ungentle art of Rugby football. Soon, we may hope to see them trip forth with girlish laughter from their theoretical study of anatomy in the lecture room, and hurl themselves with energy into the study of its practical applications in the front row of the scrum'.[101]

Although by the 1900s, women students were beginning to be a common fixture in Irish universities, some women medical students felt that not everyone was accepting of them. Writing in 1904, one female student at the Catholic University Medical School remarked:

Lady medical students are so well known nowadays in and about Dublin that they excite little or no extraordinary attention in moving through Dublin social circles; but when we return home on vacation we are often surprised at the wonder we excite. Sometimes, when we visit a family where there are grown-up daughters who have been trained to no method of earning their bread we are received with ill-concealed envy and jealousy by all its members. Again, when we visit a family whose male or female head is in touch with the advances being made by this generation, we are greatly respected by such persons.[102]

Similarly, one writer to *T.C.D.* magazine in 1924, a student at Trinity College Dublin, remarked that 'even the most serious-minded woman medical student feels at times rather left out in the cold – an outsider, unwanted by some of our professors'. Writing of one professor at Trinity, Dr O'Sullivan, she mentioned how 'his wonderful patience, his quiet word of encouragement,

---

101 'The Medicine Ball', *Irish Times*, 1 October 1943, p. 3.
102 'From the ladies' colleges', *St. Stephen's: A Record of University Life* 2(2) (February 1904), p. 44.

and his keen enthusiasm in his work were a help and an inspiration to the most diffident of us'.[103]

Indeed, heated debates held at medical student societies on the topic of women in the medical profession illuminate the fact that Victorian attitudes towards women studying medicine persisted. At a meeting of the Belfast Medical Students' Association in 1911, a debate took place on the theme 'That the opening of the medical profession to women is a failure', with two female students, Miss Stewart and Miss Robinson taking up the negative side and two male students, Mr Holmes and Mr Martin the affirmative. In arguing the affirmative, Holmes 'pointed out the various instances in which the male sex had and would always prove superior' while Mr Martin's paper, which was 'very much in favour of the exclusion of women students from the medical profession', used the argument that 'women were much more likely to become hysterical in medical cases than men'. Ending his paper 'in a very boisterous manner', he compared 'lady medicals' to mustard plasters, 'namely that they were very irritating'. In arguing for the opposition, Miss Robinson mentioned the different obstacles which prevented women from entering the medical profession and discussed the successful work conducted by lady missionaries. Miss Stewart's paper referred to Dr Elizabeth Bell as a fine example to women medical students. Following the conclusion of the papers, there was much discussion and the question was passed by 45 votes to 25.[104] A similar debate took place at the Royal College of Surgeons Biological Society in 1918; however, the debate this time was won by a majority in favour of women in the medical profession. Interestingly, the main argument by those opposing women in the medical profession was that women relied too much on sentiment to be good doctors and many gave up their careers on marriage. Those in favour pointed to the examples of good female doctors in the RAMC and the need for women to treat women patients.[105] Likewise, in 1946, the issue was still being debated at the Medical Society of University College Cork; however, in this case, it was the male students who spoke in favour of women in the profession and the female students who spoke against.[106]

In the medical student societies, women students usually conformed to typical gender roles such as making the tea for the meetings.[107] Although women were admitted to most of the medical student societies, with the

---

103 Correspondence, *T.C.D.: A College Miscellany* 30(521) (28 February 1924), p. 129.
104 First general meeting, 16 December 1911, BMSA Minute Book, 1907–32 [Royal Victoria Hospital Archives].
105 'Students' Union Notes: Biological and Debating Society', *R.C.S.I. Students' Quarterly* 2(1) (March 1918): 7–8 [RCPI Heritage Centre, TPCK/6/7/12].
106 'Medical Society', *Quarryman* (March 1946), p. 32.
107 'The Medical Society', *National Student* 1(4) (April 1911), p. 122.

exception of the Biological Association of Trinity College, which did not allow women to attend meetings until 1929, their attendance tended to have been irregular, and when they did attend it was often noted in the student press, suggesting that their presence there may have been somewhat unusual.[108] When women students did attend meetings, they were sometimes the victims of unchivalrous displays. For instance, at a meeting of the Belfast Medical Students' Association in 1915 on the topic of 'military service for junior medicals', rowdiness ensued. A Mr Wild, speaking in favour, was followed by a Miss Anderson who supported his points. Missiles were then directed at the platform which 'struck the junior secretary with unnerving precision ... in the next two minutes pandemonium prevailed in the balcony and there was such an exhibition of rowdyism as caused many of the ladies present to throw contemptuous looks at the balcony', which encouraged the male students to respond with a show of missiles directed at the women students. The chairman's appeal for order was inefficient and the speakers for the opposition were drowned out by the 'clamour of the gentlemen in the upper storey'.[109] Similarly, James Lloyd Turner Graham provided the following report of a meeting of the Biological Society of the Royal College of Surgeons in 1935: 'Stayed in town till 8:0 when I went to the Biological Society's meeting in the College. It was the usual rowdy scene and we had some fun. The fellows, of many of them are a crowd of toughs. They charged in before the women and swiped all the tea'.[110] Graham's quote suggests that medical student societies were another realm for the performance of masculinity.

In 1929, it was decided that women students at Trinity College who had reached the grade of attending hospital could become associate members of the Biological Association; this proposal was passed by 29 votes to 16. Apparently, the question had been raised ten years previously, at which point it was heavily defeated.[111] It is unclear why the Biological Association was slow to admit women, but Trinity College was the last of the Irish universities to admit women to its courses (in 1904), so it is possible that student societies, similarly, were slower to admit female students. In spite of being officially admitted, women were in fact prevented from entering the opening meeting of the association in 1931. When the students arrived at the front gate, they were told that they could not enter, owing to the six o'clock rule which prevented women from entering the Graduates Memorial Building

108 The Biological Association appears to have been exceptional in this regard.
109 First general meeting, 17 December 1915, BMSA Minute Book, 1907–32 [Royal Victoria Hospital Archives].
110 James Lloyd Turner Graham diary, 21 October 1935 [RCPI Heritage Centre, BMS/48].
111 'T.C.D. Biological Association: women students to be admitted', Irish Times, 27 November 1929, p. 8.

after this time.[112] The secretaries of the Biological Association responded to these allegations in the next issue of *T.C.D.* where they stated that although women had become eligible for membership the previous year, and special arrangements had been made for meetings to be held in the Museum Buildings, women were generally not allowed to enter the Graduates' Memorial Building after six o'clock.[113]

By the 1900s, special ladies' rooms were established for female medical students at some Irish universities. These provided women with a place to socialise separately from the male students. At Trinity College, a special reading room was constructed within the anatomy department (which also had a separate entrance for women students) for female medical students. The Royal Victoria Hospital in Belfast had a special sitting room for female students in the early twentieth century. And, from 1892, at the Royal College of Surgeons, there existed a 'suite of apartments' specifically for women medical students. There were also 'ladies' rooms' for female students at Queen's College Belfast.[114] Women medical students who did not live at home tended to live together in digs or in special accommodation for women students, such as Riddel Hall in Belfast.[115] *T.C.D.: A College Miscellany* reported in 1944 that 42 per cent of female students lived at home, 27 per cent in digs, 22 per cent in Trinity Hall and 8 per cent with relatives.[116] Similarly, at University College Cork, 30.9 per cent of female students lived in digs, with about two-thirds living either at home, with relatives or in religious houses or hostels.[117] In Dublin, in the late nineteenth century, a committee of women doctors was established by Emily Winifred Dickson to help female students in the city find appropriate accommodation.[118] At the Royal College of Surgeons, a Lady Dean of Residence was responsible for the welfare of the female students there.[119] These separate living conditions, ladies' rooms, as well as social activities, all helped to reinforce a separate identity for women medical students at Irish universities.

112 Correspondence, *T.C.D. A College Miscellany* 38(656) (5 November 1931), p. 17.
113 Correspondence, *T.C.D. A College Miscellany* 38(657) (12 November 1931), p. 30.
114 Kelly, *Irish women in medicine*, pp. 97–8.
115 Kelly, *Irish women in medicine*, pp. 99–100.
116 'Women's social survey, 1944', *T.C.D.: A College Miscellany* 51(893) (December 1944), p. 90.
117 'Our students', *Cork University Record* 1 (summer term 1944), p. 10.
118 Clara L. Williams, 'A short account of the school of medicine for men and women, RCSI', *Magazine of the London School of Medicine for Women and Royal Free Hospital*, no.3 (January 1896), p. 107.
119 *Royal College of Surgeons in Ireland: Schools of Surgery, including Carmichael and Ledwich Schools, 1948–49 handbook* (Dublin: George F. Healy & Co., 1948), p. 9.

Female medical missionary students

By the 1930s, there was still a huge demand for women doctors in India. As Janet Lee has argued in her work on single Protestant women missionaries in China, 'In essence, missionary work allowed women to stay within the confines of socially sanctioned notions of femininity, yet stretch these boundaries and experience opportunities normally reserved for men'.[120] Although Catholic orders of nuns had been involved in the provision of health care during the nineteenth century and beyond, this sphere of work had not been extended to colonial territories. The Church hierarchy believed that the chastity of priests and nuns would be endangered through medical work, and as a result members of religious orders were banned by canon law from studying medicine, practising obstetrics or coming into intimate contact with the human body.[121] Catholic nuns who provided nursing care in the missions were therefore untrained and 'as nursing became more professionalised in the late nineteenth century this meant that they were placed at a serious disadvantage against their Protestant rivals'.[122] According to David Hardiman, 'Many Catholics believed that they were losing out badly to Protestant missions through a lack of systematic work in this sphere, and demands for a change in policy began to be voiced more vociferously in the early years of the twentieth century'.[123] With the accession of Pope Pius XI in 1922, who approved of medical missionary work, came important developments in the 1920s such as a Missionary Vatican Exhibition held in Rome in 1925 that devoted a whole section to medical issues. The following year, Pope Pius published an encyclical that iterated the importance of medical work in mission activities in the European colonies and this led to the formation of a number of Catholic medical missions over the next decade.[124] In 1936, members of female orders were finally permitted to study medicine under Canon 489: Maternity Training for Missionary Sisters,

120 Janet Lee, 'Between subordination and she-tiger', p. 624, cited in Myrtle Hill, 'Gender, Culture and "the Spiritual Empire"', p. 221.
121 David Hardiman, 'Introduction', in David Hardiman (ed.), *Healing bodies, saving souls: medical missions in Asia and Africa* (Amsterdam: Rodopi, 2006), p. 24. For more on the history of Catholic women medical missionaries, see Ailish Veale, '"It's all a matter of balanced tensions": Irish medical missionaries in Nigeria, 1937–1967' (unpublished PhD thesis, Trinity College Dublin, 2014) and Ailish Veale, 'International and modern ideals in Irish female medical missionary activity, 1937–1962', *Women's History Review* 25(4) (2016), pp. 602–18.
122 D.L. Robert, *American Women in Mission: A Social History of Their Thought and Practice* (Macon, Ga.: Mercer University Press), p. 271, cited in Hardiman, 'Introduction', *Healing bodies, saving souls*, p. 24.
123 Hardiman, 'Introduction', *Healing bodies, saving souls*, p. 24.
124 Hardiman, 'Introduction', *Healing bodies, saving souls*, p. 24.

although male priests were still not allowed to attend medical schools.[125] In Ireland, one of the most important medical missionary orders, the Medical Missionary Sisters of Africa, was founded by Mother Mary Martin in 1937. According to Ailish Veale, 'The congregation's focus on mother and child medicine reflected the ambitions and interests of the Catholic Church, and the Irish state. The missionary sisters practised their own distinct brand of maternity medicine that incorporated Irish medical thought, Catholic moral doctrine, and the demands of the local women'.[126]

Austrian Anna Dengel, who went on to found the Medical Missions Sisters, trained at Queen's College Cork (graduating in 1919), and was inspired in her schooldays to take up medicine by the story of the Scottish doctor Agnes McLaren. McLaren (1837–1913) trained in Montpellier, France because British medical schools were not open to women at that time. She then moved to Pakistan where she founded a hospital for women and children and spent her life devoted to the missionary cause. Dengel initially went to stay at the Ursuline Convent in Cork to prepare for her entrance examinations for Queen's College Cork before matriculating at the medical school in 1914. She wrote that the times were hard for her financially although she did receive a yearly £50 contribution from a woman called Miss Willis. During her studies, she won a stipend of £50 but did not accept it because she was a 'foreigner and thought that this might not be accepted by the native students'.[127] Bertram Windle helped her by getting her a post working as anatomy demonstrator.[128] After graduation, Dengel worked as an assistant to two general practitioners in Claycross, near Nottingham, while she waited for her visa, which would allow her to go to India to work as a missionary.[129]

Although Dengel was exceptional, there appears to have been an acceptance of students with a religious vocation, in particular at University College Dublin and University College Cork from the 1930s. University College Dublin organised a summer training course for missionaries from 1935, which appears to have been held annually until at least 1940.[130] In 1943,

125 Hardiman, 'Introduction', *Healing bodies, saving souls*, p. 24.
126 Veale, 'International and modern ideals in Irish female medical missionary activity, 1937–1962', p. 603.
127 'Die Wege meiner Berufung' ('The path to my vocation'), dictated by Sr Anna Dengel to Sr Monica Nehaus, July–August 1969 (English translation), p. 4 [Medical Missions Sisters Archives, London, AE/5/2/liv].
128 'Die Wage meiner Berufung', p. 4.
129 'Anna Maria Dengel', q.v. Leone McGregor Hellstedt (ed.), *Women physicians of the world: autobiographies of medical pioneers* (Washington, DC and London: Medical Women's International Federation, Hemisphere Publishing, 1978), p. 93.
130 UCD Medical Faculty (Minute Book 3), November 1931–1947, Wednesday, 24 April 1935, p. 24 [UCD Archives, F8/3].

the medical faculty had discussions over the reduction of fees for medical missionaries. Agreeing that missionary work was 'exceptional', the faculty agreed to reduce fees for medical missionaries by half, subject to a 'guarantee for the refund of the balance of the full fee in the case of those missionary students who should happen to leave the order concerned within twelve months of qualification'.[131]

Catholic religious sisters became a common feature of some of the Irish medical schools following the change in canon law. Missionary orders were in frequent contact with Archbishop John Charles McQuaid in order to ensure that they were clear about the guidelines and regulations for religious sisters undertaking medical studies. Under guidelines released by Propaganda Fide in 1936, religious sisters were expected to 'attend Catholic nursing schools and universities, or, if these be wanting, then hospitals under Catholic management'. Sisters were also to attend hospitals in twos, at least, and to wear 'modest lay-dress' and live in religious houses 'where they may have daily spiritual helps and safeguards'.[132] Writing to Archbishop McQuaid in 1948, the Mother superior of the Franciscan Missionary Sisters for Africa, Sister Augustine, requested permission for two of their sisters to take a two-year course in midwifery at the Coombe Maternity Hospital. During this time, the sisters would stay with the Sisters of Charity at Seville Place.[133] McQuaid approved this request but requested that the sisters 'inform themselves accurately of the regulations binding on sisters residing in this house', particularly in regard to the hour of returning to their accommodation at night.[134] Evidently, these missionary sisters lived a disciplined existence which separated them from the rest of the medical student community, and, as the following chapter will illustrate, this was felt by contemporary students themselves.

Conclusion

In 1921, the *Irish Times*, in an article on the admission of women to the medical profession in Britain and Ireland, asserted that 'This feminine invasion of medicine is deplored by nobody except, perhaps, the oldest of

131 UCD Medical Faculty (Minute Book 3), November 1931–1947, Monday, 2 June 1943 [UCD Archives, F8/3].
132 'Instruction S. Cong. Prop.Fide: 11th February, 1936: maternity training for missionary sisters', issued to Medical Missionaries of Mary [Dublin Diocesan Archives].
133 Letter from Sister Augustine, Superior to Archbishop McQuaid, dated 18 August 1948 [Dublin Diocesan Archives].
134 Letter from Archbishop McQuaid, dated 20 August 1948 [Dublin Diocesan Archives].

old fogeys'.[135] By this point, it was generally felt that women had a right to attend Irish medical schools. Moreover, and in contrast with British medical schools, Irish medical schools had shown themselves to be surprisingly lenient with regard to the question of women's admission, albeit in some cases for financial reasons. However, in spite of this, it is clear that Victorian arguments against women studying medicine prevailed. In the student press, female medical students were presented as the 'other' and characterised as studious, bookish, cold, defeminised or alternately as obsessed or unconcerned with their appearances. It is clear that although women and men were largely educated together for all subjects, with the exception of anatomy dissections, that women occupied a separate social sphere from the male students. This was reinforced through their living arrangements and separate social activities, and also through the construction of 'ladies' rooms' by Irish universities. Within this female sphere, female medical missionary students, a significant proportion of the female medical student body from the 1940s, remained a separate group.

135 'Women doctors', *Irish Times*, 23 November 1921, p. 4.

7

Medical Education and Student Culture
North and South of the Border,
*c.*1920–1950

Writing in *Mistura*, the magazine of the Royal College of Surgeons, in 1954, a student explained that it was during the university years that

> the various attributes are formed, just as irrevocably as the adaptation of shortcomings may occur. We must envisage this undergraduate period as an era delicate in temperament, pliable in direction and pregnant with influences which will direct us ultimately either into the channel of success and accomplishment, based on the quality of our work and our attributes in general, or into an abyss of failure, not only to ourselves, but to others who depended so much on us – our fathers, our mothers and our patients.[1]

As in previous decades, the experiences of student days were thought to be fundamental in helping to shape the futures of newly qualified Irish doctors in the 1950s. After Irish independence in 1922, Irish medical education continued to be influenced by British ideas and continued to be monitored by the General Medical Council. In addition, problems with the quality of education were still prevalent and these were addressed by both the Rockefeller Foundation in the 1920s and the American Medical Association in the 1950s.

This chapter will draw on sources such as student magazines, memoirs, contemporary newspapers and medical journals in order to build a picture of what life was like for students studying at Irish medical schools from the 1920s to the 1950s. Additionally, in order to provide an added insight into

---

1 Editorial, *Mistura* 1(2) (spring term 1954), p. 2.

the experiences of Irish medical students who graduated in the 1940s and 1950s, I will draw primarily on oral history interviews which were conducted between 2013 and 2014 with graduates from Irish medical schools. These interviews provide a revealing insight into the experiences of medical students who graduated in the post-war era. Oral historians have long emphasised the value of oral history as a source and the special value which oral testimony has 'as subjective, spoken testimony'.[2] As Lynn Abrams has argued, oral history 'is a creative, interactive methodology that forces us to get to grips with many layers of meaning and interpretation contained within people's memories'.[3] Surprisingly, oral history has not been utilised by historians in trying to uncover what it was like to be a medical student in the past. As the evidence presented in this chapter will show, oral history interviews with Irish medical graduates allow a glimpse into the world of students of the past.[4] For students who attended Irish medical schools in this era, it is clear that medical study was strenuous and lecture-teaching sometimes poor, although Irish medical schools continued to have a reputation for good clinical teaching well into the twentieth century. Students' social lives were limited as a result of economic factors, while emigration was inevitable for the majority of medical graduates in this period.

The 1920s: a problematic decade for medical education

The years following Irish independence were challenging for the Irish medical profession. One of the most significant issues for Irish doctors in the 1920s was the question of the establishment of a Free State medical register which, if enacted, could have potentially impacted on the experiences of medical graduates from Irish universities. Following partition in 1922, the Irish government called for its own medical council

---

2 Paul Thompson, *Voice of the past: oral history* (Oxford: Oxford University Press, 2000), p. 118.
3 Lynn Abrams, *Oral history theory* (London: Routledge, 2010), p. 18.
4 Twenty-four oral history interviews were conducted with graduates who studied at Irish medical schools from as early as 1938 up until 1958. Of these, two were graduates from QUB, one from RCSI, one from Galway, six from TCD, nine from UCD and five from UCC. The majority of graduates were recruited through university alumni associations and through assistance from Harriet Wheelock, archivist of the RCPI Heritage Centre. Unfortunately, it was difficult to find interviewees who had attended the Royal College of Surgeons and University College Galway, perhaps owing to the fact that many of these graduates had emigrated, and in the case of the Galway medical school there would have been a much smaller number of graduates. Pseudonyms have been assigned to graduates to protect their anonymity, while their university and years of attendance are provided in brackets after their names.

and system of registration.[5] Irish doctors condemned this. An executive composed of senior members of the Irish medical profession argued in a circular forwarded to candidates of the Senate that at present 'most of our medical graduates must seek a livelihood outside the country'. Although they recognised that this fact was 'deplorable', 'to send them abroad uneducated or with an inferior status is not to provide a remedy'. Moreover, it was believed that the plans would result in the collapse of several of the Irish medical schools, as students would go to Belfast, now part of Northern Ireland and Britain, or elsewhere in Britain, for medical training instead. With the collapse of medical schools, the Irish medical profession would become 'largely deprived of the stimulus of teaching and research' and become 'isolated and retrograde'.[6] Professor C.Y. Pearson, of University College Cork, believed that the establishment of a separate register for the Free State would be detrimental to many Irish medical schools and to students who were expecting to have their names placed on the General Medical Register after graduation and thus be in a position to attain posts in Britain.[7] Considering that medical students comprised the majority of students at Irish universities in this period, the loss of fees would have been enormous for universities.[8] Moreover, not only would the move potentially result in the closure of Irish medical schools, according to Sir Thomas Myles, 'If the worst happened, the loss to the Free State would be very considerable. It would be a financial, moral and social loss – a loss in sport, a loss in everything'.[9]

Medical professors at University College Galway were much opposed to the proposals. Dr R.B. Mahon, professor of medicine, believed that 'Irish doctors at present enjoyed a status in the world of medicine because they were associated with the English medical profession' and that they would no longer enjoy that status 'if placed on a register of a country that had a population which was not as large even as a big American or English city'.[10] It was argued that there would also be important consequences for Irish hospitals where students were thought to be a great asset 'because of the spirit of competition they engender between the different hospitals, and between the individual members of the staff of each hospital'.[11] It was also

5 Greta Jones, 'A mysterious discrimination': Irish medical emigration to the United States in the 1950s', *Social History of Medicine* 25(1) (2011), p. 140.
6 'The Doctors' Case Stated', *Irish Examiner*, 29 August 1925, p. 8.
7 'Prof. Pearson's views', *Irish Examiner*, 19 August 1925, p. 6.
8 'The Medical Register', *Irish Times*, 22 August 1925, p. 8.
9 'Medical schools in the Free State', *Irish Times*, 29 May 1924, p. 5.
10 'Medical register: Galway medical men's views', *Connacht Tribune*, 22 August 1925, p. 10.
11 'Letters to the editor: the Medical Crisis', *Irish Examiner*, 3 September 1925, p. 2.

claimed that hospitals would lose the services of resident medical students.[12] Several commentators prophesied that Ireland's best professors would not remain in the country 'whilst they can go across the water to universities and schools where they can obtain a large clientele and a good salary'.[13]

Medical students actively made their feelings known on this issue. A meeting of medical students from University College Cork and University College Galway held in Cork resulted in a resolution being passed that they viewed the prospect of separation from the General Medical Council 'with alarm'. The reasons for their opposition to the proposals were, first, that Irish medical men would be cut off from 'a large field of research, employment and experience' outside the Irish Free State; secondly, that there would be a significant degree of unemployment for Irish medical graduates, and, thirdly, that 'medical science, like all other sciences, is international, not national'. The students appealed to the Irish representatives of the General Medical Council and members of the Irish government to 'do all in their power to secure that the present arrangements remain unchanged'.[14] Similarly, in August 1925, a mass meeting of Galway medical students considered the situation and unanimously adopted a resolution opposing the establishment of a separate medical register. According to M.A. Naughton, secretary of the Galway University Students' Association, 'At least ninety per cent of the medical students in the Free State colleges – and this I know for sure – when they begin their study of medicine look forward to going abroad and getting good "jobs". Otherwise most of them would never have started here at all and wasted one-third of their life studying for nothing'.[15]

The disagreements over medical registration were eventually resolved by a system of reciprocal registration.[16] Under the Medical Practitioners Act of 1927, a separate register was established for Irish doctors which was to be regulated by a body containing 'two government appointees, two members elected from the general body of Irish medical practitioners, and representatives nominated from the medical schools in independent Ireland'.[17] Irish doctors could still automatically register on the general medical register while graduates from Northern Ireland and the rest of Britain also had the right to practise medicine in the Free State.[18] As a condition of this system

12 '200 students in the hospitals', *Irish Times*, 19 August 1925, p. 5.
13 'Hospitals will suffer', *Irish Times*, 19 August 1925, p. 5.
14 'Protest by medical students', *Irish Times*, 10 December 1924, p. 7.
15 'Students to hold meetings', *Irish Times*, 26 August 1925, p. 7.
16 Jones, 'A mysterious discrimination', p. 140.
17 Greta Jones, 'The Rockefeller Foundation and Medical Education in Ireland in the 1920s', *Irish Historical Studies* 30(120) (November 1997), p. 576.
18 Jones, 'The Rockefeller Foundation', p. 576.

of reciprocal registration, the British General Medical Council continued to inspect and approve Irish medical schools both north and south of the border.[19]

In addition to the issue over medical registration, Irish medical schools were also plagued by other issues in the 1920s. In 1925, a report by Alan Gregg of the Rockefeller Foundation concerning medical education in Ireland found that 'Medical education in Ireland then is no simple educational matter but one involving some of the deepest and most sensitive and most maltreated emotions and sympathies of the Irish people'.[20] Gregg identified tensions between University College Dublin and Trinity College Dublin and the issue between denominational hospitals and medical schools.[21] It is unclear whether these denominational rivalries had a direct impact on students themselves. As later sections in the chapter will show, denominational rivalries do not appear to have been wholly important for students in the 1940s and 1950s. Gregg was also highly critical of the quality of Irish medical education, with the exception of Queen's University Belfast, although he admitted that the school did not have the potential for groundbreaking research or to be a major influence on the development of medical education in Britain.[22] Irish medical schools had suffered after the 'severing of relations with the rest of the British Isles' which had 'brought about a crisis in the funding of research'.[23] The Rockefeller Foundation's plans to help reform Irish medical education were interrupted as a result of the crisis over medical registration in Ireland in 1925, and, owing to what was perceived to be several crises affecting Irish medicine this meant that 'the resources of the Rockefeller Foundation were relatively underused, and that the impression created in the Foundation about Ireland was generally unfavourable'.[24] Evidently the 1920s proved to be a problematic decade with regard to medical education in Ireland. However, it is clear that problems with standards of medical education and student experience at Irish institutions persisted well beyond this decade.

Educational experiences, c.1930s–1950s

By the 1930s, medical students were still thought to have their own identity which separated them from the other students in the university. One

19 Jones, 'A mysterious discrimination', p. 140.
20 Alan Gregg, 'General considerations on medical education in England and Ireland' (1925), p. 266, cited in Jones, 'The Rockefeller Foundation', p. 566.
21 Jones, 'The Rockefeller Foundation', p. 566.
22 Jones, 'The Rockefeller Foundation', p. 566.
23 Jones, 'The Rockefeller Foundation', p. 566.
24 Jones, 'The Rockefeller Foundation', pp. 572–80.

piece in *T.C.D.: A College Miscellany* in 1937, for instance, described the medical student as a 'distinct species of undergraduate', describing them as 'a class outspoken and boisterous and tend[ing] to smell of ether'.[25] Certain educational practices, such as grinds, still remained. Gearoid Crookes, for instance, recalled taking a grind in anatomy in 1935, owing to time he had squandered on social activities rather than studying.[26] Similarly, James Lloyd Turner Graham, a student at the Royal College of Surgeons, recorded attending grinds with a man called Billy in 1935 who appears to have been affiliated with the college.[27] Graham, however, was more interested in describing the female students in his grind class than providing details on the teaching he received.

Students' reasons for studying medicine in the 1940s and 1950s had not changed much either. Some, like Anne (UCC, 1947–53), had family members who had been doctors. Seamus (UCD, 1942–7) stated, 'My father was a surgeon, you see, and so, there were other doctors in my family, my father and two brothers are doctors … so it was medicine in the family. And also, the thing I felt, what else would I do?' Jean (UCC, 1951–7), a religious sister from Dublin, was asked by her order if she would be interested in studying medicine, to which she replied 'I didn't mind, as long as I was doing something practical. As long as I wasn't teaching – I just wanted to do practical things'. Some graduates cited parental influence. Francis (UCC, 1943–9), whose father owned a lounge bar, stated that his father suggested that he should go and study medicine as he was 'a great admirer of my best friend, who was a year older than I, and who was a teacher's son, and he said "Jack is going up to do medicine. You should go with him"'. Others, like Seán (UCD, 1952–8), believed,

I always wanted to. I always had an interest. Even as a schoolboy … this is a strange story, I used to collect bones. I was interested in it, until one day … I think I came home one day with a skull and my mother drew a line at that. I had to abandon my bone collection very quickly. I kind of got interested in it, and I liked people and that kind of thing.

Similarly, Michael (UCD, 1951–7), whose parents had both been doctors, recalled, 'I never had any doubt that medicine was for me'.

---

25 'Advice to Freshmen', *T.C.D.: A College Miscellany* 44(763) (28 October 1937), p. 8.
26 Gearoid P. Crookes, *Far away and long ago: a memoir* (Dublin: Tudor House Publications, 2003), p. 142.
27 Diary of James Lloyd Turner Graham, entry for Friday, 28 June 1935 [RCPI Heritage Centre, BMS/48].

Mary (UCG, 1946–52), whose mother owned a pub in Co. Galway, stated, 'Because there were ten children in our family, and everybody had to go and do something, although we lived in the heart of the country'. Originally, she thought she might like to do nursing, but on the suggestion of her brother decided to study medicine instead. Martha (TCD, 1943–9), the daughter of a businessman, stated, 'In those days it was so different. If you wanted to study anything, there was a very small area you could study. I could have studied medicine or dentistry and my brother studied engineering. If you wanted to do something like history or literature, I mean everybody would simply go crazy "What do you want to do that for?"' Some graduates could not remember why they decided to study medicine. Stephen (QUB, 1942–7), responded 'I don't know. People who study medicine say "it's because I want to do good" and so forth. I don't know why because there was no history of medicine in our family'.

Complaints about the medical curriculum persisted into the 1930s. One medical student at Trinity College in 1933 argued that students spent an 'unnecessarily long time studying Botany, Zoology and Anatomy, especially the latter'. The additional time spent studying anatomy he or she felt had 'devastating results to our work in Pathology'.[28] Similarly, another student argued that the preliminary scientific course was regarded by most students as being a 'necessary evil'. The issue of students at Trinity having to take an Arts degree was also mentioned, with the correspondent arguing that 'it fails in its object (an admirable one) of ensuring that medical graduates of the University will have a fair general education and it effectively baffles those medical students (fairly large in number) who are able and anxious to obtain the advantages to be derived from systematic study under direction of "humane learning"'.[29] Another student in 1942 described the arts course in the medical school as being 'an expensive farce....at the best it is an extra degree which will impress the lay-man; at the worst it is a waste of time'.[30] Likewise, in 1956, a student at the Royal College of Surgeons explained, 'The early stages of medicine are frankly ludicrous and seem to have been devised by someone suffering from a Mack Sennett sense of humour'.[31]

The medical student's day by the 1930s and 1940s was intense, although there were still opportunities for extra-curricular activities. Noël Browne entered at Trinity College Dublin in 1933 and recalled 'The short terms,

28   Correspondence, *T.C.D.: A College Miscellany* 39(679) (2 February 1933), p. 80.
29   'The Schools: I. The Medical School', *T.C.D.: A College Miscellany* 39(682) (23 February 1933), pp. 114–15.
30   'The broad-backed hippopotamus', *T.C.D.: A College Miscellany* 49(856) (26 November 1942), p. 51.
31   'The medicine man', *Mistura* 3(1) (Christmas 1955–New Year 1956), p. 21.

crammed with lectures and clinics, and the long vacations created an exhila-
rating pattern of study of man's body and mind, in health and sickness,
interspersed with the limitless permutations of recreations and pleasures
to be found in Dublin'.[32] For Browne, entering into university life and
leaving behind the cloistered experiences of boarding school, 'was a welcome
experience of personal liberty' and he engaged in a range of activities such
as hunting, horse-racing, squash, rugby and boxing.[33] Other accounts were
less positive. A fictional account detailing a secret meeting of the 'Society
for the Preservation of Chronic Medical Students' published in *T.C.D.*
magazine in 1946, painted a dreary account of the medical student's day,
rushing to hospital in the morning where he was inflicted with the 'psycho-
logical trauma' of making an imperfect guess to the clinician's question,
suffering 'much sarcasm at the hands of the clinician, and jeering from the
keener students'. Following the clinic, the student returned to college to 'hurl
himself at his books' before a lecture at noon, lunch from 1 to 2, and another
lecture from 2 to 3, before 3 hours of study in the library.[34] At this point,
medical students themselves were calling for the 'traditional notion of the
medical student being a nuisance' to be discarded. According to an editorial
in *T.C.D.* in 1940, although medical students represented one-third of the
total student population of the university, 'very few are known on walking
through the Front Square'. Because of the fact that the course was longer
and examinations more difficult, 'the life of the student is too continuously
the passage from lecture to lecture, and from one examination to another'
meaning that students now had less time for socialising. Moreover, it was
argued that the 'medical student of today is not the noise-maker and sleep-
disturber that many people have been brought up to imagine, but a person
whose earnestness and sincerity in college should now be fully recognised'.[35]
By 1948, similar sentiments were being echoed with another *T.C.D.* piece
stating that medical students did not have the time 'to dwell on such petty
things as literature and poetry' owing to the 'rigidly practical life' of the
medical school.[36] These sentiments are backed up in some doctors' memoirs.
Thomas Hennessy, who started his studies at University College Dublin in
1951, recalled that once term began in his first year, he had four lectures
every morning and a three-hour practical four times a week. According to
Hennessy, 'If you were conscientious in finishing off this seven-hour day
with four hours' study in the evening, and if you were starting from scratch

32 Noël Browne, *Against the tide* (Dublin: Gill & Macmillan, 1986), pp. 60–1.
33 Browne, *Against the tide*, pp. 61–2.
34 'Medical news', *T.C.D.: A College Miscellany* 51(917) (8 March 1946), pp. 104–5.
35 Editorial, *T.C.D.: A College Miscellany* 46(813) (6 June 1940), pp. 181–2.
36 'What's wrong with: 4. The Medical School', *T.C.D.: A College Miscellany* 54(957) (27
    May 1948), p. 427.

as I was, you studied most of the weekend as well'.[37] Examinations were
mentally exhausting. Hennessy recalled having

> notebooks full of drawings, diagrams and graphs with which to
> revise the practicals, and voluminous lecture notes to supplement our
> textbooks. There were only a few weeks left before the exam and I
> suppose most of us felt a compulsion to use all the time available for
> revision which meant studying for nine to ten hours each day. I don't
> know about my colleagues but I certainly felt the strain.[38]

The full days of classes meant that medical students tended to socialise
together. According to Maureen (UCD, 1952–8), the medical student body
was

> Pretty separate and even when the whole college was in the terrace,
> the medical students would have been fairly separate. And I think the
> reason is that our day was very full. We had classes both mornings
> and afternoons, you know, mostly lectures in the mornings, practicals
> in the afternoons and then of course, when we started going to the
> hospitals we were out of the place. So there wouldn't have been much
> socialising at all with other students.

Opinions on medical teaching varied and oral history interviewees were
sometimes reluctant to criticise their former professors. James (UCD,
1938–44) recalled of the teaching, 'It was rather thrown at you, take it or
leave it a bit. I wouldn't want to be critical of them. They were fine men but
some were … there were, as you went on, I think, moving into the '40s, a lot
of younger specialists came into the teaching area and there were … I think
that they got the idea of how to get the message across better'. Similarly, Seán
(UCD, 1952–8) remembered, 'There wasn't this continuous assessment. You
went to lectures, it was there for you. You attended, you worked at it, it was
up to yourself. There was an exam at the end of the year. That was it, but
you were very much on your own.'
    Several respondents recalled the formal nature of teaching in Irish
medical schools. Stephen (QUB, 1942–7) remarked, 'It was, in a way, too
formal I think. That was one of the problems with universities and medical
schools 60, 70 years ago, so there's bound to be changes. But they were, in
a way, too formal. It was once you got into the ward that you really learned,

---

37 Thomas Hennessy, *My life as a surgeon: an autobiography* (Dublin: A. & A. Farmar,
    2011), p. 59.
38 Hennessy, *My life as a surgeon*, p. 66.

that's where you really [learnt] your meds and your surgery and your paediatrics'. Maureen (UCD, 1952–8), recalled,

> The discipline, you would have been a bit afraid of the professors, of being caught, and what they used to have sometimes if the few kind-of professors who weren't, maybe, so good, or spoke low, and people would start getting restless and throw things around. And they used to bring in the attendant to stand and watch the class, you know, and taking notes so it was kept fairly strict.

Student behaviour appears to have been overall good from interviewees' remembrances and according to the student press. One piece in a 1955 edition of *Snakes Alive*, the magazine of Queen's University Belfast, explained:

> One hears stories about pianos and furniture being thrown out of the East Wing, about beds being strewn all over Grosvenor Road, of men who took 10–15 years to qualify. All these are extremely funny and to the gifted raconteur provide an inexhaustible fund of stories about past medical students. To-day these could not take place, the authorities simply would not tolerate it, they cannot afford to. There are certain sections of the public who would rise up in anger if these sort of stories continually leaked out and rightly so, because it is their, the tax-payers' money, which helps to keep the fees low and equip the universities.[39]

The quote suggests that by the 1950s some students believed themselves to be better behaved than their predecessors, while it indicates that the image of the medical student of the past as being badly behaved persisted.

Some graduates were more critical of the teaching they experienced in medical school. Mary (UCG, 1946–52) recalled that the professors 'thought they were kind-of little gods ... you just ... sat, bored. And they'd be late coming in. There was no, there was no organisation ... or very little of it'. She added, 'Well, there wasn't much teaching, as such. They just read things, standing at the, I don't know what they call it, and we just took notes, that sort of thing. If anybody asked a question, it was always the professors' sons ... We never spoke'. Robert (UCD, 1939–44) explained 'We had no real proper relationship with the staff, there weren't too many students. The teaching was appalling. The teaching in the university itself during our first three years was very poor. Almost as bad as a guy can come in and read a book. Again, I would change that completely'.

---

39 'Random reflections of a medical student by Candidus', *Snakes Alive* 3(2) (March 1955), p. 15.

Increasing numbers of students also had an impact on students' educational experiences. Professor Henry Moore, professor of medicine at the Mater Hospital in Dublin, explained in 1941 that the overcrowding caused 'a great difficulty in bedside teaching because of the large classes. I have had as many as eighty students at bedside classes. Consequently, it is not an easy matter to train the student adequately in the various methods of clinical examination'.[40] Similarly, Dr Harold Quinlan, consultant physician to St Vincent's Hospital, Dublin, reported, 'It is certainly not a satisfactory condition for the teaching faculty because we find it most difficult to find accommodation for them both in the hospitals and the university. The lectures are overcrowded and so are the clinics, so much so that we have had to introduce a second lecturer'.[41] This was in contrast to conditions in the past where Irish medical schools had the advantage of small bedside classes.[42]

The provincial medical schools in Cork and Galway appear to have had particular issues. Overcrowding was a problem at University College Galway in the early 1940s, in particular in the departments of physiology and pathology, which were equipped for 40 students and 24 students respectively. Limitation of students or the duplication of practical classes were suggested as solutions to the problem but the committee agreed 'on educational and financial grounds' that the best solution was the provision of additional accommodation and assistance in teaching.[43] Similarly, in 1941, the clinical lecturers met to discuss the difficulty they were having in dealing with large clinical classes and agreed that 'if numbers exceeded twenty per year, teaching became unsatisfactory. If the number to exceed forty per year, teaching in the hospital would be impossible'.[44] At University College Cork there were similar issues with overcrowding resulting in the restriction of numbers of students there. From 1948 to 1949, University College Dublin limited the numbers being admitted to its first-year medical course, and when the number exceeded this, the selection of students was made on the basis of the marks attained in the pre-medical examinations.[45] The medical school at University College Cork had similar entrance requirements in place and from October 1948 students were only admitted to the pre-medical class after producing evidence of an elementary

40 'Are there too many doctors?', *Irish Times*, 1 November 1941, p. 6.
41 'Are there too many doctors?', p. 6.
42 'Are there too many doctors?', p. 6.
43 Meeting, 26 June 1941, Rough Minutes of Academic Council meetings, August 1941–August 1942 [NUI Galway Archives, 4/4].
44 Memo: Meeting of clinical lecturers, 30 June 1941, Minutes of meetings of Academic Council, September 1940–September 1941 [NUI Galway Archives, 4/3].
45 'Limiting the number of medicals', by President Alfred O'Rahilly, *Cork University Record* 7 (summer term 1946), p. 22.

knowledge of chemistry and experimental physics (i.e., 'having passed in these subjects at Matriculation, Leaving Certificate, Cork Technical Institute, or at a Special Test held by University College Cork').[46] This new regulation was introduced not only to limit numbers of students but also for educational reasons as it was concluded that students should have a rudimentary knowledge of the science subjects before starting their pre-medical studies.[47] Several oral history interviewees, who entered medical school before these regulations were put in place, found the first year of medical study difficult due to their lack of basic scientific knowledge. Sylvia (QUB, 1944–50) stated: 'I had to do physics, chemistry, botany and zoology, and physics was a nightmare. I hadn't done well in school'. Female respondents, in particular, remarked on having a lack of preliminary knowledge of the science subjects. Lily (TCD, 1946–53) recalled, 'well, first year, because a lot of people hadn't done physics and chemistry and botany and zoology. Those were the four, and I failed botany the first time around, but I shouldn't have, but I thought it was a load of nonsense, and it was really, really, from the lecturer's speeches to the practicals. I thought it was a waste of time'. Similarly, Mary (UCG, 1946–52) recalled 'the boys knew an awful lot more than we did [the women students], because they did chemistry and physics at school and we didn't'. UCC also introduced an 'anti-chronic' regulation whereby medical students were only given two years to pass each of their three examinations in medicine and dentistry. If a student could not pass the pre-medical, first or second examinations within a period of two sessions, it was 'a sign that he is unfit for a medical career'.[48]

Irish medical education was influenced by British ideas and continued to be so well after independence. Because of the recognition that many Irish doctors would end up going to work in the United Kingdom following graduation, changes in British medical education directly affected Irish medical schools.[49] It was therefore essential that Irish medical schools provided similar regulation of education. The Goodenough Committee, which was established in Britain in 1942 to enquire into the organisation of medical education in the country, recommended in their 1944 report that after passing his or her qualifying examination and prior to being admitted to the Medical Register, students should be required to complete a 12-month internship in a hospital so that they could be 'properly equipped for practice as family doctors'.[50]

46 'Limiting the number of medicals', p. 22.
47 'Limiting the number of medicals', p. 23.
48 'Limiting the number of medicals', p. 24.
49 Jones, 'A mysterious discrimination', p. 140.
50 'The training of doctors: report by the Goodenough Committee', *British Medical Journal*, 22 July 1944, p. 121.

An Irish committee comprised of representatives of all of the Irish medical schools, the Department of Local Government and Public Health and all of the Dublin hospitals met in 1945 to consider the report and agreed in general with the majority of the recommendations. The issue of Irish medical students having a residence in the hospital prior to qualification was discussed and it was agreed that this might have to be curtailed in future to allow for postgraduates' pre-registration residence.[51]

In December 1949, representatives from British and Irish medicine met to discuss the proposals made by the Goodenough Report.[52] It was agreed at this meeting that the existing position of reciprocal registration for Irish and British medical graduates should continue.[53] The British government introduced the 1950 Medical Act which implemented many of the recommendations of the Goodenough Report. The regulation that Irish students would have to undertake a year in a hospital in order to register was introduced for students qualifying from 1 January 1953.[54] The issue was debated in the Dáil where some TDs (Members of Parliament) disagreed with the lengthening of medical study to seven years because the cost would hinder 'ordinary people' from studying. James Dillon, TD for Monaghan from 1932 to 1969, suggested that the 'somewhat archaic requirements' of the curriculum could be eliminated, adding that 'ordinary people in a society like ours ought to have as ready access as possible to any professional vocation that they feel called upon to assume'.[55]

In discussions over the internship scheme, the Medical Faculty of University College Galway recommended that 'foreign students' should not be admitted, or at least a small number should be admitted to first year, only if they could demonstrate evidence that they would be accepted as interns elsewhere.[56] Thomas Hennessy, who graduated in the late 1950s, remarked that interns were paid £3. 2s. 6d. a week and had free board and lodging at the hospital they worked at. Without this, they would have had to have received further support from home, 'and that was unthinkable after being

51 Report of the Medical Education Investigation Committee 1945, p. 7 [RCPI Heritage Centre].

52 Jones, 'A mysterious discrimination', p. 140.

53 Dr James Ryan, speaking in Dáil Éireann Debate on Medical Practitioners Bill, 1951 – second stage, Dáil Éireann Debates, Vol.128, No.3, pp. 364–5.

54 Committee on Finance, Medical Practitioners Bill, 1951 – committee and final stages, 12 December 1951, Dáil Éireann Debates, Vol.128, No.6, p. 850.

55 James Dillon, speaking in Committee on Finance, Medical Practitioners Bill, 1951 – committee and final stages, 12 December 1951, Dáil Éireann Debates, Vol.128, No.6, p. 855.

56 Report of Medical Faculty meeting held 28 November, 1950, Rough Minutes of Governing Body Meetings, June 1950–July 1951 [NUI Galway Archives and Special Collections, 3/60].

maintained by one's parents for six years'.[57] Dr Patrick Maguire, a TD for Monaghan from 1948 to 1954, remarked of the length of the medical course that if he had 'visualised spending seven years in the university doing it, I would never have started, for the simple reason that it would probably have resulted in putting my parents in the poorhouse'.[58]

Evidence of cordial relationships between British and Irish students may be found in the example of the Irish and British Medical Students' Associations. The Irish Medical Students' Association was founded in 1944 with representatives from the medical associations of the Irish medical schools, including the Belfast Medical Students' Association, the Dublin University Biological Association, the Royal College of Surgeons in Ireland Biological Society and the Medical Societies of University College Cork, University College Dublin and University College Galway.[59] Its aims were outlined as the promotion of better relations between medical students, both in Ireland and abroad; to strive to represent the opinions of the medical students of Ireland; to promote better relations between medical students and the medical profession, both in Ireland and abroad; to research subjects of interest to medical students and disseminate the results of the same.[60]

In 1945, the IMSA affiliated with the British Medical Students' Association, forming their own region within this organisation as well as having their own independent existence.[61] This was viewed by the *Lancet* as being 'a valuable liaison for the Irish students, since 80% of them practise in Britain after qualifying'.[62] According to the *Cork University Record*, that 'the undergraduates, both of Ireland and England, are linked by ties of medical interest in a common association presages well for the future – a future in which those entrusted with the guidance of medical politics will have a sympathetic understanding of one another's difficulties'.[63] The British MSA held its three-day tenth annual meeting in Dublin at the invitation of the Irish association in 1951.[64] The IMSA had a keen interest in the medical curriculum at Irish universities and in 1948 were invited to submit a memorandum summarising the views of students of the Irish medical schools on the course of studies for submission to the committee inquiring

57 Hennessy, *My life as a surgeon*, p. 95.
58 Dr James Maguire, speaking in Dáil Éireann Debate on Medical Practitioners Bill, 1951 – second stage, Dáil Éireann Debates, Vol.128, No.3, p. 369.
59 Constitution of the Irish Medical Students' Association [RCPI Heritage centre, JF/1/4].
60 Constitution of the Irish Medical Students' Association.
61 'B.M.S.A. News', *British Medical Students' Journal* (the journal of the British Medical Students' Association), 1(2) (autumn term, 1946), p. 31.
62 'British Medical Students' Association', *Lancet*, 25 August 1945, p. 247.
63 'Medical student ambassadors', *Cork University Record* 5 (Christmas 1945), p. 9.
64 'A.G.M. Dublin – November, 1951', *British Medical Students' Journal* (the journal of the British Medical Students' Association), 6(2) (spring term, 1952), p. 16.

into reform in the curriculum.[65] The memorandum, while acknowledging that the students believed that Irish medical education was of a 'very high standard' and appreciating 'the full advantage the Dublin Schools have over the English Schools', nonetheless outlined a rigorous list of suggestions for changes with regard to each of the subjects taught during the medical degree. For many of the subjects, students requested a more practical knowledge than what was currently being taught. For instance, with regard to anatomy, it was recommended that the emphasis should be on 'the inculcation of fundamental principles and methods rather than on the acquiring of a mass of purely factual knowledge'. With regard to clinical teaching, the IMSA reported that the average attendance at a clinic in a Dublin teaching hospital was 51 students, and suggested that there should be an increase in the number of clinicians. Students also encouraged the provision of arts lectures for medical students and the use of films for teaching purposes.[66] Dr Edward Freeman, chairman of the committee, met with student representatives of the Dublin universities in April that year. The students outlined their views that the anatomy and physiology courses could be shortened and that there should be more extensive clinical teaching in the final years. They also argued that unnecessary matter should be deleted from the curriculum and that the course in mental diseases should deal with psychoses and borderline states rather than with established diseases. The students also commented on the proposed GMC regulations regarding students having to do one year's internship in a general hospital before qualification suggesting that students should be paid a salary with residential emoluments. Finally, it was suggested that the final examination should be simplified because 'at present, they are regarded more as tests of endurance than anything else'.[67]

Religion and medical school rivalries

Following the creation of the Irish Free State and the emergence of a more Catholic and conservative Ireland, Catholicism began to have a greater impact on Irish medical curricula. The *Cork University Record* proclaimed in 1944 that 'our students are over 97 per cent Catholics and we do not intend to ignore this fact. Negative undenominationalism does not appeal to us in Cork. We have always respected, and will always respect, the rights

65 Report to the students on the memorandum prepared by the IMSA for the Minister for Health's Committee enquiry into undergraduate medical education [RCPI Heritage centre, JF/1/4].
66 IMSA memorandum on the medical curriculum [RCPI Heritage centre, JF/1/4].
67 Report to the students on the memorandum prepared by the IMSA for the Minister for Health's Committee enquiry into undergraduate medical education.

of religious minorities among us. But it is no advantage to them that our Catholic Students should be subjected to a purely secularist education'. University College Cork was said to 'stand not only for a social philosophy' but also maintained specifically Catholic training for students through courses in apologetics, through the Legion of Mary, in the Sodality and in the College Retreats.[68] Specific courses in medical ethics were also provided at Irish universities from the 1940s, although some medical schools included medical ethics in their courses on medical jurisprudence prior to this.[69] At UCD, a short course was provided from 1940, 'to deal with the moral problems confronting medical graduates in the course of their practice'.[70] This course was taken in third year and students covered subjects such as euthanasia, abortion, contraception and sterilisation, where students were warned by Monsignor Horgan to 'never empty the uterus'.[71]

The introduction of courses in medical ethics appears to have been prompted by a resolution by the Irish Catholic hierarchy approving and recommending the inclusion of a course in medical ethics at institutions which were part of the National University.[72] At University College Galway, after communication from the Bishop of Galway, it was decided that a course of at least ten lectures in medical ethics were to be given to fourth-year medical students by the professor of philosophy.[73] An examination was also introduced in medical ethics and students were not to be admitted to the final medical examination without having first passed this.[74] According to a 1940 letter from Michael Browne, Bishop of Galway (who had previously been professor of moral theology at St Patrick's College, Maynooth),

Owing to the wide-spread discussion of the social and moral questions underlying medical practice and owing also to the materialistic attacks, which are so prevalent today, upon accepted moral standards, it is

68 *Cork University Record* 1 (summer term 1944), p. 3.
69 Report from Medical Faculty on matters referred by the Senate of the University or by the Standing Committee of the Senate, UCD Academic Council Minutes, vol.3 (20 June 1940), p. 504 [UCD Archives].
70 Recommendations of the Faculty of Medicine, UCD Academic Council Minutes, vol.3 (20 June 1940), p. 477 [UCD Archives].
71 Hennessy, *My life as a surgeon*, p. 83.
72 Report from Medical Faculty on matters referred by the Senate of the University or by the Standing Committee of the Senate, UCD Academic Council Minutes, vol.3 (20 June 1940), p. 504.
73 Communication from the Bishop of Galway re: medical ethics, undated, but probably 1940, Minutes of meetings of Academic Council, September 1940–September 1941 [NUI Galway Archives, 4/3].
74 Academic Council meeting, 18 June 1940, Minutes of meetings of Academic Council, September 1940–September 1941 [NUI Galway Archives, 4/3].

very widely recognised that medical students should have a full and scientific knowledge of the moral principles relating to their profession, so that they could give a rational defence of them in correlation with general ethical principles.[75]

Choice of medical school continued to remain dependent on religious affiliation in many cases. John Charles McQuaid, archbishop of Dublin between 1940 and 1971, held a huge amount of influence over the question of Catholic students attending Trinity College Dublin. Christopher (TCD, 1942–9) recalled that it was frowned upon 'for any of the faithful to attend the college for heretics, commonly called Trinity College Dublin. Which were not advantageous, or not much of an invitation – some of them would have gone in any event, but from other dioceses in Ireland, where there was no restriction, but it was, um, he was a very, very severe man'. Similarly, Thomas (TCD, 1946–52) recalled:

Most northerners who were at Trinity would not have been Roman Catholics, put it that way. And they often tended to … for start off, they come in from the north down to the south often from the country. They would have had parents that said, 'Oh, you can't go to Dublin. Terrible things happen in Dublin, you know.' And all that and the second reason is that, the Archbishop of Dublin at that time was called John Charles McQuaid, of notorious memory of many, and John Charles McQuaid thought that if anybody walked, even walked through Trinity they were committing either heinous or cardinal sin or whatever. They were going to hell and I can well remember, the rooms I had over Botany Bay, you looked out over the old fire station in Pearse Street which had a clock. This was an advantage of the room I was in. You just looked out the window. You didn't need a watch, just the clock, and, but there was also a crowd of people that got out of Pearse Street station, but they wouldn't walk through Trinity.

Seamus (UCD, 1942–7) remembered, 'And Trinity, I remember Trinity in those days. John Charles had a thing against Trinity. And he didn't want people going to Trinity. The Protestant, and in this lectern passage every year, he always brought up the subject of Trinity … you must not go without very special permission'.

75 Copy of letter from Michael, Bishop of Galway, dated 24 April 1940, Address: Mount St Mary's Galway to Rt. Rev Monsignor Hynes, MA, University College, Galway, Minutes of meetings of Academic Council, September 1940–September 1941 [NUI Galway Archives, 4/3].

There was a sense that students from different medical schools did not encounter each other or socialise too much, although they did meet each other during their hospital experience. Dan Maher, a fourth-year student at the Royal College of Surgeons believed in 1954 that 'a closer sense of friendship should exist between all Medical Schools and a more closer interrelationship should be built up. The time for petty squabbling died at the turn of the century'.[76] It was not until students began getting hospital experience that they started to meet students from the other Irish medical schools. John (RCSI, 1947–53) recalled meeting students from UCD and UCG while obtaining his hospital experience at the Richmond Hospital in Dublin, while at the Rotunda he encountered students from Edinburgh and England. Religious rivalries between the different universities appear to have been exaggerated. David (TCD, 1940–6) recalled:

UCD students coming down to Trinity and invading it, sort-of, some sort-of stupid snowballing with each other. Yes, they were competitive in a way but there wasn't any harsh stuff at all. And no, I think there was a fellow feeling ... well, of course, the hospitals were associated, six or seven small hospitals with Trinity and the Mater and Vincent's were associated mostly with UCD, but it didn't mean you couldn't go to classes there and sometimes those more adventurous people would cross over.

Similarly, Christopher (TCD, 1942–9), when asked whether he had the opportunity to mix with students from other medical schools, recalled, 'Oh yes, oh yes. They, the ecclesiastical side of it stopped short of that ... there was a bit of rivalry, all right, perhaps, but no, nothing more than that really'.

At University College Cork, owing to the influence of university president Alfred O'Rahilly in the 1940s and 1950s, student life was relatively strict. Anne (UCC, 1947–53) recalled, 'You weren't allowed to wear slacks. You had to wear stockings above your knees all the time. You weren't allowed to sit on the grass on the quad. You weren't allowed ... oceans, of oceans of things'. In the 1952 'Rules for Students' at University College Cork, women students were prohibited from smoking in the College grounds (men, on the other hand, could smoke in the Club Premises and in the laboratories and dissecting rooms 'provided the express permission of the Professor in charge is obtained', and another rule dictated, 'Women students shall not lie about on the grass'.[77] Similarly, Colm (UCC, 1949–55) recalled that at UCC:

76 'The forum', *Mistura* 1(3) (summer term 1954), p. 15.
77 'University College Cork: rules for students' (September 1952), pp. 4–5. With kind thanks to Dr Margaret O'Connor.

We – the university President, his staff and students – marched in their academic gowns to what was known as the Red Mass of St Thomas Aquinas in St Mary's Dominican church on Pope's Quay at the start of the academic year in September. It was a custom going back generations. Nothing special about it. Everyone marching was Catholic. We had two Protestants, brother and sister, in my class. We treated them, I hope, without prejudice. We had no trouble accepting them as members of our class.

Sylvia (QUB, 1944–50) remembered that religious differences became apparent when she started her clinical work in the hospitals. She recalled:

At that time there were three main hospitals, there was the Royal Victoria, there was the City Hospital and there was the Mater Hospital. I remember being shocked that I should have realised and I didn't and because in our first year, everybody was friendly and you became really close to people, and I remember talking to one girl and saying, 'Oh we're moving into clinical work' and I said, 'I'm going to the Royal, will you come to the Royal too?' She said 'No, I'm going to the Mater'. It suddenly hit me, this is what it's like. Although I had grown up understanding a fair amount about Ireland of those days, that really brought it home to me, and so I didn't really see her again.

Similarly, for students at the Dublin medical schools, religious affiliation through choice of medical school would also have impacted on choice of hospital well into the twentieth century.

Clinical experiences

Writing in 1956, a student at the Royal College of Surgeons explained: 'Dublin medical teaching has something of which it may justly be proud. The bed-side method in clinical teaching has no equal and yet Dublin is probably the last stronghold of such undergraduate tuition'.[78] By the 1950s, the clinical tradition of bedside teaching was still strong in Irish medical schools. Michael (UCD, 1951–7) stated that he admired his medical school: 'In medicine, clinical medicine was hands-on medicine. It wasn't hi-tech. There was no such thing as CAT scanners or MRI, that was all new to me in recent years. The clinicians and they were caring. They cared about their patients. They communicated, but the doctor was dominant'.

78 'Educational reform?', *Mistura* 3(1) (Christmas 1955–New Year 1956), p. 15.

Students were generally positive about the standards of clinical teaching. Sylvia (QUB, 1944–50), when asked about the standard of teaching at Queen's, recalled:

I think it was good. I think it was very good, now it must've been incredibly difficult because it was wartime. A lot of their top people were away. By the time I got to clinical work, the clinicians who had been away at the war with all that experience, and some of them doing research, and introducing new methods, some of them had done a really big job, so our teaching, the teaching was very good. You always had the odd one who wasn't up to much.

As outlined in Chapter 4, students had a range of opportunities for clinical experience, but again this varied significantly depending on one's location. Dublin remained the centre for clinical experience in Ireland, and it was common for students from Galway and Cork to go there to supplement the knowledge gained in their local hospitals. Belfast remained well-served with regard to hospitals; however, it was not unusual for some students from Queen's to obtain further clinical or obstetrical experience in Dublin.

James Lloyd Turner Graham, a student at the Royal College of Surgeons, went to the Adelaide Hospital in 1936 for his clinical lectures. Unlike some other students who revered their professors, he wrote:

Went to Adelaide Hospital this morning. A self-satisfied pup named Kinnear had the clinic. A little child was playing in the ward and he told it to shut up because it was evidently annoying him. Anyone that could do that deserves to be kicked. Nevertheless, he knew his work well. The hospital itself did not impress me. The nurses are a stiff lot who seem to be afraid to speak.[79]

Others, like Joyce Delaney, a student at UCD in the 1940s, were more impressed by their teachers. She recalled that 'Student life in the forties was so free and permissive that if you were a medical student you could wander into any Dublin hospital and attend the clinic of your choice. And the choice was dazzling'.[80] Delaney wrote that for Harry Meade's clinical lectures at St Vincent's Hospital, students

---

79 James Lloyd Turner Graham diary, Monday, 18 May 1936 [RCPI Heritage Centre, BMS/48].

80 Joyce Delaney, *No starch in my coat: an Irish doctor's progress* (London: Cox & Wyman, 1971), p. 18.

crowded into the grey cold hall of the hospital and waited till Harry's burly figure emerged from the consultants' room. Then it was like a cross-country run as we galloped down the corridors, lined with pictures of Saints and Popes and upstairs to the ward where Harry had arranged to do his clinic. Chivalry went by the board as people pushed and shoved to get into a strategic position around the patient's bed. Harry usually shoved the bed forward and stood behind the patient, arms resting on the bedhead.[81]

There was an art to choosing one's position around the bedside. According to Delaney, 'You didn't want to get too close in case Harry concentrated on making you the butt of his scathing tongue, but on the other hand you wanted him to see you because he always favoured "regulars" when it came to the examination, figuring that whatever their knowledge or lack of it at least they showed good taste!'[82] Similarly, Christopher (TCD, 1942–9) recalled:

You see, you don't, as a student, yet, as probably, maybe now it would be different, but – [get] as close to a patient as we … our professor, Professor Synge, was extremely good at talking about a patient. Maybe, I remember him, he would maybe sit down by the bedside and talk to the patient. In this case, it was a young, a young boy, but, you know, it was done in a way that didn't distress the child, or anything like that, and he asked him questions, and so on, but he had a good way with them, and uh, that sort of thing, it teaches a student more than you might think.

Ken O'Flaherty also wrote in a positive manner about the 'thrill of attending the various hospitals' in his clinical years, from 1949 on. He chose to attend the Jervis Hospital because it was smaller than the Mater or Vincent's, and had a busy casualty department, where he could see 'the action'.[83] Popular professors attracted students to their clinics. Lily (TCD, 1946–53) recalled of the clinical teaching:

It was very good, actually. They had a system where you had a card, and it had to be signed by the professor, whoever gave the lecture, or did the clinical round, and it meant the numbers would go up if a person was good, and you would tend to go to Joe Bloggs because he

81 Delaney, *No starch in my coat*, p. 19.
82 Delaney, *No starch in my coat*, p. 19.
83 Ken O'Flaherty, *From Slyne Head to Malin Head: a rural GP remembers* (Letterkenny: Browne Printers, 2003), pp. 114–15.

was better, and could teach better, and people like … the fellow who did infectious diseases, he would lie down on the floor and pretend he'd had a fit, you know?

Thomas (TCD, 1946–52) recalled the remarkable level of freedom that students in Dublin had in relation to clinical teaching:

The clinical teaching, if you picked where you went for clinics, you could go to clinicians who were good teachers and that's why the Dublin system of the small voluntary hospitals, which you know the history of all that, with their honorary consultants, so-called, attached to each. The university would pay them a small fee to give a clinic, but as well as that, of course, they did ward rounds and all. You could just walk into one of them and say, walk around with them type of thing and you could always pick the people you wanted to go with and you could always have the cards ticked for official reasons, but as well as that you could go, you went to the hospital a lot, out of hours so to speak.

Similarly, Colm (UCC, 1949–55) remembered, 'If you didn't turn up, so what. Nobody took rolls. Depends on who turned up. Very free and easy'.
Paul (UCD, 1946–52) recalled of the clinical teaching, 'Well, it was good. It was very – devoted is a good word. Really, at that stage, a patient came into the hospital because he was ill, and your job was to try and get to know him or her, carefully establish what the problems were, as best you could. And then try and fix them'. Colm (UCC, 1949–55) explained:

The level of clinical teaching medical students received would have been considered fair for the time but, as I found later in my career, inferior to the teaching provided by even the humblest of US hospitals at the time. In the relative absence of X-rays and blood tests, our senior clinicians, most of whom were in private practice and poorly motivated, taught us to rely on our senses of touch, hearing and eyes to make a diagnosis.

Similarly, Sean (UCD, 1952–8) remarked: 'There was no ultrasound then, there was no MRI, there was none of these things. It was much more based on the clinical skill of the consultant. Some, they were very astute clinicians. They could look at you, look at a patient, and say, "Yes, you want to watch that patient there now." Like a clinical antenna. It was marvellous'.
The first few weeks in the hospital proved a strain for some students. Thomas Hennessy recalled, 'During the first few weeks the unfamiliar

atmosphere of the hospital and tension created by having to perform in public and trying not to ask stupid questions overwhelmed some students and several fainted', adding that generally the students who fainted were not female, 'but hefty stalwarts from the UCD rugby team'.[84] There was also a sense of pride which went along with working in the clinical wards, with students now beginning to feel part of the medical profession. Hennessy wrote that when he and his fellow students returned to the college or went to Bewley's for coffee they 'always made sure that the earpieces of our stethoscopes were sticking out of our pockets. We also ensured that our conversation was well laced with medical terminology and anecdotes illustrating the idiosyncrasies of our clinical professors'.[85]

The practical nature of Irish medical education was a theme of several of the interviews. John (RCSI, 1947–53) recalled of the curriculum: 'Well, it was pretty ... as the curriculum is today ... some things were less embellished then because they were very embryonic. For example, biochemistry was in its infancy, immunology had not been invented at that time. And it was very simple: we saw lots of patients basically and there were less lectures. And contact with patients was greater than it is today. Thank God'.

Several interviewees also commented on the positive attitude of patients they met during their clinical experience. David (TCD, 1940–6) recalled of his experience 'on the district' as part of his midwifery training: 'The people of Dublin, the ordinary people you would learn about, were all ordinary poor patients, they were not rich people but they were very cooperative. They understood about students having to learn something and they were on the side of the students, hoping they wouldn't get failed! It was a very easy place to learn medicine I think, Dublin. The attitude of everybody was good'.

Knowledge of midwifery was another important facet of Irish medical students' education and one which brought them into direct contact with patients. It remained common for students from Cork, Galway and Belfast to go to one of the Dublin midwifery hospitals for a period to gain this experience. Anne (UCC, 1947–53) went to the Rotunda for four weeks one summer for midwifery, and remarked that although the experience was 'great', 'you had to paddle your own canoe a bit'. She recalled, 'If you went out, two students went out together, and that was frightening because you'd go, and there'd be a woman in labour, and you might have seen a woman in labour only once before, you know'. Sylvia (QUB, 1944–50), who gained her midwifery experience in Belfast, said that she would have liked to have gained some experience at the Rotunda because it provided students with

84 Hennessy, *My life as a surgeon*, p. 76.
85 Hennessy, *My life as a surgeon*, p. 76.

community experience, but she was told by her professors that 'the teaching would not meet the exam standards here':

> There would be a different approach, and you were examined in your final by the people, the consultants you'd worked with, and so I had to give up that idea. Theoretically it was possible to go, but practically it wasn't, but I would have liked to have done it, because I'd have got so much more community work. And so you were not just in touch with the woman and the baby, but the whole family if you had the whole community around you.

Ken O'Flaherty, a UCD student, in the late 1940s, undertook his obstetrical training at the Coombe, because it was smaller than the Rotunda. On entering the hospital, students were provided with 'a short introduction and training in the labour wards before going out in pairs on bicycles to the deliveries on the district which covered a large area from York Street near Stephen's Green, all the Liberties, Inchicore, Crumlin, Ballyfermot, which was still under construction, and Kilmainham'. Students were required to attend 20 deliveries in three months and to write up the details of each case.[86] The types of houses in these areas varied greatly. O'Flaherty recalled being impressed by the 'Labour' room which existed in most of the tenements, supplied with an electric ring or fire for the provision of warm water, fresh soap and towels, and occasionally a Handywoman, who would provide the obstetric history of the woman giving birth.[87]

A student from the Royal College of Surgeons, gave a similar account of being out 'on the district' in 1954:

> Your first case on district will remain prominently in your mind. A woman in her home about to have her first, fourth, or fifteenth child; the case may be one of two hours or ten hours. In time, however, the presenting part bulges the perineum, the accoucheur takes his position, and his assistants do their duty to bring into this world another of the human race. A sense of personal attachment may momentarily move you to regard this new born infant with affection and warmth. The placenta is delivered and, depending on the circumstance of the family, tea will be served for the 'Doctors'. This is most welcome as you may have missed one, or perhaps two meals, and by experience you will gather that on your return to hospital, you may or may not

---

86 O'Flaherty, *From Slyne Head to Malin Head*, pp. 123–4.
87 O'Flaherty, *From Slyne Head to Malin Head*, pp. 124–5.

get something to eat. If you do, however, it will be cold, especially if the hour is late.[88]

Students were often struck by the poverty they witnessed in the tenement houses. James (UCD, 1938–44) recalled: 'The poverty was terrible because there were large families. They were living in perhaps two bedrooms and a kitchen. Unemployment was huge, but the warmth, the welcome when you arrived and when you finished, they'd always give you a glass of whiskey or something'. Similarly, Martha (TCD, 1943–9) remembered, 'They didn't even have a gas stove to boil the water on. They heated the water on a coal fire! Can you believe it? Terrible'. Anne (UCC, 1947–53) recalled, 'Really, the poverty was horrific … and they were so nice, and the husband making cups of tea for you, and everything. They were glad that you came. They didn't know how little we knew [laughs]'.

While students were usually sent out in pairs and could phone the hospital if they encountered difficulties, some, in retrospect, felt that they were not adequately supervised. Noël Browne, who studied at Trinity College Dublin, recalled his 'sense of total helplessness' when a student 'on the district' of the Rotunda Hospital. He and another medical student were called out to what turned out to be a normal birth, however, the newborn baby experienced breathing problems and suddenly stopped breathing, dying before their eyes. Browne was greatly upset by the incident, writing in his memoirs: 'Death was the result of my inadequacy. That child should not have died. Yet surely those who devised a system where inexperienced students could be sent out in a state of ignorance were also to blame? Though I persuaded myself of this, it was of little comfort to me'.[89]

Similarly, Martha (TCD, 1943–9) recalled: 'I think I made a few mistakes. I remember being very put back once because somebody corrected me about something, but it was probably par for the course. I mean, you could call out a senior doctor if you were in trouble, but to send out a student on the district with no supervision …'

In conclusion, the hospital was often viewed by students as the place where they truly began to feel like members of the medical profession. While often challenging, students' clinical experiences, more than any other, also helped to cement a sense of collective identity and solidify friendships between students. In the words of Maureen (UCD, 1952–8), 'it was kind-of a team of friends'.

---

88 'Adventure in Obstetrics', *Mistura* 2(1) (winter term 1954), p. 17.
89 Browne, *Against the tide*, p. 69.

Emigration and immigration

Following graduation, medical graduates were limited in their options. Students were not required to undertake a compulsory internship year as part of their full medical registration until the mid-1950s.[90] However, some medical students, such as Noël Browne, undertook an intern year following graduation to gain more practical experience. On leaving Trinity in 1942, Browne entered in Dr Steevens' Hospital as a resident physician, where he was 'constantly on call on a rota system to attend at the wards and outpatients' department. There were incidents of all kinds day and night, trivial or fatal accidents and sometimes suicides'.[91] Similarly, Joyce Delaney, who graduated from UCD in 1949, entered at St Vincent's hospital as an unpaid intern for six months.[92] According to Delaney, 'the job was honorary; acceptance, in whatever capacity, on the junior staff, was considered sufficiently rewarding without looking for payment'.[93]

Prior to the introduction of compulsory internships, medical graduates would try to obtain a position as a house physician or house surgeon in the first year after graduation before entering into general practice. However, some entered into practice without having previously obtained a dedicated period of hospital experience.[94] Moreover, these house surgeon and house physician positions were extremely competitive and generally awarded to students who had done the best in examinations.[95] With the change in regulation, doctors were now unable to register without having undertaken the internship year.[96]

The emigration of newly qualified doctors to Britain remained significant from the 1920s to the 1950s. Numbers of medical students graduating from Irish universities increased significantly from the 1920s on. However, opportunities were still limited in the United Kingdom. One female doctor who qualified in Dublin, reported in 1925,

> I was qualified in Dublin, and came over to London because there was nothing to do in Ireland. Doctors are apparently the heaviest exports

---

90 Michael P. Flynn, *Medical doctor of many parts: memoirs of a public health practitioner and health manager, spanning sixty years of social change* (Dublin: Colourbooks Ltd, 2002), p. 4.
91 Browne, *Against the tide*, p. 65.
92 Delaney, *No starch in my coat*, p. 22.
93 Delaney, *No starch in my coat*, p. 22.
94 Professor Frank Kane, MD, 'The changing curriculum in medicine', *Cork University Record* 6 (Easter 1946), p. 23.
95 Flynn, *Medical doctor of many parts*, p. 4.
96 Kane, 'The changing curriculum in medicine', p. 24.

of the Free State at the moment. I know a score of girls and men who are in the same position as myself. I have haunted the registry and agencies until the shoes have been worn off my feet. Just now I have not the price of a cup of coffee in my purse. All I have on which to live is the small allowance they can send me from home, and that they cannot afford. They really did all they could for me when they paid the cost of my medical education.[97]

According to Mr Seton Pringle, President of the Royal College of Surgeons in Dublin, in 1925, it was estimated that there were 104 new medical students registered in the Free State and 61 in Northern Ireland. By 1934, this figure had risen to 383 for the Free State and 153 for Northern Ireland.[98] The increase was felt by students themselves. One medical student at University College Galway in 1931 reported that 'the numerical strength of the faculty has been given a strong upward trend' with the admission of thirty 'pre-reg.' students, compared with four or five entrants starting five years previously.[99]

Aidan MacCarthy, who qualified from University College Cork in 1938, recalled that it was difficult for new graduates to obtain medical appointments in Ireland:

because all specialised appointments were controlled by local medical professional nepotism, and the jobs were very limited in number. The situation was not helped by the fact that these so-called dispensary jobs were occupied by doctors well into their eighties – settled, well liked, and with no intention of retiring. The result was that nearly 80 per cent of newly qualified doctors had to cross the water to England and Wales, where medical work was plentiful, particularly in the armed services.[100]

Similarly, a 1936 *Irish Times* article explained that 400 new students had entered upon the books of the Medical Council during 1935, and that 'in four or five years' time, [when] they emerge as qualified doctors, the Free State will be able to absorb only fifty of them'. The high number of medical students was explained as being partly caused by the fact that many medical students had chosen that course because 'the less ambitious occupations in which normally they would have found a place have not recovered from a

---

97 'Irishwoman's bitter experiences', *Irish Examiner*, 10 February 1925, p. 6.
98 'More medical students', *Irish Press*, 18 February 1936, p. 3.
99 'Medical', *University Annual: University College, Galway* 6(7) (1931–2), p. 63.
100 Aidan MacCarthy, *A doctor's war* (Cork: Collins Press, 2005), p. 11.

period of economic stress' and that the years of training involved in medical study offered students and their parents 'a breathing space, and makes more distant the day when an overcrowded world must be faced'. The increasing number of women students was also blamed for placing stress on the medical marketplace.[101]

The situation remained the same with regard to emigration of medical graduates in the 1940s and 1950s.[102] *The Irish Press* reported in 1943 that 75 per cent of newly qualified doctors emigrated to England and the British Empire and called for a reduction in the number of medical students admitted to Irish universities.[103] Similarly, the *Cork University Record* reported in 1944 that at least two-thirds of their medical graduates (on average, 40 a year) went to England to seek work and experience.[104] England was thought to provide good opportunities in hospital work, with the post of casualty officer being the most easily obtained for new graduates and providing the best general experience.[105] Joyce Delaney recalled:

> When I qualified in 1949, it was every doctor's ambition to become a medical 'all-rounder' and for this it was necessary to get as much experience as possible. We were, like the eggs, for export to England. America, as a place of employment didn't enter most of our minds. It was associated with 'wild colonial boys' and tin trunks. Middle-class Dublin in that era rather looked down its nose at any suggestion of an American accent. As it was, the thought of going to England was frightening enough, since apart from a short trip to the Isle of Man, I had never been out of Ireland.[106]

Francis (UCC, 1943–9) recollected: 'So, my father knew I was going to emigrate, because when I was 16, he said – I was only barely 17, and I was going up to college, but the year before, he said – "You won't be living here, you won't be living in Cork, you'll be living in Dublin, or London, or someplace"'. He added, 'My mother cried when I went up to college, because, to do medicine, because she realised that I would, for certain, be emigrating'.

101 'Free State "Medicals"', *Irish Times*, 17 February 1936, p. 6.
102 For more on the emigration of Irish female doctors during the Second World War, see Jennifer Redmond, 'The thermometer and the travel permit: Irish women in the medical profession in Britain during World War Two', in D.A.J. Macpherson and Mary J. Hickman (eds), *Women and Irish diaspora identities: theories, concepts and new perspectives* (Manchester: Manchester University Press, 2014), pp. 92–111.
103 'Turning out too many doctors', *Irish Press*, 23 April 1943, p. 1.
104 'Medicus Medico', *Cork University Record* 1 (summer term 1944), p. 27.
105 'Medicus Medico', p. 27.
106 Delaney, *No starch in my coat*, p. 22.

In the ten years between 1951 and 1961, over 400,000 persons left the Republic of Ireland.[107] This was equal to almost one-sixth of the total population recorded in 1951.[108] From the post-war period up until the 1970s, at least four-fifths of these people emigrated to Britain.[109] After the war, North America and particularly the United States became another attractive option for newly qualified Irish doctors.[110] Emigration was deeply ingrained as a stage in the life-cycle of young Irish people, while the decision to emigrate also stemmed partly from the bleak domestic environment in Ireland in the 1950s.[111] As a consequence of a rise in foreign-trained medical graduates immigrating to the United States for work, the American Medical Association issued a list in 1950 of approved foreign medical schools which they believed to provide a medical education which was on par with that provided in American medical schools.[112] The medical schools of the Republic of Ireland (excluding Queen's University Belfast which was now part of Northern Ireland and the United Kingdom) were not on this list. What followed was 'an intense struggle involving diplomacy, doctor activism and political intervention on both sides of the Atlantic'.[113] This became an important issue for Irish medical schools during the 1950s and helped to draw attention to poor standards of education. The report of the American Medical Association, in addition to one produced by the General Medical Council in 1954, highlighted a range of problems with the Irish medical schools.[114] In Galway and Cork, opportunities for clinical experience were restricted, while more generally no Irish professors had 'a clinical department or laboratory in training'. Clinical pathology was neglected while libraries and museums were lacking in investment. Moreover, it was claimed that university calendars 'were often unreliable guides to the teaching programmes'.[115] This meant that graduates from Irish medical schools, as a result of not graduating from an institution on the 'approved list', were unable to emigrate to the United States until the list was done away with in 1958, and an examination offered by the Educational Commission for Foreign Medical Graduates introduced instead.[116]

107 Enda Delaney, 'The vanishing Irish? The exodus from Ireland in the 1950s', in Dermot Keogh, Finbarr O'Shea and Carmel Quinlan (eds), *Ireland: the lost decade in the 1950s* (Dublin: Mercier Press, 2004), p. 81.
108 Delaney, 'The vanishing Irish?', p. 81.
109 Delaney, 'The vanishing Irish?', p. 81.
110 Jones, 'A mysterious discrimination', p. 139.
111 Delaney, 'The Vanishing Irish?', p. 82.
112 Jones, 'A mysterious discrimination', p. 139.
113 Jones, 'A mysterious discrimination', p. 140.
114 Jones, 'A mysterious discrimination', p. 144.
115 Jones, 'A mysterious discrimination', p. 144.
116 Jones, 'A mysterious discrimination', pp. 152–4.

Emigration was not necessarily easy for Irish medical graduates. Thomas Hennessy, who graduated from UCD in 1957, recalled that after graduating he 'still had not taken it all in and I think my chief reaction was one of relief that it was all over at last. I would soon realise that this was not the end of anything, just the beginning of an even longer and rougher road'.[117] Hennessy initially worked as a trainee surgeon at St Michael's Hospital in Dun Laoghaire and at the Jervis Street Hospital before moving to Liverpool to work for three years. Anne (UCC, 1947–53) recalled her sadness at having to emigrate after her one-year internship in Ireland, explaining that there was 'terrible poverty' in Ireland in the 1950s and that 'the specialities weren't here. And ... nearly everybody went to be trained abroad, you know'. Recalling her experiences of emigrating to England, she stated, 'Yeah, it was sad going. I was very sad to emigrate, you know? I always remember the first Christmas I couldn't, I, we didn't get time off because, as junior doctor, you were the dogsbody, you stayed there all over Christmas. I was heartbroken'. Other interviewees, like Colm (UCC, 1949–54), a late entrant to his medical course, was excited about the prospect of emigration to the United States for postgraduate training, following the example of his younger brother. He recalled, 'There was a big wide open world opening up to me then. I couldn't wait to get my hands on it'. He left from Shannon on an Aer Lingus Constellation turboprop that took 14 hours, which included a stopover in Newfoundland, before arriving in Boston. His most vivid memory of his departure was waving goodbye to his father standing at the bottom of the steps leading up to the aircraft. He never appreciated, until years later, the sense of loss his father must have been experiencing at the emigration of the eldest of his two sons.

Opportunities were slim with regard to hospital appointments in Ireland in the 1940s and 1950s, and many of the interviewees remarked on nepotism in Irish hospitals. Martha (TCD, 1943–9) recollected: 'Oh you had to [emigrate]. You couldn't get a job there. Perhaps if your father was a medical man, or something, he might get you somewhere or other, you know. But I think you'd have to have influence. I don't think you'd get in. I don't know if it's still the same'. When asked about opportunities following graduation, John (RCSI, 1947–53) recalled: 'There weren't any. Absolutely not. Nepotism ruled. Unless you had somebody actually working in the hospital in a senior position you had no chance at all of getting a job in that hospital. You might as a house officer or something very junior but after that it depended on who you knew, not what you knew, it was absolutely true so ... huge emigration of course was the answer at that time. It was the only answer really at the time'. Similarly, Thomas (TCD, 1946–52) recalled: 'It was no accident that in some

117 Hennessy, *My life as a surgeon*, p. 93.

of the Dublin hospitals you had, sort of, almost family occasions. Like the
Meenans, the Meenans at St Vincent's and all that. There was about four
of them. They were consultants there, four brothers or three brothers. All
very good, it just so happened, but then you wonder to yourself, well, there
must be some place where there are four brothers that are all very bad, and
of course there are traditions'.

The Irish student body was also undergoing changes. The 1950s were
distinctive in Irish medical schools because of a decline in numbers of
Irish-born medical students and the increase in numbers of international
medical students. Writing in 1958, Professor Geoffrey Bewley, professor of
social, forensic and preventive medicine at the Royal College of Surgeons,
remarked on the change in nationality in the student body. In 1931, 'the
students were almost all Irish or of Irish descent; now they are international,
of every creed and colour, and no one who has worked in the Royal College
of Surgeons in Ireland could possibly agree to apartheid or segregation'.[118] At
UCC, the majority of international medical students came from the United
States, but the Cork medical student body also incorporated students from
Africa, the Caribbean islands and Poland.[119] Similarly, at UCG, there was
an influx of Polish medical students after the Second World War, as well
as overseas students from what was then Malaya, the United States and
Canada in the 1950s.[120] Some, like E.B. McKee, an American student from
Rhode Island, who began his studies at the Royal College of Surgeons in
1955, were inspired by family and economic factors. McKee was encouraged
to study medicine in Ireland by his aunt Bertha, and an Irish medical
degree was cheaper and offered him an escape from his tedious temporary
job as a fish cutter.[121]

After the Second World War, a number of British ex-servicemen took
up medical courses in Ireland. Sylvia (QUB, 1944–50) recalled that the
ex-servicemen were

> like something from a different world … they were, they brought a
> quality to our year, and it was mainly the year I was in, and maybe the
> next year, those two years would've had a lot of these ex-service people,
> and there were two things about it. First of all they were determined
> to rebuild their lives and make something of it. The second thing was

118 'A professor looks back', *Mistura* (summer term 1958), p. 9.
119 Denis J. O'Sullivan, *The Cork School of Medicine: a history* (Cork: UCC Medical
     Alumni Association, University College Cork, 2007), pp. 55–6.
120 James P. Murray, *Galway: a medico-social history* (Galway: Kenny's Bookshop, 2002),
     p. 196.
121 E.B. McKee, *Doc: revelations of a reluctant Yank studying medicine among the Irish*
     (Narragansett, RI: Ebook Bakery Books, 2013), p. 27.

that for the very first time they offered grants, university grants, the government were paying for them, but they weren't allowed to fail any exam, which meant that they were all hard-working students, and they pushed the standard up.

Stephen (QUB, 1942–7) recalled students interrupting their medical study to go into the army. Similarly, Ted (UCD, 1946–52), recalled there being students from Africa and India in his class as well as ex-servicemen. Because these men were older than the rest of the medical student body, they tended to socialise separately from the other students. Maureen (UCD, 1952–8) recalled two Englishmen who had served in the army, 'They wouldn't have been very integrated. They would, I mean, they seemed to me to be very old, but I suppose they were in their thirties ... But I wouldn't have said they integrated much with the teenagers, you know. The young ones, they would have had their own little group'. Thomas (TCD, 1946–52) recalled an influx of servicemen to his medical class from 1946. He also remembered three African students in his year.

The majority of students in most of the universities, however, were Irish. Paul (UCD, 1946–52) recalled that 'They were, there were a few [non-Irish students]. Some came from English schools. Usually, their parents would have been Irish, yeah. And then, we had a couple of Poles who had come across just after the War, through the Iron Curtain, and so on. The Js [Jesuits] did that, they kind of brought them in ... And, um, they had to learn the language, and it was hard on them. And one or two Americans, not more than that, I'd say'. Life could be difficult for international students. Douglas Noah, a Canadian student at University College Galway, in a letter to the Academic Council in 1954, remarked that he had felt 'especially and completely unsettled in Galway. I was unhappy there from the start, I found social conventions, habits, intellectual outlook and even clothes so completely different from my own that I always had an uneasy feeling I was being watched and criticised'. This sense of loneliness and unhappiness, Noah claimed, made it difficult for him to concentrate on his studies, and he failed two examinations. Moreover, 'the changeable Galway weather didn't help much either and I soon developed colds, headaches, and other physical ailments'. Noah requested to transfer his studies to Dublin where he felt more at home.[122] The Royal College of Surgeons tended to have a higher proportion of international students. John (RCSI, 1947–53) recalled that:

---

122 Letter dated 14 December 1954 to Professor Mitchell, Registrar, University College Galway from Douglas J. Noah, Eustace House, 69 Lower Leeson Street, Dublin. Rough Minutes for Academic Council meetings, September 1954–1955 [NUI Galway Archives and Special Collections, 4/17].

There was always a contingent from Nigeria, always. I think they were supported by the British Foreign Office financially, and there were always about, I'd say, ten Nigerians per year, you know, and apart from that a few New Zealanders, one Australian perhaps in my time, some Jamaicans, and that was very nearly – there would be nobody from continental Europe, for example. There might be a few Poles, particularly more or less refugees after the Second World War, they would have, they appeared. Indeed. And that was it.

Oral history interviewees also recalled that international students tended to socialise separately from the Irish students.

It is clear that by the 1950s the student body was more diverse than it had been for previous generations. International students now made up a greater proportion of the student body, although Irish students were still in the majority. As the following section will illustrate, women students also continued to be an important part of the student body although it is arguable whether their experiences changed significantly.

Women's experiences

It appears that even in the 1950s women medical students were ridiculed in the student press in the same way that their predecessors had been. In a 1953 issue of *Snakes Alive*, the magazine of Queen's College Belfast, a student wrote that there were only four female students in third year, in contrast with greater numbers in fifth year. The author remarked: '!Is this the sign of a straying trend? 5th Year contains about three dozen of the pests – sorry – pets. As the 5 Year mortality (marriage) is about 75% and the State is paying large sums annually for their stay at Medical School, and as only a small proportion are suited for the profession anyway, let us hope so'.[123] The March issue of the magazine in the same year included a cartoon showing two glamorous women medical students with the caption: 'How did you do in the oral?' 'Quite well. The Professor proposed to me.'[124] Female students remained in the minority at Irish medical schools in the 1940s and 1950s, although numbers were gradually increasing from the lows of the post-First World War period.

Clair Callan, who began her studies at UCD in 1957, for instance, recalled that of the 120 students beginning in her class that year, there were 20 women students. She recalled the lecture halls having tiered seats

123 *Snakes Alive* 1(3) (June 1953), p. 2.
124 *Snakes Alive* 1(2) (March 1953), p. 22.

with numbers on them and students being assigned numbers. In her words, 'The boys far outnumbered the girls, and the first three rows of any lecture theatre were reserved for the girls. But we never filled them all and had lots of space to spread out after the roll was taken'.[125] Religious sisters comprised a significant proportion of the female student body at UCD and UCC. According to Callan, of the 20 female students in her year, 12 were nuns from the religious orders who 'kept to themselves and remained steadfastly serious, as though smiles were against their rules. If they didn't have their noses in books, they were simply coming up for air before sticking them back down again'. In contrast, the 'eight-person secular girl group' chatted and gossiped amongst themselves before lectures began.[126] Similarly, Ted (UCD, 1946–52) remembered there being nuns from the Holy Rosary Sisters convent in Killeshandra, Co. Cavan, in his year, and that these religious sisters 'kind of kept to themselves'. Jean (UCC, 1951–7), a religious sister, stayed with other sisters from her order who were studying at UCC at a Domincan Hostel in Cork, and although she did not mix too much socially with the other students in her class, she stated, 'I felt at home with them'. In spite of some negative representations in the student press, all of the female medical graduates interviewed responded that they did not experience significant differences in their treatment compared with the male students. Sylvia (QUB, 1944–50) remarked, 'We were totally acceptant of each other'. Maureen (UCD, 1952–8) recalled:

> I wouldn't have been conscious of any difference now, I mean we were treated, you know, very much as a student, and there wasn't any kind of problem being a woman. In fact, we might have been treated more politely by, say, particularly the clinical doctors at the lectures, whereas they'd bawl out – have a roar at the man if he was doing something wrong. They'd be a little bit, you know, more polite to the young ladies. And you were called 'Miss Murphy' and 'Miss this'. But I wouldn't have been conscious at all of any problem being a woman medical student or doctor though I think maybe, as it went on, I could see there is more of a struggle to, kind-of, make it, but there was great camaraderie, I think.

Male students similarly reported a lack of difference in experiences between men and women. Christopher (TCD, 1942–9) recalled that the female students 'were mostly, you know, very industrious, and very good. A

---

125 Clair M. Callan, *Standing my ground: memoir of a woman physician* (Bloomington, Ind.: Archway Publishing, 2014), p. 31.
126 Callan, *Standing my ground*, p. 31.

lot of swots [laughs]'. When asked whether women and men medical students socialised together, John (RCSI, 1947–53) remarked:

> A bit, but there was an unwritten law that they did not have romantic attachments with each other because being together for, shall we say, six years, there was a guarantee that it would probably disintegrate with corresponding embarrassment to the whole lot, you know. So I think there was an unwritten law that they did their courting, as it was innocently called, outside the College.

Other students, such as Andrew (UCD, 1949–55), however, recalled, 'Yeah, well, there were some lines going on. I mean, some members of the class married other members if I remember rightly'. Paul (UCD, 1946–52) recollected, 'But they all sat in the front rows, which I resented, because you went alphabetically [by surname] up the, you know, and I was M, so I was at the very top of the, trying to hear what was going on, and these women were all down in front, because they were women'.

Some female students seem to have also been particularly vulnerable with regard to family issues in relation to pursuing their medical studies. Mary Coyne, a student at University College Galway, wrote to the Academic Council in 1953 stating that she had failed the second medical examination three times, with one of these occasions being on account of her grandfather dying suddenly and Coyne having to look after the family and six boarders while her mother was away in Donegal for the funeral.[127] Similarly, Lucy Hornsby wrote to the Academic Council in 1954 requesting an opportunity to take her second medical examination again. Owing to her mother's illness, Hornsby had been called back to her homeland in England, explaining that since then her mother 'has been a semi-invalid and I have been prevented from studying wholeheartedly in my effort to help her'.[128]

Nevertheless, while most oral history interviewees recalled that men and women were largely treated as equals, female students appear to have been targets of student pranks and teasing. Lily (TCD, 1946–53) recalled, 'No, I would find the boys would rag you, you know, as usual. If you did well at hockey, you know ... or something, and the press had written it up, you, you might be, they might tease you'. Similarly, Mary (UCG, 1946–52) recalled, 'They were very nice. The odd, you know, there'd be jokes and things. But

---

127 Letter from Mary B. Coyne, dated 1 April 1953, Academic Council Rough Minutes, June 1952–September 1953 [NUI Galway Archives, 4/15].
128 Letter from Lucy Cecilia Hornsby, dated 3 February 1954, Rough Minutes of Meetings of Academic Council September 1953–August 1954 [NUI Galway Archives, 4/16].

they were very innocent really'. She added 'Occasionally, there'd be a bit, they'd look and say "Mm I like your coat", or, you know, something like that, which didn't happen often because we never had new coats anyway!' Stephen (QUB, 1942–7) recalled how the male medical students in his class would sometimes sing a song about each of the female medical students as they waited for them to come into class and sit at the front before John Henry Biggart's pathology lecture. According to Stephen, 'That was quite an occupation, of course. We made up very nice, and sometimes not very nice songs, as each of them came. We had a very good attitude towards them, they were medical students as we were. As far as we were concerned they weren't any different from we, apart from difference in sex'. Similarly, Una (UCC, 1951–7) remembered, 'Oh there was no problem ... well, we were separated in that, well, not separated, but we were put in the front row. Which had its disadvantages. Not the least of which if you weren't watching, they'd come in and take all your shoes off and the lecturer would come in to lecture to twelve barefoot women, well with the exception of the nun, they wouldn't do it to her!'

Female students at Trinity College appear to have been more restricted. Martha (TCD, 1943–9) explained, 'There weren't many [female students]. There was only four women in my year, in a hundred men. So, I mean, you were in a very, very tiny minority, really. You probably didn't get as much out of it as the men did, you know, because you [were] very constrained'. She recalled that students were 'constricted' at Trinity with regard to behaviour because of issues such as having to sign in to get into the college. Remarking, 'You weren't allowed to do anything, basically ... you had to behave yourself or they'd throw you out, I'm quite sure'. Thomas (TCD, 1946–52) remembered:

> the constraints of women in Trinity were amazing at that time. They amazed even me ... it was very restrictive. You weren't allowed to entertain a girl in any sense of the word. You weren't allowed to entertain a girl in your rooms. You had to get the permission of the junior dean, who's in charge of rooms and you have to write him a nice note and say that you're having a sort of having a moment with Miss So-and-so, gabble gabble or something like that and he would give permission or not as the case may be.

He also remembered there being a special building for the women students. 'They had to come in and go straight up number 6. They could walk through to the library of course and walk to the lectures, and then to the engineering building and to the medical school, obviously, but that was where they congregated'. In his view, there seemed to be no effort made at, to bring men and women together, in any way, socially or any other. Only in the lecture theatre, we always sat down in alphabetical order of surname in the first two or three years, two years, but for the convenience of the person who kept the attendance, because you had a number, you see, behind you, and it was 'uncovered' obviously if you were not there.

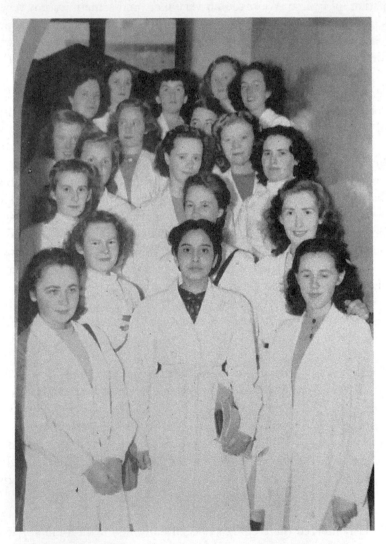

10   'A bevy of first years on the way to the anatomy room'.
Photograph from L.E. McLoughlin (ed.), *Surgeon's log, annals of the schools of surgery, Royal College of Surgeons in Ireland* (Dublin: Regal, 1949). Courtesy of the RCSI Heritage Collections.

Beulah Bewley, who studied at Trinity in the late 1940s and early 1950s, recalled in her memoirs one instance where a professor of psychiatry, during a lecture on female disorders, stated that he 'did not like the smell of menstruating women'. All of the women immediately left the lecture in protest, but this was the only incident of disrespect on the part of a professor which Bewley noted.[129]

Although women and men continued to enjoy generally similar educational experiences, it is clear that in the 1950s divisions still remained between the two groups. This was particularly the case at Trinity College. Religious sisters, a significant part of the female student body from the 1940s, were another segregated group. It appears likely, however, that the separation of male and female students was in part a conscious decision by the students themselves rather than something enforced by Irish universities.

Social life

Possibly the most amazing object in College is the Med. He is in every club, society and poker game in the place. He is strewn along the Quad; he is talking in the Library; he is guzzling in the Rest; he is hoofling in the Guild Council and boozing in the Oyster. Seldom, if ever, does he work, because, sound man that he is, he knows there is no need for it. It is an indisputable fact that anyone with the brain of a gnat and the hide of a rhinoceros can fly through his Med exams ... nothing disturbs his joyous life but an occasional lack of cash – which defect is quickly remedied by hocking his pal's coat or his landlady's blankets. He is the smug bug in the rug; he is the happy parasite whose capacity for porter is only equalled by his incapacity for work.[130]

This extract from an article in a 1950 issue of the *Quarryman*, a student magazine of University College Cork, highlights the important role that the medical student continued to play in the social life of the university. Such representations were not uncommon. A cartoon in *Mistura* magazine, published in 1955, illustrated the medical student in a variety of guises: as he appeared to his landlady (covered in money), to his father (as a devil-horned poker-playing, smoking and drinking character), to his mother (with a halo around his head), to 'the girlfriend' (as a suave and refined looking gentleman), to 'pre-reg.' students (the bottom half of a student's body is

---

129 Beulah Bewley and Susan Bewley (eds), *My life as a woman and doctor* (Bristol: Silverwood Books, 2016), p. 55.
130 'The Med', *Quarryman* (Easter 1950), unpaginated.

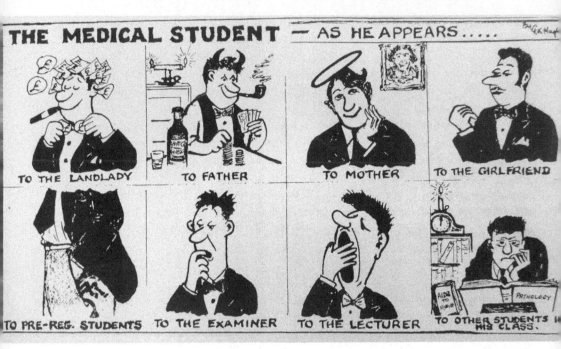

11 'The Medical Student as he appears…'.
Cartoon drawn by George K. Maharaj (LRCP & SI, 1957) from *Mistura*
(summer term 1955). Courtesy of the RCSI Heritage Collections.

shown with a stethoscope hanging out of the pocket), to the examiner (foolish-looking and struggling to answer a question), to the lecturer (yawning) and to other students in his class (as a conscientious individual studying late into the night). The prevalence of these types of sources suggests that the multiple representations of medical students which had been in existence since the nineteenth century still persisted.

With regard to their social lives, it is evident that socialising was limited for medical students in the 1940s and 1950s owing to increasing hours of study and a lack of money. Ted (UCD, 1946–52) remembered: 'I think an awful lot of us knew that there wasn't an awful lot of money behind us, and we had to get our exams, and go through, and get on, and felt that we were quite privileged anyway.' Most interviewees mentioned going to the cinema (or 'the pictures'). Anne (UCC, 1947–53) recalled: 'The great thing was going to the pictures … Going to the movies. That was a great thing. They were cheap, they were great, they were warm, and there was a good story. So, it, and money was very scarce, you know? You got one outfit at the beginning of the year, and you did, you had your previous clothes … there was no, no big spending, like there is now'. Sylvia (QUB, 1944–50) recalled:

'After the war, things were difficult. There wasn't a lot of money around. There wasn't the same social life that your generation is used to. It wasn't like that. The University put on a number of formal dances and my husband would have come up and gone with me to those, and so he came as often as he could, but I couldn't expect it to happen too much.' She also mentioned her involvement with the church and the student representative council, but remarked that once students 'went into clinical work, you couldn't keep up university things. You were most of the time in the hospital anyway, and it was just too much pressure, and I didn't want to start failing exams again'. Thomas (TCD, 1946–52) recalled: 'Money was very scarce … I mean, I considered myself about average and I, virtually, by moderate standards, had no money at all. I mean, you went to the pictures on Friday night as a great treat, 9 pence, back row of the Metropole or something like that, or the Savoy or wherever'.

The consumption of alcohol does not appear to have been prevalent among the cohort that were interviewed. When asked about this, most graduates responded that students did not have the money to indulge in drinking or referred to the fact that drinking was simply not a part of student culture in Ireland of the 1940s and 1950s. Seamus (UCD, 1942–7) recalled: 'Some of them did, but drinking … none of my friends drank at all. Some of them did go to the pubs, that's true.' Drinking tended to revolve more so around rugby matches or regattas, while some Dublin graduates recalled that there were divisions between those who drank and those who did not. Paul (UCD, 1946–52), when asked about whether students went to pubs much, recalled: 'Well, you either did or you didn't … Now, funnily enough, when we formed a table, our own table, for the Hall dance, there would be six boys, who would ask six girls. There was no drink at the table. At our table … But then, there was another crowd, who had been to Hartigan's first, you know?' Similarly, Andrew (UCD, 1949–55) recalled: 'Pub culture, again, was very much focused around the rugby team'. Maureen (UCD, 1952–8) remembered: 'There were always the few wild ones and alcohol was the big one – Hartigan's, the pub on the corner, was a great medical students' pub, and there was always the few that would skip lectures and be in Hartigan's. But there were an awful lot of teetotallers as well, you see, in those days, both men and women who wouldn't have started drinking maybe until they were into their twenties, because I know in my class there would have been a lot, including myself, that didn't drink alcohol until we were much older'. John (RCSI, 1947–53) recalled:

Yes, well, there was obviously a certain amount of drunkenness, you know, basically. And in those days, I think, when people drunk, people were sort-of heroes. I think that was a little bit of the wrong atmosphere at the time, but there was very little violence compared to today where things are concluded with knives, and little things like that. There might be the odd punch-up but nothing awful. I mean nobody was, as it were, knocked out or indeed killed, thank God, you know.

Most students acknowledged that there was a certain amount of drinking that went on, but that there was little drunkenness because students did not have the money to afford it. Colm (UCC, 1949–55) recalled that students 'couldn't afford it', and 'I never remember drinking or having a drink in sight. All soft drinks or tea and biscuits. That was about as much. Nothing to be served. Of course, there was smoking'.

Involvement in charity work became more significant for students in the 1940s and 1950s. At Queen's University Belfast, a Hospital Fund was established as part of the university's Students' Day in 1935 while a Compassionate Guild was founded at the Royal College of Surgeons in 1944 which provided assistance and care to the poor in Dublin.[131] John (RCSI, 1947–53) recalled: 'We had an organisation known as the Compassionate Guild which helped the poor people of Dublin. And we used to have a flag day once a year and that was well supported. And also the students, they went and visited the homes of these people. So there was a good social sort-of ethic there from day one'. Interviewees also recalled dances and hops and that these served as a means for men and women to socialise, while medical societies also provided a social outlet for students from the 1930s to the 1950s.

Sport remained an important part of medical student life in the 1940s and 1950s. Ristéard Mulcahy, who studied at UCD between 1939 and 1944, recalled getting involved in rowing and cycling. However, he gave up rowing in his final years of medical study so as to allow more time for clinical experience in the hospital and studying.[132] Similarly, David (TCD, 1940–6) recalled that students were interested in sport because 'it all made sense from a health point of view: if you're athletic you're more likely to be healthy. And, but, more a social thing, more a kind-of addiction'.

It is clear, however, that financial considerations restricted students in the 1940s and 1950s with regard to their social lives. Representations of medical students as drunken and more interested in socialising than in their

131 'Students' Day Hospital Fund', *New Northman* 3(3) (summer term 1935): p. 24; *Royal College of Surgeons in Ireland: Schools of Surgery, including Carmichael and Ledwich Schools, 1947–48 handbook* (Dublin: George F. Healy & Co., 1948), p. 28.
132 Ristéard Mulcahy, *Memoirs of a medical maverick* (Dublin: Liberties Press, 2010), pp. 48–54.

academic pursuits were evidently not based in reality, while graduates of the post-war era appear to have been more focused and serious in their academic pursuits.

Conclusion

Writing in 1957, a student at Queen's University, Belfast explained:

> Whatever the stories are and will be, one thing is certain – the life of the medical student does not change very much, it is only people who change. One of our graduates who is still alive told us that when he graduated at the turn of the century his constant worry was – 'What shall I do – there are no jobs'. To-day, 50 years later, this is still a worry to medical students.[133]

To what extent had medical student life in Ireland changed by the 1950s? Although representations of medical students as boisterous and rowdy persisted in the student press, it is clear from oral history interviews that such representations were simply fictions, and did not have a sound basis in reality. Although reasons for studying medicine did not change significantly, medical students of the period from the 1930s to the 1950s largely appear to have been focused on passing their examinations and dealing with a more strenuous curriculum. Clinical experience persisted as the most important part of medical education, while students' obstetrical experience placed them in direct contact with patients, often without much supervision. The provincial medical schools continued to be critiqued by outside bodies while damning reports by the American Medical Association suggested that Irish medical education was not up to international standards. Evidently, emigration remained an important part of medical graduate life and was seen by most students as being the probable outcome of medical study.

The Irish student body does not appear to have been particularly cohesive. Owing to their long hours, medical students tended to stick together and continued to have a separate identity from the rest of the students. Although rivalries between different medical schools were not very significant, medical students did not tend to socialise with students outside of their university until they gained hospital experience. Fundamentally, however, educational experiences continued to help cement a sense of institutional identity. As David (TCD, 1940–6), explained: 'These different medical

133 'Random reflections of a medical student by Candidus', *Snakes Alive* 3(2) (March 1955), p. 15.

schools – we were all like men in football clubs, you got to know your own friends and everything and I mean if you're six years working in a medical school you get rather stuck with them and get to know them well'. Women students continued to be a separate part of the student body, while this was also further complicated by the introduction of religious sisters to many Irish medical schools from the 1940s, who tended to socialise separately. International students and ex-servicemen were increasingly prevalent at Irish medical schools in the post-war period, and it appears that these students formed another separate group within the student body. Finally, it is clear that links between British medical education and Irish medical education persisted even after Irish independence in 1922.

Conclusion

A piece in *Mistura* in 1954 explained the transition from student to doctor in the following way:

> This mode of life persists until the metamorphosis into 'Doctor'. This latter change occurs very suddenly. One moment the Medical Student is standing in a black gown; then he mutters some words under his breath, and lo and behold – 'Doctor'. 'Doctors' are characterised by their brusque manner, lots of money, little hair and by the fact that they never speak to Medical Students.[1]

This book has explored the experiences of medical students studying at Irish universities in the nineteenth and twentieth centuries. Although it is clear that medical education went through some significant changes during this period, with a shift, broadly speaking, from the medical apprenticeship system of the early nineteenth century, to a greater focus on clinical and bedside medicine in the mid-nineteenth century, to attempts to make medicine more scientific in the late nineteenth to early twentieth century, it is clear that medical students of the past and of today share many of the same concerns.

Irish medical schools continue to be 'exporting schools'.[2] A recent study conducted on emigration and Irish medical graduates found that emigration was on the minds of a significant proportion of the medical student body. Of the 2,273 medical students interviewed, 88 per cent indicated that they were definitely migrating or considering migrating following graduation or completion of their pre-registration intern year, with factors such as career opportunities, working conditions and lifestyle being important factors in

1 'The medical student or Apollo with a scalpel', *Mistura* 2(1) (winter term 1954), p. 5.
2 Greta Jones, '"Strike out boldly for the prizes that are available to you": medical emigration from Ireland, 1860–1905', *Medical History* 54(1) (2010), p. 74.

their decision to leave.[3] Similarly, a report published by the Royal College of Surgeons in Ireland found that the falling income levels for junior doctors in Ireland, excessive working hours and an uncertain career pathway were important push factors, while the prospect of a better work–life balance in countries such as Australia, New Zealand, the UK and the United States, was an important pull factor.[4] Moreover, the introduction of the HPAT (Health Professions Admissions Test) in Ireland in 2009 suggests that the Irish medical profession remains concerned with ensuring that potential students possess what are viewed as being suitable traits. The test, which has generated much debate since its introduction, assesses the suitability of potential medical students by assessing their logical and non-verbal reasoning as well as inter-personal understanding. Additionally, it is clear that women have made significant progress in the Irish medical profession. Today female students predominate in medical school applications in Ireland, a pattern which is mirrored by medical schools internationally. In 2009, for instance, women students represented 50 per cent of entrants to Irish medical schools, while in 2010, 60 per cent were female.[5] However, recent concerns about the 'feminisation' of medicine and reports of a gender bias in favour of male students in the Irish HPAT entrance examination suggest that the 'historic relative over-representation of females in medical school is a sensitive and emotive issue'.[6] There are new concerns too, such as 'burn-out' among stressed medical students, which led UCC's medical school to introduce a cognitive behavioural coaching programme called SAFEMED in 2013 to help protect students' emotional well-being and prepare them for the pressures of a career as a medical practitioner.[7] The working pressures faced by junior doctors in Ireland have recently received much attention, with the Irish Medical Organisation reporting in 2013 that junior doctors were working on average 63 hours a week, with some working over 100.[8] This resulted in a strike by junior doctors in October 2013, putting pressure on the Health Service Executive to ensure that all Irish hospitals comply with

3 Pishoy Gouda et al., 'Ireland's medical brain drain migration intentions of Irish medical students', *Human Resources for Health* 13(11) (2015).

4 Lavanya Chalikonda, 'Why are Irish doctors emigrating?', *Royal College of Surgeons in Ireland Student Medical Journal* 6(1) (2013), pp. 93–8.

5 Siun O'Flynn, Anne Mills and Tony Fitzgerald (National research group evaluating revised entry mechanisms to medicine), 'Interim report: school leaver entrants' (July 2012), pp. 16–17: www.ucd.ie/t4cms/HPAT-report-July2012.pdf.

6 Siun O'Flynn, Anne Mills and Tony Fitzgerald, 'Entry to Medical School, the gender question: what has happened?', *Irish Medical Journal* 106(8) (September 2013), pp. 230–1.

7 Catherine Shanahan, 'Medical graduates get antidote to stress', *Irish Examiner*, 31 May 2013.

8 Helen Jacques, 'Irish doctors to strike over "dangerous" working hours', *BMJ Careers*, 6 September 2013.

the European Union's Working Time Directive which provides for the right
to work no more than 48 hours a week.

I have previously argued that it is important for historians to 'think about
Ireland as having a distinctive history of medical education and, indeed,
history of medicine from that of Britain'.[9] Although this is certainly true
with regard to women's experiences within Irish medical schools, where
women appear to have been more readily accepted than in Britain, it is clear
that for the nineteenth century, and much of the twentieth century, the
British and Irish medical professions were inextricably linked and had much
in common. And, in common with their counterparts in Britain, elsewhere
in Europe, and in the United States, Irish medical students were warned
about the importance of cultivating diligence and good behaviour and
avoiding the company of idle students in an effort to improve the reputation
of medical students, who conventionally were viewed as badly behaved:
an image which persisted into the twentieth century. As reports of bad
behaviour by medical students began to decline, their image was remoulded
into a more respectable one by the late-nineteenth century. Traits such as
nobility and heroism became more important, thus reinforcing ideals about
medicine being a 'manly' profession, particularly significant as women began
to be part of the student body in Ireland from the 1880s.

Considering that a high proportion of Irish medical graduates emigrated
to Britain after finishing their study, Irish medical schools continued to be
surveyed by the General Medical Council well into the twentieth century.
However, Irish medical education had its own distinctive character and set of
problems. Much attention has been paid to the distinctive elements of Irish
medical education, in particular, bedside teaching as spearheaded by Robert
Graves at the Meath Hospital in the early nineteenth century. However,
although clinical teaching remained a distinctive part of Irish medical
education, teaching more generally was of a poor standard for much of the
nineteenth and twentieth centuries. On top of this, Irish medical schools
were beset with economic difficulties which meant that practices such as
night classes, grinding and the issue of sham certificates were common.
Moreover, owing to increased competition between medical schools, Irish
students had a huge amount of power as consumers in the period. Medical
students were not passive consumers either. Students also actively began to
get involved in the concerns of the profession in the nineteenth century too
and their complaints highlight not only the inadequacies of teaching at Irish
schools but also that students were beginning to see themselves as part of
the profession and therefore felt entitled to get involved in such discussions.

9 Laura Kelly, *Irish women in medicine, c.1880s–1920s: origins, education and careers*
(Manchester: Manchester University Press, 2012), p. 195.

Medical student experience was not homogenous and was shaped by a variety of factors, including location and gender. Female medical students, although largely treated in an egalitarian and paternalistic manner by Irish medical schools, had quite a different social experience compared with their male counterparts. Even by the 1950s, women medical students, though now an accepted part of the student body for over 70 years at this point, were still a separate group within the student body. Within the female student body, there was also segregation as well. Medical missionary nuns, who began to be part of the student body following the 1936 change in canon law, were a very visible but separate part of the female medical student body.

It is clear that medical students of the past stood out within the medical body and had their own sense of identity. This is evident from how they are represented in student magazines from the period. Moreover, the lengthy period of study and long hours spent daily together in the lecture theatre and hospital helped to cement cohesive bonds. Medical students did not mix a great deal with students from other faculties owing to the strenuous nature of their studies. Again, this helped to separate them from their counterparts in other faculties across the university. Although it is evident that there was a large amount of sectarianism within the Irish medical profession in both the nineteenth and twentieth centuries, this does not appear to have affected Irish students' experiences, while oral history respondents who studied in the 1940s and 1950s did not recall major rivalries between the different institutions. Moreover, one's identity as a medical student appears to have been more important than one's religious affiliation. Religious affiliation did, however, often influence one's choice of medical school and hospital for clinical experience.

Social class and mobility are also crucial in understanding the history of the Irish medical profession. Given the length of a medical degree, students in the period examined in this book were generally of social backgrounds that could afford to pay for five to six years of education in addition to living costs, although in contrast with British medical schools, many Irish students could economise by living at home while attending university. Having a doctor in the family in both nineteenth- and twentieth-century Ireland provided social capital and brought prestige on some families. It is evident that the middle classes dominated entrants to Irish medical schools from the mid-nineteenth to the early twentieth century although there were important distinctions between the social backgrounds of students attending Trinity College and the Queen's Colleges. Religion was also an important factor in choice of medical school, and although Catholics began to increase in number in the medical profession from the mid-nineteenth century they still continued to attend the Catholic University and the Queen's Colleges rather than Trinity College. For generations of Catholic students in the mid-twentieth century, University College Dublin and the Queen's Colleges were preferred.

Although educational experiences at Irish medical schools did not significantly change from the 1880s to the 1920s, it is clear that the educational sphere of the hospital was regarded as more important than the lecture theatre and laboratory by students and professors alike. Various aspects of medical education and student culture were couched in a highly masculine rhetoric in the student press and subsequently in doctors' memoirs. While women attending Irish institutions from the 1880s to the 1930s were treated in a fair manner, it is clear that the masculinisation of the medical student experience served as a means of segregating male and female students. Many of the problems associated with Irish medical schools persisted into the twentieth century, while the medical profession was faced with new concerns such as critical reports by the Rockefeller Foundation and the American Medical Association. By this stage, the student body had started to change, with the introduction of increasing numbers of international students. From interviews conducted with graduates of the period it is clear that educational experiences were prioritised over social activities as the medical curriculum became more intense. Emigration has always been a significant factor in Irish medical schools. Many medical students realised that emigration was the only way they would be able to pursue a medical career after graduation. For a lot of students, England was the main choice. However, in the 1940s and 1950s, the United States and Canada became common destinations for Irish medical graduates, but following the damning report by the American Medical Association on Irish medical schools in the 1950s, students' opportunities to work in the United States were significantly reduced.

To conclude, this book has encouraged a different methodological approach from that previously utilised by historians of higher education and medical education. Through its emphasis on sources written by students and former students, it has aimed to give a 'bottom-up' view of university life, histories of which have tended to be dominated by a focus on university staff. The main contribution of this book is, I hope, to reinstate the voices of Irish medical students, who have generally been left out of the historical narrative on medical education. It is clear that the concerns of the medical profession do not change significantly over time: the modern Irish medical student arguably shares many of the same anxieties and experiences as his or her predecessors, while the medical school continues to be one of the most important agents of professionalisation.

Bibliography

Manuscript sources

Dáil Éireann Debates
Debate on Medical Practitioners Bill, 1951, Second Stage, Vol.128, No.3.
Committee on Finance, Medical Practitioners Bill, December 1951, Vol.128, No.6.

Dublin Diocesan Archives
'Instruction S. Cong. Prop. Fide: 11th February 1936: maternity training for missionary sisters', issued to Medical Missionaries of Mary.
Letter from Sister Augustine, Superior to Archbishop McQuaid, dated 18 August 1948.
Letter from Archbishop McQuaid, dated 20 August 1948.

Harry Ransom Center, Texas
Diaries of Alexander Porter, 1861–4.

Medical Missions Sisters Archives, London
'Die Wege meiner Berufung' ('The path to my vocation'), dictated by Sr Anna Dengel to Sr Monica Nehaus, July–August 1969 (English translation) [AE/5/2/1iv].

National Archives of Ireland
Meath Hospital Medical Board Minutes (Rough), 30 October 1879–27 November 1902.
Meath Hospital Medical Board Minute Book, 1879–99.
Meath Hospital Medical Board Minute Book, 1899–1937.
Rules and regulations of the City of Dublin Hospital (Dublin: Browne & Nolan, 1896).

National Library of Ireland
1901 and 1911 Census Records
Letters from Patrick McCartan to Joseph McGarrity [MS 17,457].

National University of Ireland, Galway, Archives and Special Collections
Academic Council Correspondence, March–April 1923 [1/23].
Academic Council Minutes, 1930 [1/47].

Rough Minutes of Governing Body Meetings, June 1950–July 1951 [3/60].
Minutes of Meetings of Academic Council, September 1940–September 1941 [4/3].
Rough Minutes of Academic Council Meetings, August 1941–August 1942 [4/4].
Rough Minutes of Meetings of Academic Council, September 1953–August 1954 [4/15].
Rough Minutes of Meetings of Academic Council, September 1953–August 1954 [4/16].
Special report of the professor of anatomy and physiology, 10 March 1908 [BU/B/274].
University College Galway: Report on the Galway Medical School (Galway: O'Gorman
    Printing House, 1925).
Student matriculation registers for Queen's College Galway/University College Galway,
    1861–1917.

Public Records Office of Northern Ireland
Florence Stewart memoirs [PRONI D/3612/3/1].
Letter from Willie Stewart to his mother, dated 18 November 1876 [PRONI D/953/3].

Queen's University Belfast Special Collections
Belfast Medical Students' Association Minute Book, November 1898–November 1907.

Queen's University Belfast Student Records Office
Student matriculation registers, 1850–1917.

Royal College of Physicians of Ireland Heritage Centre
Diary of James Lloyd Turner Graham, 1933–6 [BMS/48].
Diary of James Little [TPCK/6/5/10].
Dublin Clinical Hospitals Standing Committee [DCHC/2].
Dublin Hospital Football Union Minute Book, 1884–1901 [BMS/2/3].
Papers of John Fleetwood [JF/1/].
Kirkpatrick collection [TCPK/6 and TCPK/7].
Sir Patrick Dun's Hospital papers [PDH].

Royal College of Surgeons in Ireland Heritage Collections
Emily Winifred Dickson papers [RCSI/IP/Dickson].
John Kirby, *Theatre of anatomy and school of surgery, Peter-Street, Dublin, established in
    the year, 1810* (Dublin: Hodges and McArthur, 1827).
Testimonial for Dr Thomas Mulhall Corbet by George H. Porter, dated 22 January
    1887.
Testimonial for Thomas Mulhall Corbet by Edwin Lapper, dated 25 January 1887, and
    by Thomas P. Mason, dated 24 January 1887.

Royal Victoria Hospital, Belfast
Belfast Medical Students' Association Committee Minute Book 1899–1925.
Belfast Medical Students' Association Minute Book, General Meetings, 1907–32.
Royal Victoria Hospital, Medical Staff Minutes, 1875–1905.

Trinity College Dublin Manuscripts
Adelaide Hospital Medical Board Minute Book, 17 September 1875–8 May 1880 [IE
    TCD MS 11270/2/3/3/2].

Adelaide Hospital Medical Board Minute Book: 5 May 1880–7 June 1900 [IE TCD MS 11270/2/3/3/3].
Annual Reports of Adelaide Hospital, 1858–65 [IE TCD MS 11270/11/1/1].
Student matriculation registers for Trinity College Dublin, 1850–1913.
TCD Biological Association Minute Book 1, November 1879–May 1885.
TCD Biological Association Minute Book 2, February 1894–December 1899.
TCD Biological Association Minute Book 4, March 1904–December 1908.
TCD Biological Association Minute Book 6, November 1921–October 1929.

University College Cork University Archives
Copy of Resolutions from QCCMSA Meeting, 13 February 1895, and Copy of Resolutions from QCCMSA Meeting, 26 February 1896 [UC/COUNCIL/1/1/].
Handwritten report of the Extraordinary Visitation of QCC, 15–16 May 1884 [UC/PRESIDENT/5/10(1)].
Letter: Professor of Zoology, 9 March 1897, QCC [UC/COUNCIL/19/364].
Letter: Dublin Medical Students Club to the President of Queen's College Cork (undated but approximately 1882–3) [UC/COUNCIL/16/43].
Letter from QCCMSA, dated 18 January 1899, addressed to Alex Jack esq. [UC/COUNCIL/18/38(i)].
Letter from Medical Students Association [UC/COUNCIL/21/32].
Letter to the Council of QCC, dated 20 March 1896 [UC/COUNCIL/19/165].
Letter, dated 16 December 1896, from QCC Medical Students' Association to College Council [UC/COUNCIL/19/296].
Rugby Football Club Minutes, QCC 1905–12 [UC/MB/CS/RF/1].
'The Cork School of Medicine: Queen's College, Cork and Associated Hospitals' (Cork: George Purcell & Co., undated) [UC/Council/4/46(4)].
Student matriculation registers for Queen's College Cork/University College Cork, 1850–1917.

University College Dublin Archives and Special Collections
Catholic University School of Medicine Governing Body Minute Book, 1892–1911 [CU/14].
William Doolin, 'Medical education, reprinted from "Studies"', September 1925, UCD Special Collections.
UCD Medical Faculty Minute Book 3, November 1931–47 [F8/3].

Wellcome Library, London
Royal College of Surgeons in Ireland: Schools of Surgery, including Carmichael and Ledwich Schools (Dublin: Ponsonby and Gibbs, 1938–9).
Papers of Robert Jones relating to his studies in Dublin at the Royal College of Surgeons in Ireland and the Meath Hospital, 1836–7 [MSS 6061–6062].
Testimonial for Robert Jones by William Henry Porter, dated 11 January 1840 [MSS 6061–6062].

Contemporary medical journals

British Medical Journal
Dublin Journal of Medical Science
Dublin Medical Press
Irish Journal of Medical Science
Irish Medical Journal
The Lancet
London Medical and Physical Journal
Medical Press and Circular
Ulster Medical Journal

Contemporary periodicals

Belfast News-Letter
Connacht Tribune
Fermanagh Herald
Freeman's Journal
Irish Examiner
Irish Independent
Irish Press
Irish Times
Weekly Irish Times

Contemporary student periodicals

Alexandra College Magazine
The British Medical Students' Journal (the journal of the British Medical Students' Association)
Cork University Record
Fravlio-Queens
Galway University College Magazine
Hermes: An Illustrated University Literary Quarterly
Magazine of the London School of Medicine for Women and Royal Victoria Hospital
Mistura
The National Student
The New Northman
The Northman
Q.C.B.
Q.C.C.
Q.C.G.
The Quarryman
R.C.S.I.: A Students' Quarterly
Snakes Alive
St. Stephen's: A Record of University Life
T.C.D.: A College Miscellany

Contemporary publications

Robert Adams, 'Richmond, Whitworth and Hardwicke Hospitals: introductory lecture delivered on Thursday, November 1st, 1860' (Dublin: J.M. O'Toole, 1860).

John T. Banks, 'Introductory address delivered on the opening of the medical session, 1st November 1883 at the Richmond, Whitworth and Hardwicke Government Hospitals' (Dublin: Gunn & Cameron, 1883).

W. Battersby, '"Medical education", an address delivered in the dining hall of Trinity College at the opening meeting of the second session of the Dublin University Medico-Chirurgical Society, November 27th, 1868 by the auditor W.E. Battersby, B.A. Med. Sch.' (Dublin: M. & S. Eaton, 1868).

Charles Benson, 'Address delivered to the students in the City of Dublin Hospital on Tuesday, November 8th, 1859' (Dublin: Fannin and Co., 1859).

—— 'A lecture introductory to the course of clinical instruction in the City of Dublin Hospital, for the session 1844–45' (Dublin: Medical Press Office, undated).

Charles A. Cameron, *History of the Royal College of Surgeons in Ireland and of the Irish Schools of Medicine including numerous biographical sketches; also a medical bibliography* (Dublin: Fannin & Co., 1886).

Dominic Corrigan, 'Introductory lecture, winter session 1858–9, Richmond, Whitworth and Hardwicke Hospitals' (Dublin: J.M. O'Toole, 1858).

James Craig, 'Introductory address delivered at the opening of the session of 1893–4 in the theatre of the Meath Hospital' (Dublin: John Falconer, 1893).

Henry Curran, 'The introductory lecture of the winter session 1858–59 delivered in the Carmichael School of Medicine on Tuesday, November 2nd, 1858' (Dublin: Browne & Nolan, 1858).

The Dublin University Calendar for the year 1885 (Dublin: Hodges, Figgis and Co., 1885).

Arthur Wynne Foot, 'An address delivered in the theatre of the Royal College of Surgeons in Ireland at the opening of the session, October 29, 1883' (Dublin: John Falconer, 1883).

—— 'An introductory address delivered at the Ledwich School of Medicine, November 1st, 1873' (Dublin: John Falconer, 1873).

Kendal Franks, 'Introductory address delivered at the opening of the session of 1889–90 at the Adelaide Hospital' (Dublin: John Falconer, 1889).

Robert J. Graves, *Clinical lectures on the practice of medicine*, 2nd edn, ed. J. Moore Neligan, MD MRIA, vol.1 (Dublin: Fannin & Co., 1848).

Guide for medical students, more especially for those about to commence their medical studies, by the registrar of the Catholic University School of Medicine (Dublin: Browne & Nolan, 1892).

Guide to the Belfast Medical School for session 1903–4 (Belfast: A. Mayne and Boyd, 1903).

Edward Hamilton, 'Royal College of Surgeons inaugural address, session 1885–86' (Dublin: Gunn & Cameron, 1885).

William Hemming, 'The medical student's guide: or, plain instructions as to the best course to be pursued by those entering the medical profession', reprinted from the *Student's Journal and Hospital Gazette* (London: Bailliere, Tindall, & Cox, 1876).

H.A. Hinkson *Student life in Trinity College, Dublin* (Dublin: J. Charles & Son, 1892).

Thomas S. Holland, 'The Irish School of Medicine as it is and as it ought to be; an address: introductory to a course on pathological anatomy and histology in relation to the practice of medicine and surgery delivered at the Royal Cork Institution by Thomas S. Holland MD' (Cork: George Purcell & Co., 1853).

Alfred Hudson, '"The study of clinical medicine": a lecture delivered in the Meath Hospital at the opening of the session 1864–5' (Dublin: William McGee, 1864).

'The Introductory lecture delivered by Doctor Jacob at the Royal College of Surgeons for the session 1844–45' (Dublin: Medical Press Office, 1844).

'The Irish medical student's guide: an epitome of medical education in Ireland and the public medical services' (Dublin: Office of the Medical Press and Circular, 1872).

Sophia Jex-Blake, *Medical women: two essays* (Edinburgh: William Oliphant & Co., 1872).

Charles Bell Keetley, FRCS, *The student's guide to the medical profession* (London: Macmillan and Co., 1878).

Thomas Laffan, '"The medical profession in the three kingdoms in 1887", the essay to which was awarded the Carmichael Prize of £100 by the Council of the Royal College of Surgeons, Ireland, 1887' (Dublin: Fannin & Co., 1888).

Alfred H. McClintock, 'Introductory lecture delivered at the Lying-in Hospital, Rutland-Square, session 1857–8' (Dublin: Browne & Nolan, 1857).

Rawdon Macnamara, 'A lecture introductory to the session 1881–1882 delivered in the Royal College of Surgeons' (Dublin: J. Atkinson & Co., 1881).

—— 'An address, introductory to the session 1884–1885, delivered in the theatre of the Meath Hospital and County of Dublin Infirmary' (Dublin: J. Atkinson & Co., 1884).

H. Macnaughton Jones, *Clinical teaching in hospitals* (Cork: George Purcell & Co., 1877).

E.D. Mapother, *First Carmichael Prize: the medical profession and its educational and licensing bodies* (Dublin: Fannin & Co., 1868).

Sir John W. Moore, *'Clinical case-taking', reprinted from the Dublin Journal of Medical Science, November 1905* (Dublin: John Falconer, 1905).

Robert Murray, 'An inaugural address delivered at the opening of the Dublin Students' Medico-Chirurgical Society, on Wednesday, January 9, 1850 by Robert Murray, President' (Dublin: Browne & Nolan, 1850).

Sir Lambert Ormsby, *Medical history of the Meath Hospital and County Dublin Infirmary from its foundation in 1753 down to the present time; including biographical sketches of the surgeons and physicians who served on its staff; with the names of apprentices, resident pupils, clinical clerks, and prizemen; also all students who studied at the hospital from the year 1838*, 2nd edn (Dublin: Fannin & Co., 1892).

NUI Calendar 1909.

Ella G.A. Ovenden, MD, 'Medicine' in Myrrha Bradshaw (ed.), *Open doors for Irishwomen: a guide to the professions open to educated women in Ireland* (Dublin: Irish Central Bureau for the Employment of Women, 1907).

Regulations for the Officers' Training Corps, 1912 (London: Harrison and Sons, 1912).

Report on Medical School, University College Galway, 1925 (Galway: O'Gorman Printing House, 1925).

Walter Rivington, '"The medical profession of the United Kingdom", being the essay to which was awarded the First Carmichael Prize by the Council of the Royal College of Surgeons in Ireland, 1887' (Dublin: Fannin & Co., 1888).

Royal College of Surgeons in Ireland Calendar, January 1886 (Dublin: Fannin & Co., 1886).

Royal College of Surgeons in Ireland: Schools of Surgery including Carmichael and Ledwich Schools, 1948–49 handbook (Dublin: George F. Healy & Co., 1948).

Royal College of Surgeons, Ireland, Officers' Training Corps, handbook, July 1913 (Dublin: Alex. Thom & Co., Abbey Street).

Philip Crampton Smyly, '"Is it true?" An address delivered in the theatre of the Meath Hospital and Co. Dublin Infirmary on Monday, October 3, 1890, introductory to the session of 1890–91' (Dublin: John Falconer, 1890).

William Stokes, '"Medical ethics": a discourse delivered in the theatre of the Meath Hospital, November 1, 1869' (Dublin: McGlashan and Gill, 1869).

—— 'An address delivered to the class of the Meath Hospital and County of Dublin Infirmary, session 1858–1859' (Dublin: Browne & Nolan, 1858).

—— 'Medical education, a discourse delivered at the Meath Hospital' (Dublin: Hodges, Smith and Co., 1861).

—— 'Medical education in the University of Dublin, a discourse delivered at the opening of the School of Physic in Ireland session 1864–65' (Dublin: Printed at the University Press by M.H. Gill, 1864).

R.F. Tobin, 'An address delivered at St Vincent's Hospital, Dublin, introductory to the medical session 1887–8' (Dublin: John Falconer, 1887).

Frederic W. Warren, 'Inaugural address delivered in the theatre of the Adelaide Hospital, introductory to the session 1883–84' (Dublin: George Healy, 1883).

J.H. Wharton, 'Introductory address to students at the Ledwich School of Medicine' (Dublin: 1860).

E. Wooton, *A guide to the medical profession: a comprehensive manual conveying the means of entering the medical profession in the chief countries of the world* (London: L. Upcott Gill, 1883).

R. Temple Wright, M.D., late scholar of King's College, London, 'Medical students of the period: a few words in defence of those much maligned people, with digressions on various topics of public interest connected with medical science' (Edinburgh and London: William Blackwood and Sons, 1867).

Doctors' memoirs

J. Johnston Abraham, *Surgeon's journey: the autobiography of J. Johnston Abraham* (London: Heinemann, 1957).

Beulah Bewley and Susan Bewley (eds), *My life as a woman and doctor* (Bristol: Silverwood Books, 2016).

Colonel Robert J. Blackham, *Scalpel, sword and stretcher: forty years of work and play* (London: Sampson Low, Marston & Co. Ltd., 1931).

Noël Browne, *Against the tide* (Dublin: Gill & Macmillan, 1986).

Clair M. Callan, *Standing my ground: memoir of a woman physician* (Bloomington, Ind.: Archway Publishing, 2014).

Dr A.D. (Louis) Courtney, … *I go alone: memoirs of a rural Irish doctor, 1878–1985* (Nenagh: Tipperary Manuscript, 2007).

Gearoid P. Crookes, *Far away and long ago: a memoir* (Dublin: Tudor House Publications, 2003).

Sidney Elizabeth Croskery, *Whilst I remember* (Dundonald: Blackstaff, 1983).

Joyce Delaney, *No starch in my coat: an Irish doctor's progress* (London: Cox & Wyman, 1971).

Michael P. Flynn, *Medical doctor of many parts: memoirs of a public health practitioner and health manager, spanning sixty years of social change* (Dublin: Colourbooks, 2002).

Thomas Garry, *African doctor* (London: John Gifford, 1939).

Oliver St John Gogarty, *It isn't this time of year at all! An unpremeditated autobiography* (London: Sphere Books, 1983).

Thomas Hennessy, *My life as a surgeon: an autobiography* (Dublin: A. & A. Farmar, 2011).

William M. Hunter, 'Private life of a country medical practitioner' (Private memoir courtesy of the Hunter family).

John Lyburn, *The fighting Irish doctor (an autobiography)* (Dublin: Morris & Co., 1947).

Aidan MacCarthy, *A doctor's war* (Cork: Collins Press, 2005).

E.B. McKee, *Doc: revelations of a reluctant Yank studying medicine among the Irish* (Narragansett, RI: Ebook Bakery Books, 2013).

Aubrey Malone, *A life in medicine: a biography of Malachy Smyth, MD, FACS, FRCS* (Baldoyle: Colour Books, 2005).

Ristéard Mulcahy, *Memoirs of a medical maverick* (Dublin: Liberties Press, 2010).

James Mullin, *The story of a toiler's life* (Dublin and London: Maunsel & Roberts, 1921).

Ken O'Flaherty, *From Slyne Head to Malin Head: a rural GP remembers* (Letterkenny: Browne Printers, 2003).

Bethel Solomons, *One doctor in his time* (London: Christopher Johnson, 1956).

R.W.M. Strain, *Les neiges d'antan; a two–part story: recollections of a medical student at the Queen's University of Belfast, 1924–30 and of a houseman, the Royal Victoria Hospital, Belfast, 1930–31* (Truro: R. Strain, 1982).

Michael Taaffe, *Those days are gone away* (London: Hutchinson, 1959).

Novels about medical student life

Oliver St John Gogarty, *Tumbling in the hay* (London: Sphere Books, 1982).

G.M. Irvine, *The lion's whelp* (London: Simpkin, Marshall, Hamilton, Kent & Co. Ltd., 1910).

Official reports

Queen's College Galway Report of an Extraordinary Visitation of Queen's College Galway held in Dublin Castle on 30th and 31st March 1870 (Dublin: Alexander Thom, 1870).

Report of the Royal Commissioners appointed to inquire into the Medical Acts, with minutes of evidence, appendices, and index (1882) [C.3259-I].

Report on the Department of Midwifery and Gynaecology, 1924–25.

Special Report from the Select Committee on the Medical Act (1858), Amendment (no.3) Bill [Lords] (1878–9) (320).

Oral history interviews

John (RCSI, 1947–53). Interviewed 3 October 2013.
David (TCD, 1940–6). Interviewed 4 October 2013.
Robert (UCD, 1939–44). Interviewed 26 August 2013.
Maureen (UCD, 1952–8). Interviewed 10 October 2013.
Seamus (UCD, 1942–7). Interviewed 11 October 2013.
Mary (UCG, 1946–52). Interviewed 2 February 2014.
Michael (UCD, 1951–7). Interviewed 4 February 2014.
Sean (UCD, 1952–8). Interviewed 4 February 2014.
Paul (UCD, 1946–52). Interviewed 5 February 2014.
Andrew (UCD, 1949–55). Interviewed 5 February 2014.
James (UCD, 1938–44). Interviewed 6 February 2014.
Lily (TCD, 1946–53). Interviewed 15 February 2014.
Martin (TCD, 1944–50). Interviewed 15 February 2014.
Martha (TCD, 1943–9). Interviewed 16 February 2014.
Anne (UCC, 1947–1953). Interviewed 7 April 2014.
Una (UCC, 1951–7). Interviewed 8 April 2014.
Colm (UCC, 1949–55). Interviewed 8 April 2014.
Francis (UCC, 1943–9). Interviewed 12 April 2014.
Ted (UCD, 1946–52). Interviewed 14 April 2014.
Stephen (QUB, 1942–7). Interviewed 19 April 2014.
Jean (UCC, 1951–7). Interviewed 6 May 2014.
Christopher (TCD, 1942–9). Interviewed 19 May 2014.
Thomas (TCD, 1946–52). Interviewed 19 May 2014.
Sylvia (QUB, 1944–50). Interviewed 21 August 2014.

Unpublished dissertations

Clara Cullen, 'The museum of Irish industry (1845–1867): research environment, popular museum and community of learning in mid-Victorian Ireland' (PhD thesis, University College Dublin, 2008).
Ann Daly, 'The Dublin Medical Press and medical authority in Ireland, 1850–1890' (PhD thesis, National University of Ireland Maynooth, 2008).
David Durnin, 'Medical provision and the Irish experience of the First World War, 1912–1925' (PhD thesis, University College Dublin, 2015).
Florent Palluault, 'Medical students in England and France, 1815–58: a comparative study' (DPhil. thesis, University of Oxford, 2003).
Ailish Veale, '"It's all a matter of balanced tensions": Irish medical missionaries in Nigeria, 1937–1967 (PhD thesis, Trinity College Dublin, 2015).

Secondary sources

Lynn Abrams, *Oral history theory* (London: Routledge, 2010).

Marcus Ackroyd, Laurence Brockliss, Michael Moss, Kate Retford and John Stevenson, *Advancing with the army: medicine, the professions and social mobility in the British Isles, 1790–1850* (Oxford: Oxford University Press, 2007).

Sarah Jane Aiston, "'A woman's place … '": male representations of university women in the student press of the University of Liverpool, 1944–1979', *Women's History Review* 15(1) (2006): 3–34.

R.D. Anderson, *British universities past and present* (London: Hambledon Continuum, 2006).

—— *Universities and elites in Britain since 1800* (Cambridge: Cambridge University Press, 1992).

Ruth Barrington, *Health, medicine and politics in Ireland, 1900–1970* (Dublin: Institute of Public Administration, 1987).

Alison Bashford, *Purity and pollution: gender, embodiment and Victorian medicine* (London: Macmillan, 1998).

A.W. Bates, 'Dr Kahn's museum: obscene anatomy in Victorian London', *Journal of the Royal Society of Medicine* 99(12) (2006): 618–24.

—— "'Indecent and demoralising representations'": public anatomy museums in mid-Victorian England', *Medical History* 52(1) (2008): 1–22.

Denis Biggart, *John Henry Biggart: pathologist, professor and Dean of Medical Faculty, Queen's University, Belfast* (Belfast: Ulster Historical Association, 2012).

Sharon R. Bird, 'Welcome to the men's club: homosociality and the maintenance of hegemonic masculinity', *Gender & Society* 10(2) (1996): 120–32.

Catriona Blake, *Charge of the parasols: women's entry into the medical profession* (London: Women's Press, 1990).

Thomas Neville Bonner, *Becoming a physician: medical education in Britain, France, Germany and the United States, 1750–1945* (Oxford: Oxford University Press, 1995).

James Bradley, Anne Crowther and Marguerite Dupree, 'Mobility and selection in Scottish university medical education, 1858–1886', *Medical History* 40 (1996): 1–24.

Eileen Breathnach, 'Women and higher education in Ireland (1879–1914)', *Crane Bag* 4(1) (1980): 47–54.

Michael Brown, "'Like a devoted army'": medicine, heroic masculinity and the military paradigm in Victorian Britain', *Journal of British Studies* 49(3) (2010): 592–622.

—— *Performing medicine: medical culture and identity in provincial England, c.1760–1850* (Manchester: Manchester University Press, 2011).

Janet Browne, 'Squibs and snobs: science in humorous British undergraduate magazines around 1830', *History of Science* 30(3) (1992): 165–97.

Stella V.F. Butler, 'A transformation in training: the formation of university medical faculties in Manchester, Leeds and Liverpool, 1870–84', *Medical History* 30 (1986): 115–32.

W.F. Bynum, *Science and the practice of medicine in the nineteenth century* (Cambridge: Cambridge University Press, 1994).

Manuel Castells, *The power of identity* (Oxford: Blackwell, 1997).

Lavanya Chalikonda, 'Why are Irish doctors emigrating?', *Royal College of Surgeons in Ireland Student Medical Journal* 6(1) (2013): 93–8.

Richard Clarke, *The Royal Victoria Hospital, Belfast: a history, 1797–1997* (Belfast: Blackstaff Press, 1997).

Davis Coakley, *Medicine in Trinity College Dublin: an illustrated history* (Dublin: Trinity College Dublin, 2014).

Aidan Collins, *St Vincent's hospital, Fairview: celebrating 150 years of service* (Dublin: Albertine Kennedy Publishing, 2007).

Timothy Collins, 'Dodos and discord: a biographical note on A.G. Melville of Queen's College Galway', *Journal of the Galway Archaeological and Historical Society* 50 (1998): 90–111.

R.W. Connell, *Masculinities*, 2nd edn (Berkeley: University of California Press, 2005).

R.W. Connell and James W. Messerschmidt, 'Hegemonic masculinity: rethinking the concept', *Gender & Society* 19(6) (2005): 829–59.

A. M. Cooke, 'Queen Victoria's medical household', *Medical History* 26(3) (1982): 307–20.

Catherine Cox, 'Access and engagement: the medical dispensary service in post-Famine Ireland', in Catherine Cox and Maria Luddy (eds), *Cultures of care in Irish medical history, 1750–1950* (Basingstoke: Palgrave Macmillan, 2010), pp. 57–78.

—— 'The medical marketplace and medical tradition in nineteenth-century Ireland', in Ronnie Moore and Stuart McClean (eds), *Folk healing and health care practices in Britain and Ireland: stethoscopes, wands and crystals* (New York: Berghahn Books, 2010), pp. 55–79.

—— *Negotiating insanity in the southeast of Ireland, 1820–1900* (Manchester: Manchester University Press, 2012).

Catherine Cox and Maria Luddy (eds), *Cultures of care in Irish medical history, 1750–1970* (Basingstoke: Palgrave Macmillan, 2009).

Anne Crowther and Marguerite Dupree, *Medical lives in the age of surgical revolution* (Cambridge: Cambridge University Press, 2007).

Clara Cullen, 'The museum of Irish industry, Robert Kane and education for all in the Dublin of the 1850s and 1860s', *History of Education* 38(1) (2009): 99–113.

Enda Delaney, 'The Vanishing Irish? The exodus from Ireland in the 1950s', in Dermot Keogh, Finbarr O'Shea and Carmel Quinlan (eds), *Ireland: the lost decade in the 1950s* (Dublin: Mercier Press, 2004), pp. 77–89.

John Demos and Virginia Demos, 'Adolescence in historical perspective', *Journal of Marriage and Family* 31(4) (1969): 632–8.

Paul R. Deslandes, 'Competitive examinations and the culture of masculinity in Oxbridge undergraduate life, 1850–1920', *History of Education Quarterly* 42(4) (2002): 544–78.

—— *Oxbridge men: British masculinity and the undergraduate experience, 1850–1920* (Bloomington: Indiana University Press, 2005).

David Dickson, *Dublin: the making of a capital city* (London: Profile Books, 2014).

Anne Digby, *Making a medical living: doctors and patients in the English market for medicine, 1720–1911* (Cambridge: Cambridge University Press, 1994).

—— 'Shaping new identities: general practitioners in Britain and South Africa', in Kent Maynard (ed.), *Medical identities: health, well-being and personhood* (New York: Berghahn Books, 2007), pp. 14–35.

Virginia G. Drachman, 'The limits of progress: the professional lives of women doctors, 1881–1926', *Bulletin of the History of Medicine* 60(1) (1986): 58–72.

Carol Dyhouse, *Students: a gendered history* (London: Routledge, 2005).

Lindsey Earner-Byrne, 'Moral prescription: the Irish medical profession, the Roman Catholic Church and the prohibition of birth control in twentieth-century Ireland', in Catherine Cox and Maria Luddy (eds), *Cultures of care in Irish medical history, 1750–1950* (Basingstoke: Palgrave Macmillan, 2010), pp. 207–28.

Heather Ellis, '"Boys, semi-men and bearded scholars": maturity and manliness in early nineteenth-century Oxford', in S. Brady and J.H. Arnold (eds.), *What is masculinity? historical dynamics from antiquity to the contemporary world* (Basingstoke: Palgrave Macmillan, 2011), pp. 263–82.

Gerard M. Fealy (2006) *A history of apprenticeship nurse training in Ireland* (New York: Routledge).

Harry Ferguson, 'Men and masculinities in late-modern Ireland', in Bob Pease and Keith Pringle (eds), *A man's world?: changing men's practices in a globalized world* (London: Zed, 2001), pp. 118–34.

Irene Finn, 'Women in the medical profession in Ireland, 1876–1919', in Bernadette Whelan (ed.), *Women and Paid Work in Ireland, 1500–1930* (Dublin: Four Courts Press, 2000), pp. 102–19.

Abraham Flexner, *Medical education: a comparative study* (New York: Macmillan, 1925).

Catriona Foley, *The last Irish plague: the great flu epidemic in Ireland, 1918–19* (Dublin: Irish Academic Press, 2011).

Peter Froggatt, 'Competing philosophies: the "preparatory" medical schools of the Royal Belfast Academical Institution and the Catholic University of Ireland, 1835–1909', in Greta Jones and Elizabeth Malcolm (eds), *Medicine, disease and the state in Ireland, 1650–1940* (Cork: Cork University Press, 1999), pp. 59–84.

—— 'The distinctiveness of Belfast medicine and its medical school', *Ulster Medical Journal* 54(2) (1985): 89–108.

—— 'The first medical school in Belfast, 1835–49', *Medical History* 22 (1978): 237–66.

—— 'The response of the medical profession to the Great Famine', in Margaret Crawford (ed.), *Famine: the Irish experience, 900–1900: subsistence crises and famines in Ireland* (Edinburgh: John Donald Publishers Ltd., 1989), pp. 134–56.

Louise Fuller, *Irish Catholicism since 1950: the undoing of a culture* (Dublin: Gill & Macmillan, 2002).

James Garner, 'The great experiment: the admission of women students to St Mary's Hospital Medical School, 1916–1925', *Medical History* 41 (1998).

Delia Gavrus, 'Men of dreams and men of action: neurologists, neurosurgeons and the performance of professional identity, 1920–1950', *Bulletin of the History of Medicine* 85(1) (2011): 57–92.

Laurence M. Geary, *Medicine and charity in Ireland, 1718–1851* (Dublin: University College Dublin Press, 2005).

Toby Gelfand, 'The history of the medical profession', in Roy Porter and W.F. Bynum (eds), *Companion encyclopedia of the history of medicine*, vol.2 (London: Routledge, 1993), pp. 1119–50.

John R. Gillis, *Youth and history: tradition and change in European age relations, 1770–present* (New York: Academic Press, 1974).

John D. Goldthorpe, *Social mobility and class structure in modern Britain*, 2nd edn (Oxford: Oxford University Press, 1987).

Pishoy Gouda, Kevin Kitt, David S. Evans, Deirdre Goggin, Deirdre McGrath, Jason Last, Martina Hennessy, Richard Arnett, Siun O'Flynn, Fidelma Dunne and Diarmuid O'Donovan, 'Ireland's medical brain drain migration intentions of Irish medical students', *Human Resources for Health* 13(11) (2015).

David Hardiman (ed.), *Healing bodies, saving souls: medical missions in Asia and Africa* (Amsterdam: Rodopi, 2006).

Judith Harford, 'The movement for the higher education of women in Ireland: gender equality or denominational rivalry?', *History of Education* 35 (2005): 497–516.

—— *The opening of university education to women in Ireland* (Dublin: Irish Academic Press, 2008).

T.M. Healy, *From sanatorium to hospital: a social and medical account of Peamount, 1912–1997* (Dublin: A. & A. Farmar, 2002).

E.A. Heaman, *St. Mary's: the history of a London teaching hospital* (Liverpool: Liverpool University Press, 2003).

Hanora M. Henry, *Our Lady's hospital, Cork: history of the mental hospital spanning 200 years* (Cork: Haven Books, 1989).

Matthew Hilton, *Smoking in British popular culture, 1800–2000* (Manchester: Manchester University Press, 2000).

Myrtle Hill, 'Gender, Culture and "the Spiritual Empire": the Irish Protestant female missionary experience', *Women's History Review* 16(2) (2007): 203–26.

Richard Holt, *Sport and the British: a modern history* (Oxford: Oxford University Press, 1990).

Helen Lefkowitz Horowitz, *Campus life: undergraduate cultures from the end of the eighteenth century to the present* (Chicago: University of Chicago Press, 1988).

Matt Houlbrook, 'Cities', in H.G. Cocks and Matt Houlbrook (eds), *Palgrave advances in the modern history of sexuality* (Basingstoke: Palgrave Macmillan, 2006).

Tom Hunt, *Sport and society in Victorian Ireland: the case of Westmeath* (Cork: Cork University Press, 2007).

John Hutchinson, *The dynamics of cultural nationalism: the Gaelic revival and the creation of the Irish nation state* (London: Allen & Unwin, 1987).

Tom Inglis, *Moral monopoly: the Catholic Church in modern Irish society* (Dublin: Gill & Macmillan, 1997).

Tomás Irish, 'Fractured families: educated elites in Britain and France and the challenge of the Great War', *Historical Journal* 57(2) (2014): 509–30.

—— *Trinity in war and revolution, 1912–1923* (Dublin: Royal Irish Academy, 2015).

L.S. Jacyna, 'The laboratory and the clinic: the impact of pathology on surgical diagnosis in the Glasgow Western Infirmary, 1875–1910', *Bulletin of the History of Medicine* 62(3) (1988): 384–406.

Pat Jalland (ed.), *Octavia Wilberforce: the autobiography of a pioneer woman doctor* (London: Cassell, 1994).

N.D. Jewson, 'The disappearance of the sick-man from medical cosmology, 1770–1870', *Sociology* 10(2) (1976): 225–44.

Colin Jones, 'Montpellier medical students and the medicalisation of eighteenth-century France', in Roy Porter and Andrew Wear (eds), *Problems and methods in the history of medicine* (London: Croom Helm, 1987), pp. 57–80.

Greta Jones, *Captain of all these men of death: the history of tuberculosis in nineteenth- and twentieth-century Ireland* (Amsterdam: Rodopi, 2001).

—— '"A mysterious discrimination": Irish medical emigration to the United States in the 1950s', *Social History of Medicine* 25(1) (2011): 139–56.

—— 'The Rockefeller Foundation and medical education in Ireland in the 1920s', *Irish Historical Studies* 30(120) (1997): 564–80.

—— '"Strike out boldly for the prizes that are available to you": medical emigration from Ireland, 1860–1905', *Medical History* 54(1) (2010): 55–74.

Greta Jones and Elizabeth Malcolm, 'Introduction: an anatomy of Irish medical history', in Greta Jones and Elizabeth Malcolm (eds), *Medicine, disease and the state in Ireland, 1650–1940* (Cork: Cork University Press, 1998).

Ludmilla Jordanova, 'Medical men, 1780–1820', in Joanna Woodall (ed.), *Portraiture: facing the subject* (Manchester: Manchester University Press, 1997), pp. 101–15.

Laura Kelly, 'Anatomy dissections and student experience at Irish universities c.1900s–1960s', *Studies in History and Philosophy of Biological and Biomedical Sciences* 42:4 (2011): 467–74.

—— '"Fascinating scalpel-wielders and fair dissectors": women's experience of medical education, c.1880s–1920s', *Medical History* 54(4) (2010): 495–516.

—— *Irish women in medicine, c.1880s–1920s: origins, education and careers* (Manchester: Manchester University Press, 2012).

—— 'Migration and medical education: Irish medical students at the University of Glasgow, 1859–1900', *Irish Economic and Social History* 39(1) (2012): 39–55.

—— '"The turning point in the whole struggle": the admission of women to the King and Queen's College of Physicians in Ireland', *Women's History Review* 22(1) (2013): 97–125.

Daniel Kilbride, 'Southern medical students in Philadelphia, 1800–1861: science and sociability in the "Republic of Medicine"', *Journal of Southern History* 65(4) (1999): 697–732.

T.P.C. Kirkpatrick, *History of the medical teaching in Trinity College Dublin and of the School of Physic in Ireland* (Dublin: Hanna and Neale, 1912).

Christopher Lawrence, 'Incommunicable knowledge: science, technology and the clinical art in Britain 1850–1914', *Journal of Contemporary History* 20(4) (1985): 503–20.

—— 'The shaping of things to come: Scottish medical education, 1700–1939', *Medical Education* 40(3) (2006): 212–18.

S.C. Lawrence, *Charitable knowledge: hospital pupils and practitioners in eighteenth-century London* (Cambridge: Cambridge University Press, 1986).

Colm Lennon (ed.), *Confraternities and sodalities in Ireland: charity, church and sociability* (Dublin: Columba Press, 2013).

Sonja Levsen, 'Constructing elite identities: university students, military masculinity and the consequences of the Great War in Britain and Germany', *Past & Present* 198 (2008): 147–83.

Irvine Loudon, *Medical care and the general practitioner, 1750–1850* (Oxford: Oxford University Press, 1986).

Maria Luddy, *Women and philanthropy in nineteenth-century Ireland* (Cambridge: Cambridge University Press, 1995).

B. Lyons, *The quality of Mercer's: the story of Mercer's hospital, 1734–1991* (Dublin: Glendale, 1991).

J.B. Lyons, *The irresistible rise of the RCSI* (Dublin: Royal College of Surgeons, 1984).

Donal McCartney, *UCD: a national idea: the history of University College, Dublin* (Dublin: Gill & Macmillan, 1999).

Patrick F. McDevitt, 'Muscular Catholicism: nationalism, masculinity and Gaelic team sports, 1884–1916', *Gender & History* 9(2) (1997): 262–84.

R.B. McDowell and D.A. Webb, *Trinity College Dublin, 1592–1952: an academic history* (Cambridge: Cambridge University Press, 2004).

Leone McGregor Hellstedt (ed.), *Women physicians of the world: autobiographies of medical pioneers* (Washington, DC and London: Medical Women's International Federation, Hemisphere Publishing, 1978).

Yvonne McKenna, *Made holy: Irish women religious at home and abroad* (Dublin: Irish Academic Press, 2006).

Elizabeth Malcolm, *Swift's hospital: a history of St Patrick's hospital, Dublin, 1746–1989* (Dublin: Gill & Macmillan, 1989).

J.A. Mangan, *Athleticism in the Victorian and Edwardian public school* (London: Frank Cass, 2000).

——— *The games ethic and imperialism: aspects of the differences of an ideal* (Harmondsworth: Viking, 1986).

Kathleen Manning, *Rituals, ceremonies and cultural meaning in higher education* (Westport, Conn.: Bergin & Garvey, 2000).

F.O.C. Meenan, 'The Catholic University School of Medicine 1860–1880', *Studies: An Irish Quarterly Review* 66(262–3) (1977): 135–44.

——— *Cecilia Street: the Catholic University School of Medicine, 1855–1931* (Dublin: Gill & Macmillan, 1987).

——— *St Vincent's Hospital, 1834–1994: an historical and social portrait* (Dublin: Gill & Macmillan, 1994).

Michael A. Messner, 'Like family: power, intimacy and sexuality in male athletes' friendships', in Peter M. Nardi (ed.), *Men's friendships* (Newbury Park, Calif.: SAGE, 1992).

T.W. Moody, 'The Irish university question of the nineteenth century', *History* 43(148) (1958): 90–109.

T.W. Moody and J.C. Beckett, *Queen's, Belfast, 1845–1949: the history of a university* (London: Faber & Faber, 1959).

Dermot Moran, 'Nationalism, religion and the education question', *Crane Bag* 7(2) (1983): 77–84.

Regina M. Morantz-Sanchez, *Sympathy and science: women physicians in American Medicine* (Chapel Hill: University of North Carolina Press, 1985).

Ellen Singer More, *Restoring the balance: women physicians and the practice of medicine, 1850–1995* (Cambridge, Mass.: Harvard University Press, 1999).

John A. Murphy, *The College: a history of Queen's/University College, Cork, 1845–1995* (Cork: Cork University Press, 1996).

——— *Where Finbarr played: a concise illustrated history of sport in University College Cork, 1911–2011* (Cork: University College Cork, 2011).

James Murray, *Galway: a medico-social history* (Galway: Kenny's Bookshop and Art Gallery, 1994).

John Nauright and Timothy J.L. Chandler (eds), *Making men: rugby and masculine identity* (London: Routledge, 1999).

Sioban Nelson, *Say little, do much: nursing, nuns and hospitals in the nineteenth century* (Philadelphia: University of Pennsylvania Press, 2003).

Charles Newman, *The evolution of medical education in the nineteenth century* (Oxford: Oxford University Press, 1957).

Robert A. Nye, 'Medicine and science as masculine "Fields of Honor"', *Osiris* 12 (1997): 60–79.

Bridget O'Brien (Carroll), 'In Dublin's fair city', in Anne Macdona (ed.), *From Newman to new woman: UCD women remember* (Dublin: New Island, 2001).

Eoin O'Brien, *The Royal College of Surgeons in Ireland, 1784–1984* (Dublin: Eason, 1984).

Ulick O'Connor, *Oliver St John Gogarty* (London: Mandarin, 1990).

T.F. O'Higgins, *A double life* (Dublin: Town House, 1996).

C.D. O'Malley (ed.), *The history of medical education* (Berkeley: University of California Press, 1970).

Ciaran O'Neill, *Catholics of consequence: transnational education, social mobility, and the Irish Catholic elite, 1850–1900* (Oxford: Oxford University Press, 2014).

Ronan O'Rahilly, *Benjamin Alcock: the first professor of anatomy and physiology in Queen's College Cork* (Cork: Cork University Press, 1948).

—— *A history of the Cork medical school, 1849–1949* (Cork: Cork University Press, 1949).

Denis J. O'Sullivan, *The Cork School of Medicine: a history* (Cork: UCC Medical Alumni Association, University College Cork, 2007).

Gearoid O'Tuathaigh, 'The establishment of the Queen's Colleges: ideological and political background', in Tadhg Foley (ed.), *From Queen's College to National University: essays on the academic history of QCG/UCG/NUI Galway* (Dublin: Four Courts Press, 1999), pp. 1–15.

Roberta Park, '"Mended or ended?": football injuries and the British and American medical press, 1870–1910', *International Journal of the History of Sport* 18(2) (2001): 110–33.

Susan M. Parkes, *A danger to the men: a history of women in Trinity College Dublin, 1904–2004* (Dublin: Lilliput Press, 2004).

—— 'Higher education, 1793–1908', in W.E. Vaughan (ed.), *A new history of Ireland*, vol.6, *Ireland under the Union II, 1870–1921* (Oxford: Clarendon Press, 1996), pp. 539–70.

Susan M. Parkes and Judith Harford, 'Women and higher education in Ireland', in Deirdre Raftery and Susan M. Parkes (eds), *Female education in Ireland, 1700–1900: Minerva or Madonna* (Dublin: Irish Academic Press, 2007), pp. 105–43.

Noel Parry and José Parry, *The rise of the medical profession: a study of collective social mobility* (London: Croom Helm, 1976).

Senia Pašeta, 'The Catholic hierarchy and the Irish university question, 1880–1908', *History* 85(278) (2000): 268–84.

—— 'Trinity College, Dublin, and the education of Irish Catholics, 1873–1908', *Studia Hibernica* 30 (1998–9): 7–20.

Harold Perkin, *The rise of professional society: England since 1880* (London and New York: Routledge, 1989).

M. Jeanne Peterson, *The medical profession in mid-Victorian London* (Berkeley: University of California Press, 1978).

Vike Plock, *Joyce, medicine and modernity* (Gainesville: University Press of Florida, 2010).

Alessandro Portelli, 'What makes oral history different', in Robert Perks and Alistair Thomson (eds), *The oral history reader* (London and New York: Routledge, 2003).

Roy Porter, 'Before the fringe: "quackery" and the eighteenth-century medical market', in Roger Cooter (ed.), *Studies in the history of alternative medicine* (Basingstoke: Macmillan, 1988), pp. 1–25.

—— *The greatest benefit to mankind* (London: HarperCollins, 1997).

—— 'The patient's view: doing medical history from below', *Theory and Society* 14(2) (1985): 175–98.

Theodor Puschmann, *A history of medical education* (New York: Hafner, 1966).

W.J. Reader, *Professional men: the rise of the professional classes in nineteenth-century England* (London: Cox & Wyman Ltd., 1966).

Jennifer Redmond, 'The thermometer and the travel permit: Irish women in the medical profession in Britain during World War Two', in D.A.J. Macpherson and Mary J. Hickman (eds), *Women and Irish diaspora identities: theories, concepts and new perspectives* (Manchester: Manchester University Press, 2014), pp. 92–111.

Jonathan Reinarz, 'The age of museum medicine: the rise and fall of the medical museum at Birmingham's School of Medicine', *Social History of Medicine* 18(3) (2005): 419–37.

—— *Health care in Birmingham: the Birmingham teaching hospitals, 1779–1939* (Woodbridge: Boydell Press, 2009).

Ruth Richardson, *Dissection, death and the destitute* (Chicago: University of Chicago Press, 2000).

Shirley Roberts, *Sophia Jex-Blake: a woman pioneer in nineteenth-century medical reform* (London: Routledge, 1993).

Lisa Rosner, *Medical education in the age of enlightenment: Edinburgh students and apprentices, 1760–1826* (Edinburgh: Edinburgh University Press, 1991).

—— 'Student culture at the turn of the nineteenth century', *Caduceus* 10(2) (1994): 65–86.

Paul Rouse, *Sport and Ireland: a history* (Oxford: Oxford University Press, 2015).

Judith Rowbotham, '"Soldiers of Christ"? images of female missionaries in late nineteenth-century Britain issues of heroism and martyrdom', *Gender & History* 12(1) (2000): 82–106.

Michael Sappol, 'The odd case of Charles Knowlton: anatomical performance, medical narrative, and identity in antebellum America', *Bulletin of the History of Medicine* 83(3) (2009): 460–98.

Mary Semple, 'Going hatching', in Anne Macdona (ed.), *From Newman to new woman: UCD women remember* (Dublin: New Island, 2001), p. 13.

Christopher Shephard, '"I have a notion of going off to India": Colonel Alexander Porter and Irish recruitment to the Indian Medical Service, 1855–96', *Irish Economic and Social History* 41(1) (2014): 36–52.

Steve Sturdy, 'The political economy of scientific medicine: science, education and the transformation of medical practice in Sheffield, 1890–1922', *Medical History* 36 (1992): 125–59.

Paul Thompson, *Voice of the past: oral history* (Oxford: Oxford University Press, 2000).

John Tosh, 'What should historians do with masculinity? Reflections on nineteenth-century Britain', *History Workshop* 38 (1994): 179–202.

G. van Heteren, 'Students facing boundaries: the shift of nineteenth-century British student travel to German universities and the flexible boundaries of a medical educational system', in V. Nutton and R. Porter (eds), *The history of medical education in Britain* (Amsterdam: Rodopi, 1995), pp. 280–340.

Ailish Veale, 'International and modern ideals in Irish female medical missionary activity, 1937–1962', *Women's History Review* 25(4) (2016): 602–18.

Ivan Waddington, *The medical profession in the industrial revolution* (Dublin: Gill & Macmillan, 1984).

Keir Waddington, 'Mayhem and medical students: image, conduct, and control in the Victorian and Edwardian London teaching hospital', *Social History of Medicine* 15(1): 45–64.

—— *Medical education at St Bartholomew's Hospital, 1123–1995* (Woodbridge: Boydell Press, 2003).

John Harley Warner, *Against the spirit of system: the French impulse in nineteenth-century American medicine* (Baltimore, Md.: Johns Hopkins University Press, 1998).

—— 'A Southern medical reform: the meaning of the antebellum argument for Southern medical education', *Bulletin of the History of Medicine* 57(3) (1984): 364–81.

—— *The therapeutic perspective: medical practice, knowledge and identity in America, 1820–1885* (Princeton, NJ: Princeton University Press, 1997).

John Harley Warner and Lawrence J. Rizzolo, 'Anatomical instruction and training for professionalism from the 19th to the 21st centuries', *Clinical Anatomy* 19(5) (2006): 403–14.

John Harley Warner and James M. Edmondson, *Dissection: photographs of a rite of passage in American medicine, 1880–1930* (New York: Blast Books, 2009).

Andrew Warwick, *Masters of theory: Cambridge and the rise of mathematical physics* (Chicago: University of Chicago Press, 2003).

Mark. W. Weatherall, *Gentlemen, scientists and doctors: medicine at Cambridge, 1800–1940* (Woodbridge: Boydell Press, 2000).

—— 'Making medicine scientific: empiricism, rationality and quackery in mid-Victorian Britain', *Social History of Medicine* 9(2) (1996): 175–94.

J.D.H. Widdess, *A history of the Royal College of Physicians of Ireland, 1654–1963* (Edinburgh: E. & S. Livingstone, 1964).

—— *The Royal College of Surgeons in Ireland and its medical school* (Edinburgh: E. & S. Livingstone, 1967).

G. Wilson, *Victorian doctor: being the life of William Wilde* (London: Metheun, 1946).

Anne Witz, *Professions and patriarchy* (London: Routledge, 1992).

Index